TESTING PRAYER

TESTING PRAYER

Science and Healing

CANDY GUNTHER BROWN

Harvard University Press

Cambridge, Massachusetts

London, England

2012

Library of Congress Cataloging-in-Publication Data

Brown, Candy Gunther.
Testing prayer : science and healing / Candy Gunther Brown.
    p.   cm.
Includes bibliographical references (p.) and index.
ISBN 978-0-674-06467-6 (alk. paper)
1. Spiritual healing—Pentecostal churches.   2. Toronto blessing.   I. Title.
BR1644.7.B76 2012
234'.131—dc23
2011041928

With love and gratitude

for my husband, Josh, and daughters, Katrina and Sarah

Contents

Abbreviations

AN	ambient noise
ANGA	Apostolic Network of Global Awakening
CABG	coronary artery bypass graft
CAM	complementary and alternative medicine
CDC	Centers for Disease Control
BERA	brainstem evoked response audiometry
dBHL	decibels hearing level
dBSPL	decibels sound pressure level
GA	Global Awakening
GPCH	*Global Pentecostal and Charismatic Healing*
HIPAA	Health Insurance Portability and Accountability Act
IAHR	International Association of Healing Rooms
IM	Iris Ministries
IMT	international ministry trip
IP	intercessory prayer
IR	interaction ritual
MRSA	methicillin-resistant Staphylococcus aureus
MS	multiple sclerosis
NIHR	National Institute for Healthcare Research
NOMA	nonoverlapping magisteria
PIH	Partners in Harvest
PIP	proximal intercessory prayer
PTA	pure-tone average
RCT	randomized controlled trial

SMJ   *Southern Medical Journal*

STEP   Study of the Therapeutic Effects of Intercessory Prayer

STEPP   Study of the Therapeutic Effects of Proximal Intercessory Prayer

TACF   Toronto Airport Christian Fellowship

TAV   Toronto Airport Vineyard

TMJ   temporomandibular joint disorder

WCDN   World Christian Doctors Network

TESTING PRAYER

Introduction

The Magisteria of Science and Religion

$\cdot \! \star \! \cdot$

Public opinion polls report that most Americans believe in the healing power of prayer. In a 1996 Gallup Poll, 77 percent of respondents agreed that "God sometimes intervenes to cure people who have a serious illness," and 82 percent affirmed "the healing power of personal prayer." Of those queried in a 1997 national survey, 91 percent said that when they think of God, the image of a healer is either "extremely likely" (70 percent) or "somewhat likely" (21 percent) to come to mind. In 2003, 72 percent of those polled attested that "praying to God can cure someone—even if science says the person doesn't stand a chance." A 2007 survey concluded that 23 percent of Americans believe they personally have "witnessed a miraculous, physical healing." Such beliefs are not restricted to less educated or economically disadvantaged individuals. According to a 1997 survey, 94 percent of health maintenance organization executives think that personal prayer can aid medical treatment and accelerate recovery. Even more striking is 2004 survey data suggesting that 73 percent of U.S. medical doctors believe that miraculous healing occurs today.[1]

When people get sick, and especially when modern medicine cannot help, prayer for healing is a typical response. Even people who are not otherwise religiously active pray for their health, reasoning that prayer might help, and it probably will not hurt. A 1998 national survey reported that 75 percent of Americans prayed for their health, and 22 percent prayed for the improvement of specific conditions. A Centers for Disease Control (CDC) survey noted a dramatic increase in the use of prayer as a therapeutic intervention—rising from the least common to the most common form of complementary and alternative medicine (CAM)—between 1990 and 2002. During the twelve months prior to the CDC study, 43 percent of those polled had prayed for their own health, and 24 percent had solicited intercessory prayer for their health from others. In a 2005 study of fibromyalgia patients receiving conventional medical therapies at the Mayo Clinic, 98 percent had used some form of CAM in the previous six months; 45 percent had used "spiritual healing (prayers)"—the second most common CAM intervention (after exercise). Such findings suggest that people are most likely to resort to prayer for conditions that respond poorly or not at all to conventional medical treatments.[2]

Should Scientists Test Prayer?

Given the prevalence of prayer for health, it is not surprising that certain scientists have attempted to study whether prayer for healing exerts any empirical effects—and that other scientists have resisted the very notion of such studies. The Harvard researcher Herbert Benson attracted *New York Times* coverage when his 2006 study challenged the truism that prayer must be good for one's health. Heart patients who received *distant intercessory prayer* fared no better, but actually worse if they knew they were the objects of special prayer. Responding to the limitations of Benson's and other researchers' methodologies, I collaborated with biomedical scientists to study the effects of what I conceptualize as *proximal intercessory prayer*, or PIP.[3]

Like Benson's study, my research group's article, published in the peer-reviewed *Southern Medical Journal* in 2010, generated media interest. Better than two hundred news articles could be Googled within the week, some fifty of them in languages other than English. The *Los Angeles Times* published a favorable story, and NBC News released a syndicated television segment. Reporters and news anchors from Puerto Rico, Canada, Britain, France, and South Africa called requesting interviews, several of which aired live on radio. CNN scheduled an interview of me by the surgeon general nominee Sanjay Gupta (but pulled the story at the last minute due to breaking news). A producer for

Oprah Winfrey's *Miracle Detectives* phoned several times sniffing out material for a TV episode.[4]

With interest comes controversy. One entrepreneurial Internet blogger violated the terms of our article's press embargo—which set a date and time before which stories could not ethically be released—to post a vitriolic attack on the study. This particular unrefereed blog, written by a self-described "godless liberal" with an explicit ideological commitment to the defense of atheism, received more attention than it would have otherwise because for twenty-four hours (during which other reporters respected the embargo) this was the only public notice given to the study. Another zealous blogger offered to run me over with a car. Perhaps 1 percent of public responses to the study were negative and—this is the key point—strikingly more ad hominem and dogmatic than substantive. This public controversy suggests that in asking about the empirical effects of religious practices I hit on a subject that according to certain people's views of legitimate scientific inquiry was taboo.[5]

Controversies over biomedical tests of prayer have a lengthy and interesting history. For now, it is important that many people have perceived a conflict between science and religion—although the membrane dividing these fields has always been permeable. *Science* and *religion* are umbrella concepts that encompass diverse beliefs and practices. To draw a basic distinction, we may say that science uses observation and experimentation to test hypotheses of how things happen in the natural world. In contrast, religion is concerned less with falsification than with questions of meaning and ultimate purpose and causality. Such questions may lead to efforts to gain knowledge of natural or suprahuman forces believed to influence the world. In seeking this knowledge, religious practitioners sometimes claim to use scientific methods. Late-nineteenth- and early twentieth-century movements such as Christian Science, spiritualism, chiropractic, and Pentecostal divine healing all employed scientific language—although what members of these groups meant by "science" often would not have passed muster with conventionally trained scientists. It is important to note that both science and religion are ways of constructing what is "real" in the world rather than offering transparent windows onto reality.[6]

Until the modern period (and still today in certain cultures), religious leaders set the rules for pursuing knowledge of diverse subjects, including sickness and health. The myth of the rise of modern science is that theology first had to be dethroned before scientific progress became possible, because as long as people entertained supernatural explanations they were unlikely to investigate natural causal relationships. Research in the history of science reveals that some of the most influential leaders in the Renaissance and Enlightenment were Christians who hoped to use empirical investigations to provide evidence of the existence and nature of God—even as these same scientists engaged in metaphysical explorations of alchemy, astrology, numerology, and cabalistic mysticism, which today are generally understood to be pseudoscientific (as well as at odds with orthodox Christianity). Some historians have dared to suggest that the rise of modern science depended in part on the metaphysical leanings of revered scientific pioneers. At the same time, most scholars also agree that modern biomedical science achieved privileged cultural status because of its success in treating health problems that traditional religious healing had failed to resolve.[7]

Certain modern scientists implicitly and sometimes explicitly worry that empirical studies of prayer might be seen as validating religious healing claims. The fear is that studies seeming to show positive effects from prayer could bolster the cultural authority of religious institutions, thereby eclipsing the last two centuries of scientific progress and propelling a return to a superstitious past in which irrational, supernatural explanations hampered scientific inquiry. A 2005 editorial by *Science* magazine's editor in chief, Donald Kennedy, warns that

> the present wave of evangelical Christianity, uniquely American in
> its level of participation, would be nothing to worry about were it a
> matter restricted to individual conviction and to the expressions of
> groups gathering to worship. . . . But U.S. society is now experiencing
> a convergence between religious conviction and partisan loyalty . . .
> when the religious/political convergence leads to managing the
> nation's research agenda, its foreign assistance programs, or the high-
> school curriculum, that marks a really important change in our

national life. Twilight for the Enlightenment? Not yet. But as its beneficiaries, we should also be its stewards.

Very much alive in the minds of scientists such as Kennedy is a past era (which he fears could return) when religious institutions sometimes wielded their financial and political power to squelch scientific inquiry.[8]

In a widely heralded attempt to avoid a war between science and religion, in 1997, the Harvard University professor of paleontology and evolutionary biology Stephen Jay Gould proposed the concept of *nonoverlapping magisteria*, or NOMA. According to this principle, "the net of science covers the empirical universe: what is it made of (fact) and why does it work this way (theory). The net of religion extends over questions of moral meaning and value. These two magisteria do not overlap." Gould, a self-described Jewish agnostic, drew the conclusion that NOMA "permits—indeed enjoins—the prospect of respectful discourse, of constant input from both magisteria toward the common goal of wisdom." Yet some writers inspired by the NOMA principle have gone a step beyond Gould in construing his concept to imply that all rigorous, scientific study of the empirical effects of religious practices is off limits and that all theological inquiry is irrelevant to the practice of science. In this drawing of the boundaries, separate is inherently unequal. Thus, rather than pursuing the respectful dialogue enjoined by NOMA, those anxious to avoid inappropriate overlaps between science and religion have missed opportunities to garner insights from both magisteria in service of the common goal of wisdom.[9]

From War to Dialogue between Science and Religion

I begin with the premise that the boundaries between the magisteria of science and religion can be respected while engaging in dialogue. I ask empirical questions about the effects of religious practices on culture and society, including physical health, and I draw insights from theological analysis that are useful in developing more robust scientific inquiries. Indeed, I argue that theological understanding is essential to designing studies that have both *construct validity* and *ecological validity*—in other words, studies that isolate the intended phenomenon and study it as it naturally occurs.[10]

The Dalai Lama's interaction with the neuroscience community offers an instructive model. At first glance, what neuroscientists would hope to gain from studying the effects of mystical practices by Buddhist monks is not obvious. Nevertheless, in the late 1980s, a group of scientists began to engage with the Dalai Lama, resulting in the formation of the Mind and Life Institute to advance a dialogue between neuroscience and Buddhism, and catalyzing a series of studies of the effects of Buddhist meditation on brain structure and function. This dialogue between religion and science has worked surprisingly well, apparently because both sides benefit, and neither side feels threatened by the other. The Buddhists provide case studies of meditation experiences, the scientists study the practices as they actually occur, and the Buddhists help to ensure construct and ecological validity. The Buddhists gain an increased understanding of their own practices, without feeling threatened by potentially reductionist interpretations of science, because the Buddhists retain their magisterial prerogative to interpret their experiences according to their own religious views. The scientists likewise do not feel threatened, because they retain their magisterial prerogative to propose and pursue their own theories about the material effects of Buddhist practices on the brain as a biological system. The dialogue has been so fruitful that in 2005, with only minimal controversy, the thirty-thousand-plus-member Society for Neuroscience invited the Dalai Lama to give a keynote address at its annual meeting in Washington D.C. To me, all of this suggests the possibility of a similarly fruitful dialogue between religion and science on the topic of prayer for healing.[11]

Following the example above, in this book I likewise draw the magisterial boundary between faith and reason such that empirical questions (even about matters involving religious practice) are valid topics for empirical study (including falsification). But the magisterial boundary I respect is the *interpretation* of what the empirical findings mean for matters of religion. As subsequent chapters will explain, it is ironic that some of the voices most adamant in opposing such investigations proceed from a priori theological assumptions that because there is no supernatural, empirical investigations of religion are pointless; or that it is theologically unethical to test and potentially falsify tenets of faith on the basis of empirical evidence.

I approach the subject of theology, defined as the study of religious ideas, from the nonsectarian, academic perspective of religious studies. I do not assume the existence or nonexistence of a deity or other suprahuman forces. What I argue is that people's religious beliefs often have real-world effects that can be studied empirically. The well-known Thomas Theorem in sociology posits that if people "define situations as real, they are real in their consequences." The *perceptions* of religious practitioners—whether or not they align well with scientific *measurements* of phenomena—matter to individual and group beliefs and behaviors, and sometimes these effects are quite enduring.[12]

In his classic *Varieties of Religious Experience: A Study in Human Nature* (1902), the Harvard psychologist of religion William James criticized the "too simple-minded system of thought," what he called "medical materialism," that reduces complex religious experiences to merely biological phenomena:

> Medical materialism finishes up Saint Paul by calling his vision on the road to Damascus a discharging lesion of the occipital cortex, he being an epileptic. It snuffs out Saint Teresa as an hysteric, Saint Francis of Assisi as a hereditary degenerate. George Fox's discontent with the shams of his age, and his pining for a spiritual veracity, it treats as a disordered colon. Carlyle's organ-tones of misery it accounts for by a gastro-duodenal catarrh. All such mental overtensions, it says, are, when you come to the bottom of the matter, mere affairs of diathesis (auto-intoxications most probably), due to the perverted action of various glands which physiology will yet discover.

James's point is that such physiological processes may indeed be in play, but they cannot fully explain religious experiences. In pretending to do so, such reductionist theories obfuscate as much as they clarify. A more open-ended, agnostic stance encourages consideration of biomedical and sociological models while also asking what the details of how people perceive their situations reveal about religious experience and the effects of experience on attitudes and behaviors.[13]

A crucial limitation of many studies of healing prayer is that researchers—motivated by the admirable goal of wanting to provide comprehensive explanations—often attempt to use one type of data or method to answer questions that can be addressed better by a different kind of data or analytic approach. The subject of prayer for healing invites multidimensional investigations by raising questions of theology and religious practice, culture and social behavior, and biomedicine and public health. The research that went into this book ranged widely to include the literatures and methods of history, religious studies, sociology, anthropology, and biomedical and clinical science.

This research began with an exploratory weeklong visit to the Toronto Airport Vineyard Church in January 1995, shortly after I first heard of the Vineyard movement or the *Toronto Blessing* revivals then in full swing while I was taking courses in graduate school at Harvard University. What caught my attention, amid the general pandemonium of the raucous and very lengthy services, was the succession of testimonies by visitors from around the world who claimed healing through prayer from all manner of physical and emotional problems. I had until this point never visited a Pentecostal or Charismatic church, and I had only a slight idea of what one was. Although by this time I was writing a dissertation on nineteenth-century evangelical print culture, I began to read more about twentieth-century religious developments.

In 2003, as I put the finishing touches on the book that emerged from my dissertation, *The Word in the World: Evangelical Writing, Publishing, and Reading in America, 1789–1880*, I reflected on the limitations of that project. I had argued—and I stand by this argument—that "sanctification," also known as "holiness," or freedom from "sin" and its consequences—was a major theme in the development of evangelicalism, one that few scholars had fully appreciated. But I increasingly realized that I had overemphasized one strand of nineteenth-century discussions of holiness—a Calvinist focus on the value of suffering in purifying the soul by disciplining the body. Even more significant for twentieth-century cultural developments was the Wesleyan idea— indeed a view common to many cultures worldwide—that purification of the soul and the body are complementary rather than antagonistic. I also came to realize that my graduate studies in the History of American Civilization program—an amalgam of religious history and American studies—had made me myopic about the multidirectional global cultural flows that are critical to understanding modern religious movements.[14]

I concluded that if I wanted to trace the story of "holy bodies" from the nineteenth century to the present, I needed to learn about Pentecostal and Charismatic Christianity not only in the United States but also around the world. I also needed to supplement my familiar tools of historical and literary analysis with the ethnographic approaches of written surveys, oral interviews, and participant observation; qualitative and quantitative data analysis including statistics; and—as I discovered the centrality of healing to pentecostalism—biomedical and clinical methods. As the complexity of this subject unfolded, I drew on the expertise of researchers in a variety of natural and social science disciplines and learned to employ the broad range of methodologies necessary for studying such a multifaceted topic as religious healing. Although this book is primarily the product of my own research program, and the writing (and any errors) are my own, in appreciation of contributions made by numerous consultants, colleagues, and research assistants, as described in the acknowledgments, this book makes occasional use of the first-person-plural pronoun *we*.

We have been conducting research on pentecostal offshoots of the Toronto Blessing since 2003. This project singles out for in-depth analysis the healing-prayer practices of *pentecostals*—an umbrella term that encompasses Pentecostal and Charismatic Christians who emphasize gifts of the Holy Spirit—because pentecostals give special attention to healing prayer, and these movements are growing because many people—accurately or inaccurately—perceive these prayers to be effective. The global pentecostal networks that emerged from Toronto offer a convenient laboratory, though by no means the only possible setting, for exploring the questions about prayer and science that drive this book. My hope is that this book's focus on a subgroup of pentecostals will provide a foundation for my own and other scholars' investigations of other spiritual healing practices—for example, forms of "energy" healing rooted in Taoist, Hindu, and Buddhist traditions. The current research involved textual analysis of printed, online, and audiovisual publications, as well as regular attendance and observation at a large number of Toronto-influenced events in the United States (California, Florida, Illinois, Indiana, Massachusetts, Missouri, North Carolina, Ohio, Pennsylvania, Texas, and Washington), Canada (British Columbia, Ontario), Brazil (Maranhão, Minas Gerais, Pará, Paraná, Rio de Janeiro, São Paulo), and Mozambique (Cabo Delgado). In the Brazilian and Mozambican cases, I have for the present volume focused primarily on survey and clinical data (complemented by short-term observation and single interviews) rather than conducting long-term ethnographic research. As will become apparent, we encountered many challenges in pursuing each avenue of empirical investigation. This book is not intended as a final word on any of the subjects addressed but as an invitation to a process of dialogue among scientists and religious practitioners from diverse traditions.[15]

This book argues that researchers can and should use empirical methods to study prayer for healing, and it proposes a four-prong model for doing so. First, the collection and analysis of medical records from before and after prayer for healing may indicate whether people claiming healing exhibited any observable improvement in their conditions for which there is no obvious medical or natural explanation. Second, survey research offers insight into how individuals perceive their experiences of healing prayer. Third, prospective clinical trials can demonstrate whether prayer practices result in measurable changes in certain conditions. Finally, multiyear follow-up observations and interviews of individuals who claim healing investigate any lasting effects of healing experiences.

Can Science Prove or Disprove the Healing Power of Prayer?

Even if researchers employ a range of methodological perspectives and explanatory models, there are inherent limits to what scientific testing can prove. Scientific studies of religious practices can neither prove nor disprove the existence of the divine or suprahuman. Empirical research can measure only certain effects of religious practices and illumine how religious practitioners—as well as scientists—construct their understandings of these practices. Although this book will argue that it is impossible to present definitive scientific proof of the healing power of prayer, the same could be said of many important questions in science.

A revealing exchange in *Science* magazine in 2011 illustrates the elusiveness of scientific proof. The editors published a news report titled "At Long Last, Gravity Probe B Satellite Proves Einstein Right." A letter to the editor objected to this "title misstep" because "science doesn't 'prove' theories. Scientific measurements can only disprove theories or be consistent with them. Any theory that is consistent with measurements could be disproved by a future measurement." The editors responded with a one-line concession that the criticism was "completely correct" and "we blew it." When scientists investigate a variety of phenomena, they look for evidence to disprove—rather than prove—hypotheses and theories that might explain those phenomena. A purpose of statistical analysis is to weigh the relative probabilities—not to prove—that effects that appear to exist are not merely the product of chance. In this way, a medical treatment (for example) can be accepted as effective if the probability that it is ineffective is sufficiently low, but this is not the same as conclusively proving its effectiveness. In practice, many common pharmaceuticals and medical procedures are appropriately accepted as the standard of care on the basis of statistical inference despite the absence of conclusive proof of how or even that they work.[16]

Many people assume that science, unlike religion, provides an objective lens for viewing reality. Yet Thomas Kuhn's classic *The Structure of Scientific Revolutions* (1962) argues that the major "paradigm" shifts in science are "not the sort of battle that can be resolved by proof." This is because researchers invested in the current paradigm greet "novelty" in scientific research with "resistance" since the new paradigm threatens to invalidate much of the research conducted under the old paradigm. For this reason, the medical anthropologists Elliot Mishler and Robert Hahn have proposed that the "biomedical model" be treated not as "*the* representation or picture of reality," but as "*a* representation," one that is, like all other ethnomedicines, "rooted in cultural presuppositions and values, associated with rules of conduct." The sociologists Meredith McGuire and Debra Kantor urge setting aside the assumption that "the medical reality, as promulgated by the dominant health specialists in this culture, is necessarily the 'true' reality. From a sociological perspective, this medical definition of reality must be seen as one among many competing conceptions of illness, its causes, and treatment. Medical reality, too, is socially constructed." An important implication of this "relativistic stance toward the 'truth' of biomedicine" is that biomedicine "cannot be used to explain nonmedical healing. One paradigmatic system cannot really explain another, although the comparison may be useful as a legitimating device." This proposal that comparison be used not for proof but as a means of corroborating particular claims is a valuable one that I employ in subsequent chapters.[17]

Just as theological understanding can help scientists to steer clear of methodological pitfalls in the study of prayer, empirical studies can help theologians avoid erroneous reasoning. Scientific investigation protects against the *post hoc, ergo propter hoc* fallacy to which healing practitioners are susceptible—that people who receive prayer for healing and then recover can attribute their newfound health to prayer. There is empirical evidence that as many as 90 percent of sick people recover regardless of treatment, as long as the healer does not do something actively to make the patient worse. Even diseases of unknown causation, especially infections, are often self-limiting once the body's immune system kicks into gear. And cancers, which are poorly understood, may grow or stop growing or even regress without any clear explanation. It is often by chance that the "last practitioner who treats the patients before recovery gets the credit." Yet the body has an astounding natural capacity for self-healing.[18]

Religious believers may protest that God created the body's ability to heal itself, but this is a separate claim, not easily subject to empirical verification. Pentecostals typically interpret a healing as "divine" if it occurs more rapidly or with fewer complications than predicted by doctors. But doctors are not psychics, and they often over- (or under-) estimate the time required for healing. Many cancer patients receive medical and alternative therapies, including prayer. When patients defy the statistics and recover despite a poor prognosis, they often claim a "miracle." In such cases, a simpler explanation is that the medical treatments administered—which were, after all, prescribed because they have been empirically demonstrated to be effective in many cases—achieved their intended effects. These treatments may have worked better than hoped, but it is well known that some people respond better or worse to such treatments for unpredictable but nonmiraculous reasons. God may, as is often claimed, have healed divinely through the means of chemotherapy, but this takes us back to the category of unverifiable ontological claims. Similarly, if someone claims to have been healed divinely of an intestinal problem because God "told" the person to fast from food, should the healing be attributed to the physical benefits of the fast or to divine revelation? In such a situation, it may be relatively easy to ascribe healing to a physiological mechanism, but the healing still may appear to be divine in the eyes of the beholder. When scientists seek to explain religious-healing claims, they often posit such factors as "placebo effect," "spontaneous remission," or the "power of suggestion." The use of such labels can disregard more than explain unexpected recoveries, yet biomedical and clinical scientists are all the time gaining new insights into possible mechanisms by which mental states may influence physical health.[19]

What Happens When People Pray for Other People's Healing?

An important subtheme of this book is that pentecostal Christianity has emerged as a major social (and indeed political) force on the world scene in large part because it places particular emphasis on intercessory prayer for healing, and many people have perceived themselves healed through the prayers of pentecostals. From a handful of adherents at the turn of the twentieth century, pentecostals now account for more than a quarter of the world's 2 billion Christians. By one count, 80 million people in the United States—36 percent of the adult population—self-identify as pentecostals. Aware that prayer for healing played some role in the rise of global pentecostalism, I collaborated with seventeen anthropologists, historians, political scientists, sociologists, and religion scholars to write *Global Pentecostal and Charismatic Healing* (2011). The collective force of our research is that the single most significant factor that explains the growth of pentecostalism is the frequency of the perception among both new converts and long-time adherents that they have received divine healing.[20]

The pattern that emerges in the following chapters is that individuals perceive themselves healed through prayer by members of their social networks. Those who experience healing attribute their recoveries to divine love and power and consequently feel motivated to express love for God and other people in part by praying for others' healing. The effects of even a single healing experience reverberate across global networks, as recipients of healing turn their attention to others and become partners and leaders of efforts to expand the reach of healing prayer. Such efforts are self-perpetuating because individuals both disburse and draw emotional energy—or love energy—from social interactions in which recipients, partners, and leaders all experience love through their involvement in healing rituals. Because pentecostals perceive God to be an unlimited source of love and power, they are emboldened to expend rather than conserve energy. The resultant social interactions replenish rather than deplete the energy available for ongoing healing exchanges.

Broadly speaking, this project engages with scholarship on the emotions, altruism, lived religious experience, practices, social behavior, and the role of the human body in religious life. Traditional theology privileges intellectual understanding, doctrine, and belief, but since the late twentieth century religious studies scholars have shifted their attention toward how religious ideas and feelings play out in people's lives. A complementary move in sociology pioneered by Peter Berger and Thomas Luckmann is known as *social constructionism*. To put it simply, people—including both religious practitioners and scientists—construct their understandings of reality in the context of social interactions. It is possible to study the processes through which people decide what is real and act on their perceptions, regardless of the ultimate validity of their worldviews.[21]

The processes by which certain pentecostals construct healing prayer can be studied in the context of globally diffuse social networks. The term *network*, which many modern pentecostals use frequently, refers to nonhierarchical, relational connections among groups with partially overlapping values and sense of mission. The origins of pentecostal networks can be traced back to the Protestant Reformation's emphasis on the priesthood of all believers and the fellowship of like-minded Christians, and to the impact of the printing and transportation revolutions on fostering a translocal sense of community membership. Informal networks, adjacent to denominational structures, played a significant role in the first and second Great Awakenings of the eighteenth and nineteenth centuries, and in the divine-healing movement that gathered momentum in the late nineteenth century. Since the ecumenical Charismatic revivals of the 1960s, the shift away from denominationally organized religion toward relational networks has increased. Although denominational bureaucracies have not disappeared, individuals and congregations may retain their denominational affiliations while participating in larger-than-denominational alliances.[22]

There is also a vibrant field of social network theory in the social and behavioral sciences, although scholars in these fields usually pay little attention to religious (as opposed to family, neighbor, work, etc.) networks. This study draws several insights from this body of scholarship. Most basically, individuals influence each other's behavior in important ways through their social interactions. Even weak social ties can be significant in forming bridges among dense clusters of close friends who would not otherwise be connected. The network perspective also recognizes the importance of relationships among interacting units larger than individuals, the activities of which are interdependent rather than fully autonomous. An important function of networks is facilitating the flow of information and other material or nonmaterial resources, thereby constituting the foundation of social capital.[23]

Of particular relevance is the sociologist Randall Collins's concept of *interaction ritual* chains, or IR theory. Building on the classic social theories of Émile Durkheim as articulated in *Elementary Forms of Religious Life* (1912), IR postulates that the chains of social situations in which individuals participate shape beliefs and behaviors. From their participation in rituals, individuals can acquire a "morally

suffused" form of "emotional energy" that is highly motivational, leading toward boldness in taking actions that feel morally valuable. In
the language of Durkheim, participation in religious rituals produces
an *effervescence* that motivates and sustains religious behavior. The
accumulation of emotional energy may lead individuals to altruistic
behavior that is, for demonstrable physiological reasons, beneficial to
the altruist's own physical and emotional health. Such a chain reaction
is captured by the title of Stephen Post and Jill Neimark's book *Why
Good Things Happen to Good People: The Exciting New Research That
Proves the Link between Doing Good and Living a Longer, Healthier,
Happier Life* (2007).[24]

Pitirim Sorokin, the founder of Harvard University's department of
sociology, explored the potentially beneficial effects of social interactions. Echoing Durkheim's concept of effervescence, Sorokin spoke
of a *love energy* that is "produced by the interaction of human beings"
and, like other forms of energy, can be stored, distributed, and become capable of doing work. Sorokin has been understandably controversial because of his theistic assumptions about the source of love
energy. But one can use Sorokin's concept while instead taking an agnostic stance that focuses on the emotional energy of social exchanges.
Sorokin suggested the intriguing possibility of developing empirical
measures of the *intensity, extensity, duration, purity,* and *adequacy* of
socially expressed love energy. For example, does one give away a few
pennies or give more sacrificially? Is love directed only toward one-
self? Or does it extend beyond one's own family and nation? Does one
behave heroically for a moment or express devotion over a span of years?
Are acts of benevolence undertaken for personal gain or for altruistic
reasons? Do subjectively loving intentions produce desirable or adverse consequences? Sorokin noted that particular expressions of love
may be evaluated as "high" in terms of one measure and "low" in terms
of another; indeed, one measure, such as intensity, may vary inversely
with another measure, such as extensity. This book's conclusion applies these five empirical measures to pentecostal prayer.[25]

Drawing on Sorokin's ideas of love energy, the sociologists Margaret Poloma, Matthew Lee, and their collaborators developed the theoretical model of *Godly Love*. They define this concept as "the dynamic

interaction between divine and human love that enlivens and expands benevolence." It is crucial that Godly Love models a *"perceived* inter-action" (emphasis mine) and does *not* imply the actual existence or activity of "God" or any other suprahuman force. The Godly Love model can be applied to examine how perceptions affect behaviors and to study the processes through which "benevolent service becomes an emergent property." Building on IR theory, Lee and Poloma argue that "exemplars of Godly Love . . . draw energy both directly from their perceived interactions with God as well as their interactions with col-laborators and the people who benefit from their benevolent service." Such interactions involve not only individuals but also interdependent social units. Because individual actions are embedded in larger rela-tional connections,

> repeated interactions develop structures that, in turn, regularize and institutionalize particular kinds of interaction, thereby in-creasing, storing, and transmitting love energy across time and space. The idea of structured action directs our attention to the ways in which social structures both constrain and facilitate the diffusion of certain kinds of love energy throughout social networks.

Thus, the Godly Love model has implications for understanding not only individual human behavior but also the larger dynamics of how cultural influences spread (or are constrained from spreading) through social networks.[26]

Toronto Blessing pentecostals, both in North America and world-wide, place a high value on participating in social networks that are both locally and globally defined—most broadly as encompassing the "church universal" or the "body of Christ." Although disavowing hi-erarchical authority chains, the pentecostals studied envision several discrete roles that participants in social interactions occupy. It is im-portant that the same individuals can inhabit multiple roles sequen-tially or even simultaneously. To extend the Godly Love framework, there are *leaders*, or exemplars, who intentionally set an example for others to emulate—and whom other pentecostals recognize as model-ing exemplary behavior. Leaders may include clergy but also laity, and indeed women, children, and members of socioeconomic and ethnic groups with low secular social status who are recognized within their religious networks as exhibiting high levels of the "gifts" and "fruits" of the Holy Spirit. Pentecostals envision themselves as belonging to a social "body," the members of which work in concert; thus leaders need ministry *partners*, or collaborators. Partnership may include pursuing similar or complementary activities or giving financial or prayer support to the work of ministry leaders. Leaders and partners direct much of their energy toward seeking to benefit other people who may or may not be members of their social networks. Thus, *recipients*, or beneficiaries, occupy an essential role as targets of pentecostal attention. The efforts of leaders and partners to benefit recipients may take the form of proselytism (generally described as "evangelism" or the sharing of "good news"); meeting practical needs such as food, shelter, and financial resources; and concern for physical and emotional health, expressed through prayers for healing, provision of supportive care to sick persons and their families, or help in obtaining medical assistance. Finally, pentecostals hypothesize a fourth role occupied by God as both the ultimate *source* of resources distributed among actors in the other three roles and as the central *object* of devotion. In pentecostal (and more broadly Christian) vernacular, God *is* love, and the two greatest God-given commandments are to love God and to love one's neighbor.[27]

Many individuals who understand themselves to be recipients of divine healing construct their experiences as an expression of God's love for them. A perceived experience of divine healing often motivates individuals to seek to express greater love for God and for other people—not only family and friends but sometimes even total strangers, perhaps from another culture. Individuals seek to express this love by working with partners to help other recipients experience healing and/or by engaging in other forms of benevolent service, such as providing for the needs of those who are economically poor and politically powerless. According to IR theory, *any* partner or recipient who participates in healing rituals can be transformed by their social interactions into a leader—including orphaned children and other previously nameless members of the two-thirds-world poor. Because many pentecostals participate in dense global networks, one individual's healing experience can influence pentecostals living on the opposite side of the world. Thus, the effects of healing practices can be diffused widely throughout pentecostal networks and, through a series of mutually interdependent interactions, stimulate the global expansion of pentecostalism.

Bringing Scientific Perspectives on Prayer into Focus

To draw a modern analogy to explain my approach to integrating the study of science and religion, the Hubble Space Telescope, launched in 1990—four years before the Toronto Blessing—takes extraordinarily revealing pictures by using several different types of cameras. In this analogy, each chapter in this book is like one particular sort of camera, offering a distinctive perspective on healing prayer practices. When viewed together, this combination of vantages offers a more complete picture than could be provided by any single lens of, first, how scientists and religious practitioners construct healing prayer and, second, the empirical outcomes of praying for other people's healing.

Chapter 1 tells the story of how protracted religious meetings dubbed the Toronto Blessing (1994–2006) at a mid-sized Ontario church birthed a transnational web of pentecostal networks—prominently including the Apostolic Network of Global Awakening and Iris Ministries—whose healing practices are contributing to the global spread of Christianity. The next two chapters consider the history of controversies, in chapter 2, over biomedical tests of prayer; and in chapter 3, concerning the value and limitations of medical documentation in examining healing claims. Each of the following three chapters assesses the effects of healing practices from distinct, complementary angles—using a combination of quantitative and qualitative empirical methods informed by theological analysis of how prayer is understood and practiced. Chapter 4 analyzes written survey data collected from pentecostal conference participants to explore perceptions of illness and healing. Chapter 5 develops the concept of proximal intercessory prayer and assesses prayer outcomes through a prospective clinical trial of the measurable effects of PIP on hearing and vision. Chapter 6 asks what if any lasting effects healing experiences may have on the individuals who claim them and on other members of their social networks. The conclusion draws together findings from preceding chapters to evaluate intersections between perceptions and measurements of healing and to interpret the effects of prayer practices.

Various readers may feel especially drawn to certain chapters. Chapters 1 and 6 consist of interlocking stories; some readers may wish to skip around and begin with these narratives. The second and third chapters can be likened to historical detective novels, brimming with surprising twists and intrigues. The fourth and fifth chapters are richly quantitative.

Can scientific tests prove or disprove the healing power of prayer? As this book will show, my answer to this question is "no, but." Empirical research can reveal much about prayer for healing—just as studies of prayer can disclose much about science—by embracing the kind of dialogue between science and religion that this book develops.

CHAPTER 1

From Toronto Blessing to Global Awakening

Healing and the Spread of Pentecostal-Charismatic Networks

✦

On January 20, 1994, Randy Clark, the pastor of a Vineyard church in St. Louis, Missouri, traveled to Toronto, Ontario, at the invitation of John Arnott, the pastor of the Toronto Airport Vineyard Church, to preach four services. What happened surprised everyone, not least Clark and Arnott. About 160 people attended the first service. When Clark said, "Come Holy Spirit," people shook, fell down, produced deep belly laughs, felt peaceful, or acted intoxicated. Some converted to Christianity, testified to physical and emotional healing and deliverance from demons, or dedicated their lives as missionaries to bringing good news to the nations of the world. Most controversial were a few people who made loud, animal-like noises such as the roar of a lion. The participants in the Toronto meetings interpreted this unusual behavior as indicating that the Holy Spirit had accepted the invitation to come.[1]

As news of this revival spread, people came from all over North America and eventually from every continent, representing many racial and ethnic groups, searching for physical and emotional healing or spiritual renewal. Arnott extended the plan for nightly services indefinitely, persuading Clark to stay for forty-two of the first sixty meetings; many other visiting church leaders also took turns preaching. For the first several months, reports of healing in the Toronto meetings were scattered, but over time the frequency of healing claims increased. Services continued six evenings a week—often for six or more hours per night—until 2006, making what was dubbed the "Toronto Blessing" the longest revival meeting in North American history. Indeed, it may be that even as of 2011, the Toronto revivals have not so much waned as decentralized, becoming a less significant pilgrimage destination as its influences have become globally diffused. The Toronto meetings drew an estimated 3 million people, including Catholics, Orthodox, and every Protestant denomination. Approximately fifty-five thousand churches around the world were affected in just the first year as visitors returned home to their own congregations and avowedly brought the "revival fires" with them. Churches all over the world began to report phenomena similar to those occurring in Toronto shortly after a pastor or a few lay members returned from a pilgrimage.[2]

Not every Christian observer—let alone the secular press—concluded that the presence of the Holy Spirit explained the Toronto Blessing. Within weeks, critics questioned whether the Toronto Blessing was a genuine revival that produced the fruit of conversions to Christianity, increased holiness in the lives of Christians, and outreach beyond the church in missionary evangelism and social benevolence. Some suggested that runaway emotionalism, hypnotic suggestion, pseudo-miraculous psychosomatic healings, or demonically inspired witchcraft constituted more plausible explanations. In his book *Counterfeit Revival* (1997), the popular evangelical author and radio personality Hank Hanegraaff interpreted Toronto as the epitome of a false revival. Even John Wimber, founder of the Vineyard movement, and the entire twenty-member oversight board of the Association of Vineyard Churches were so disturbed—especially by reports of "exotic" and "extra-biblical" animal noises—that they "disengaged" the Toronto church in December 1995. Shortly before taking this disciplinary action, Wimber had written an endorsement for John Arnott's book *The Father's Blessing* (1995), which justified the avowedly rare animal sounds as prophetic expressions; later, Wimber denied having read that part of the book.[3]

The Toronto Blessing and the Vineyard movement split their paths. The Toronto Airport Vineyard (TAV) Church was renamed the Toronto Airport Christian Fellowship (TACF). Clark himself was able to keep his St. Louis church and its new missions arm, Global Awakening, in the Vineyard movement. Wimber even encouraged Clark to develop an international healing ministry. Reflecting on his eventual distancing from the Vineyard in a 2005 interview, Clark said that at first he had hoped that Global Awakening could function like one of the Catholic orders, such as the Benedictines, in pushing the Vineyard toward recapturing the movement's original vibrancy. Clark was disappointed when Wimber seemingly rejected his efforts at revitalization—although Clark also claims that Wimber, near the end of his life (he died in 1997), expressed regret at his decision to disfellowship TAV.[4]

One of the Toronto Blessing's severest critics, the Reverend Canon Martyn Percy, a professor of theological education at King's College London, characterized the Toronto Blessing as theologically "dubious" and "offensive." Percy was particularly troubled because those who claimed that the Holy Spirit had descended on Toronto seemed to assume that God would "indulge a small, Caucasian-based, international and mainly middle-class group with great blessings, whilst leaving the lot of the poor largely untouched." Percy concluded in 1998 that there was "just no evidence of that event signifying a global revival." From the historical vantage of thirteen years since Percy's assessment, this chapter argues that the Toronto Blessing has significantly influenced the spread of global Christianity—including in the two-thirds world—by increasing the prevalence of prayer for healing and multiplying the number and influence of divine healing claims.[5]

Toronto-Blessing Pentecostals as a Case Study of Healing Prayer

The frequency with which Pentecostals and Charismatics claim healing through prayer distinguishes these groups from other Christians. This may be a surprising claim to those who associate pentecostalism with such practices as speaking in tongues; snake handling; or boisterous, televised appeals for "seed-faith" giving as the ticket to financial prosperity. A 2006 study found that 62 percent of U.S. Pentecostals—compared with 29 percent of the total population—claimed to have "experienced or witnessed a divine healing of an illness or injury." The same study, conducted by the Pew Forum on Religion & Public Life, surveyed not only the United States but also nine other countries in Latin America, Africa, and Asia (table 1.1). The study found sizable percentages of the general population, and even higher percentages of Pentecostals and Charismatics, claiming to have had personal divine healing experiences. Pentecostals are not the only people who pray for healing, but if the goal is to study claims of healing through prayer, pentecostalism is a good place to begin.[6]

The concept of prayer, even if restricted to Christian prayer, encompasses a wide variety of practices. For example, prayer may be liturgical, conversational, meditative, or petitionary. Pentecostals (like other Christians) may spend time quietly "soaking" in God's presence or contemplating Bible verses or may combine prayers of adoration and thanksgiving with petitions on the worshiper's own behalf, intercession for other people, and even commands issued to physical conditions or spiritual entities. A basic theological premise held by many pentecostals is that a personal God responds to prayers in the name of Jesus by the power of the Holy Spirit—although certain individuals and ways of praying are widely considered more effective than others (varying, for instance, by degrees of "faith," or expectancy). This and subsequent chapters will flesh out this broad-stroke overview through specific examples of how pentecostals may articulate prayers for healing in particular situations.[7]

Table 1.1.   Percentages Reporting Previous "Divine Healing" Experiences.

	U.S.	Brazil	Chile	Guatemala	Kenya	Nigeria	South Africa	India	Philippines	South Korea
Total population	29	38	26	56	71	62	38	44	38	10
Pentecostals	62	77	77	79	87	79	73	74	72	56
Charismatics	46	31	37	63	78	—	47	61	44	61
Other Christians	28	32	24	47	47	75	32	55	30	20

Source: Data summarized from Luis Lugo et. al, *Spirit and Power: A 10-Country Survey of Pentecostals* (Washington, DC: Pew Forum on Religion & Public Life, October 2006).

When pentecostals pray for *divine healing*, they often have in mind both a physical *cure* from disease or disability and a more holistic healing process that produces a sense of emotional and spiritual wholeness. Modern pentecostals are not unique in envisioning healing as benefiting body, mind, and spirit—concerns that are shared by nonpentecostal Christians as well as by participants in holistic healing movements rooted in other religious traditions. Yet many pentecostals do distinguish divine healing from a recovery expected through the regular operation of natural processes. The healing may not be instantaneous or spectacular or appear to violate natural laws—and thus be classified as a *miracle*. However, divine healing is often understood to proceed more rapidly than usual (as when a tumor dissolves in ten minutes) or under circumstances in which healing would not otherwise be expected (for instance, disappearance of cancer that has already metastasized). In practice, the distinction between divine and natural healing can easily blur. Pentecostals may pray for God to guide the hands of surgeons, make medicines efficacious, or work through psychological counseling, and then credit God for any healing achieved. In the pentecostal worldview, God, as well as angels and demons, may intervene in the natural world by working against—or through—biomedical or psychosomatic processes. The same healing, depending on whether interpreted through a worldview constructed by pentecostals or scientific naturalists, may appear to reflect divine or natural activity.[8]

The pentecostal networks that emerged from Toronto provide an apt case study for exploring larger questions about healing prayer. As healing became an increasingly prominent theme of the Toronto Blessing, the movement touched off a chain of events that made expectant prayer for healing more common in many Christian churches worldwide. A renewed emphasis on healing prayer—coupled with the widespread perception that such prayers result in divine healing—has contributed to the global spread of Christianity. This is not to say that the Toronto revivals are *sui generis,* or even that they are the most influential stream of pentecostal Christianity. Yet prayer for healing—accompanied by an expectation that prayer should and often does produce observable results (even if such results are perceived to be more common in the global South)—is a notable feature of Toronto-influenced pentecostalism. Moreover, the fact that healing prayer is practiced in the context of globalized relational and institutional networks facilitates study through the collection of before-and-after medical records, the implementation of survey and clinical research, and long-term follow-up with individuals reporting healing or indirectly affected by healing practices.

I focused my empirical research on two groups, first the Apostolic Network of Global Awakening, headquartered in Mechanicsburg, Pennsylvania but active in thirty-six countries (most often Brazil), and directed by Randy Clark, a U.S. citizen. The second group is Iris Ministries (IM), which has its headquarters in Pemba, Cabo Delgado, Mozambique, with branches in twenty-five countries; it is directed by Rolland and Heidi Baker, expatriate U.S. citizens naturalized as Mozambicans. Both organizations grew out of Toronto and belong to the same overlapping, globally diffuse pentecostal networks. Randy Clark (born in 1952) and Heidi Baker (born in 1959), who is more of a public figure than is Rolland Baker, are dynamic leaders who are respected and emulated by members of their own networks and more broadly by many pentecostals and other Christians around the world. Clark and Heidi Baker each spend approximately half the year traveling to pentecostal conferences in other states, provinces, and countries. Both of their organizations place great emphasis on prayer for divine healing in day-to-day operations and articulations of vision. Both Clark and the Bakers point to dramatic healing experiences in their own lives that motivate their unconventional lifestyles.[9]

This chapter sets the stage for the empirical perspectives on healing prayer that are explored in the rest of this book. The narrative begins by contextualizing Toronto-influenced pentecostal prayer within a longer history of Christian prayer for healing and the emergence of global pentecostalism. The Toronto meetings did not occur in a vacuum but grew out of a dense network of institutional and relational connections. The Toronto revivals produced a thickening of those network connections, notably through Clark's founding of the Apostolic Network of Global Awakening (hereafter abbreviated as ANGA when referencing the larger-than-organizational network, and as

GA when referring to Clark's own ministry entity). This chapter argues that ANGA-bridged networks—though not coterminous with global pentecostalism—exemplify the multidirectional, global patterns of cultural exchange through which healing prayer feeds pentecostal growth. Participation in network activities, notably conferences and international ministry trips, builds a sense of global community. North American ANGA affiliates borrow from pentecostals in countries they visit (such as Brazil, Mozambique, and India) heightened expectation of divine intervention in the natural world, particularly through healing. By emphasizing the capacity of ordinary Christians to become agents of healing, North American pentecostals facilitate the democratization of global healing practices. The interplay of supernaturalism and democratization accentuates the prominence of healing prayer in ANGA-brokered networks, fanning the revivalist expansion of Christianity set ablaze by the Toronto Blessing.

Prayer for Healing in the Context of Global Pentecostal Networks

Prayer for healing is not unique to pentecostalism or even to Christianity. Because sickness and death are universal human experiences, it is not surprising that many of the world's religious traditions appeal to suprahuman sources of healing energy. Extra-empirical understandings of "energy" are central to healing practices such as acupuncture, tai chi, yoga, Reiki, and Therapeutic Touch that draw on traditions that include Taoism, Hinduism, and Buddhism. Although there are many revealing parallels between pentecostal love energy and other models of energetic healing, the important project of comparison has been reserved for a subsequent book (now in progress).[10]

The present volume lays the foundation for future comparative work through an in-depth consideration of Christianity, which has aptly been characterized as a "religion of healing." The religion's founder, Jesus of Nazareth, reputedly exercised an extraordinary capacity to heal—often by "laying his hands" on the sick—and he commissioned his followers to heal likewise. New Testament instructions for church practice advise that if anyone is sick, "let them call the elders of the church to pray over them and anoint them with oil in the name of the Lord. And the prayer offered in faith will make the sick person well" (James 5:14–15). Historical records indicate that prayer for healing was a common feature of church practice for at least several hundred years. Over time, the emphasis on healing prayer diminished for a variety of reasons, including a theological refashioning of sickness as an aid to holiness, but the practice of praying for healing never disappeared completely. At the time of the Reformation, during the sixteenth century, the Catholic Church continued to practice healing prayer, whereas the emerging Protestant movement took a more skeptical stance toward the availability of divine healing in the postbiblical era.[11]

Scattered reports of healing through prayer can be found throughout church history. The number and geographic reach of publicized healings increased greatly in the modern era. The dissemination of newspapers and improved travel technologies made it more likely that activities in one locality would influence events at the opposite end of the globe. News of healings circulated during the Great Awakenings, the transatlantic religious revivals of the eighteenth and nineteenth centuries. John Wesley, the English leader of the eighteenth-century Methodist revivals, recorded numerous instances of healing in response to prayer, most famously the healing of his horse. The best-known evangelist of the First Great Awakening, England's George Whitefield, claimed that he himself, after prayer, arose from his deathbed to preach the gospel. Charles Grandison Finney, the foremost revivalist of the Second Great Awakening in the antebellum United States, encouraged his congregations to pray expectantly for healing. Contemporaneous with Finney, Edward Irving of the National Scottish Church proclaimed the renewal of healing gifts to audiences numbering over ten thousand. Johann Christoph Blumhardt in Germany and Dorothea Trudel and Otto Stockmayer in Switzerland attracted international attention in the 1840s and 1850s when each of them established "healing homes," residences where the sick could stay and receive prayer over an extended period of time; newspapers and books carried reports of miraculous cures throughout Europe and around the world. Numerous international visitors traveled to the European healing homes to investigate for themselves, many of them going on to found similar healing homes in their own countries. The American homeopathic physician and Episcopal layman Charles Cullis publicized the European precedents in the 1870s and 1880s through his publishing company, the Willard Tract Repository, which produced a score of major publications and dozens of tracts on divine healing.[12]

By the third quarter of the nineteenth century, divine healing was a frequent, albeit controversial, theme in the many international conferences of the Holiness, Higher Christian Life, and Keswick revival movements. Healing evangelists, many of whom itinerated internationally, included the Englishwoman Elizabeth Baxter, the Americans A. J. Gordon, Maria Woodworth-Etter, and Carrie Judd Montgomery, the African American Elizabeth Mix, the Canadian A. B. Simpson, and a Scottish Australian immigrant to the United States, John Alexander Dowie. A significant marker of an emerging, global divine healing movement, the International Conference on Divine Healing and True Holiness met in London in 1885, attracting nearly two thousand attendees from at least nine countries and three continents.[13]

Healing prayer played a central role in the emergence of global pentecostalism in the twentieth century. The term *globalization* refers, on a basic level, to the widespread perception that the world seems increasingly interconnected. It is important to note that disease spreads more rapidly in an interrelated, urbanizing world. At the same time, fear is itself contagious as information and misinformation about disease spreads through global communication networks. Globalization heightens both the actual threat and the fear of disease, thereby fueling the growth of religious movements such as pentecostalism for which healing is a central concern.[14]

The term *pentecostal* refers to the Jewish holiday of Pentecost, which falls fifty days after Passover. According to the New Testament account in Acts 2, Jesus's disciples received the Holy Spirit on the first Pentecost after Jesus's Crucifixion. The apostle Paul's first letter to the Corinthians lists nine *charisms* (the root of the word *Charismatic*), or gifts, of the Holy Spirit: the word of wisdom, word of knowledge, faith, gifts of healing, the working of miracles, prophecy, the discerning of spirits, divers kinds of tongues, and the interpretation of tongues. As used here, the capitalized *Pentecostal* refers to self-described Pentecostal denominations such as the Assemblies of God or the Church of God in Christ. Many Pentecostals insist that glossolalia—speaking in tongues—is the initial evidence of Spirit baptism, whereas Charismatics generally allow that Spirit baptism may or may not be accompanied by glossolalia. The lower-case pentecostal encompasses Pentecostals, Charismatics, and other Christians who emphasize gifts of the Holy Spirit.[15]

Scholars of pentecostalism often refer to three waves of modern interest in the Holy Spirit and spiritual gifts such as healing. The first is identified primarily with revivals that began on Azusa Street, in Los Angeles, California in 1906 and quickly fanned out globally; the second with the ecumenical Protestant and Catholic Charismatic renewals of the 1960s and 1970s; and the third with the Signs and Wonders and neo-pentecostal movements of the 1980s and 1990s. This "third wave" was epitomized by the Toronto Blessing revivals that began in 1994 and birthed a dense, globally diffused web of overlapping pentecostal networks that aim to promote a worldwide revival of Christianity by means of healing evangelism.[16]

Many United States denominational Pentecostal historians have traced the origins of Pentecostalism to Topeka, Kansas, where Agnes Ozman, a student in Charles Parham's Bible school, claimed to speak in tongues in 1901. The Azusa Street revivals, under the leadership of the African American William Seymour—who had audited Parham's Bible classes from a segregated seat—spread Pentecostal revivals globally. Participant accounts of the Azusa Street revivals indicate that healing, more than glossolalia, constituted the primary draw for outsiders. Testimonies ranged from relief from minor pains to cures for blindness, deafness, cancers, paralysis, re-creation of missing body parts, and resurrections from the dead. "Trophies" of healing such as discarded crutches lined the walls of Azusa Street's Apostolic Faith Mission. Seymour gained a worldwide audience by publishing a periodical, *The Apostolic Faith*, that claimed an international circulation of fifty-thousand by 1908. Simultaneously, dozens of missionaries set out from Azusa to found Pentecostal churches in fifty countries.[17]

There is evidence that the origins of pentecostalism are more global than center-periphery accounts of U.S. influence assert. The Welsh revivals of 1904–1905, during which one hundred thousand people allegedly had Christian conversion experiences, produced reports that spread worldwide. Korean revivals birthed in a prayer meeting in 1903 intensified in 1907, after a U.S. missionary, Howard Agnew Johnston, brought back news of revivals in Wales and India. Word of the Welsh revivals had reached India shortly before revivals began there in 1905. Pandita Ramabai, a high-caste Brahmin convert to Christianity, had already been closely following reports of revival in Australia in 1903, and had sent her daughter and Minnie Abrams, an American missionary in her employ, to investigate. Reporting on the transnational revivals, Abrams wrote a book, *Baptism of the Holy Ghost and Fire* (1906), that circulated worldwide. An American missionary to Chile, Willis Hoover, read Abrams's book shortly before he disseminated news of the Chilean revivals of 1908–1909. Two Americans, F. B. Meyers and Joseph Smale, visited Wales and brought reports to Los Angeles before the Azusa Street revivals began in 1906.[18]

Pentecostalism took root on every continent during the first half of the twentieth century. There is historical evidence of pentecostal growth, for example, in Korea, China, India, Ghana, Nigeria, South Africa, Australia, Germany, Sweden, Argentina, Brazil, Colombia, Mexico, and Puerto Rico, and among Native Americans, Latinos/as, and African Americans in the United States. From 1947 to 1958, the Voice of Healing revivals, named for an influential magazine of that title, swept the United States and stimulated a new wave of foreign missionary activity. It was significant that several of the most influential twentieth-century U.S. healing evangelists, including John G. Lake, T. L. Osborn, Derek Prince, C. Peter Wagner, and the Catholic Francis MacNutt, all spent time as missionaries in Latin America, Asia, or Africa (and the naturalized American healing evangelist Mahesh Chavda was born a Hindu in Kenya), where they not only disseminated pentecostal ideas but also learned from local cosmologies—particularly concerning the role of Satan and demons as agents of disease.[19]

The ecumenical Charismatic renewals of the 1960s and 1970s ushered belief in divine healing into mainstream Protestant and

Catholic churches worldwide, especially as pentecostals—notably the Americans Kathryn Kuhlman (1907–1976) and Oral Roberts (1918–2009)—exploited print, radio, and television technologies. The Catholic Charismatic renewal had diverse international sources, including the Cursillo movement, which originated in Spain in 1944; the Jamaa movement in the Belgian Congo in the 1950s; and Hungary's Social Mission Society, founded in 1908, and the Holy Spirit Society, established in the 1930s. Begun in the 1960s, the *Word of Faith* movement (which correlates healing and prosperity with speaking words of faith) was led by Kenneth E. Hagin's Rhema Bible Institute in Tulsa, Oklahoma. Its media personalities, such as Kenneth and Gloria Copeland, the African Americans Frederick Price and T. D. Jakes, and the Bahamian Myles Munroe, also succeeded in reaching extensive international audiences. At the same time, pentecostals from the global South, such as the Nigerian David Oyedepo, the Indian Mathew Naickomparambil, and the Argentinian Carlos Annacondia, influenced the global North as international conference speakers and producers of widely circulated media offerings.[20]

By the mid-1960s, traditional barriers between Protestant denominations and even between Protestants and Catholics had begun to break down, to be replaced by a new polarity between churches that either affirmed the ongoing operation of gifts of the Holy Spirit or took the "cessationist" stance of insisting that spiritual gifts had ceased in the postapostolic era. The Third Wave Charismatic renewals of the 1980s and 1990s brought about a further shift away from denominational structures in favor of looser relational connections. A leader in the Jesus movement of the 1960s, Kenn Gulliksen, started the first Vineyard church in Los Angeles, California in 1974 as a home Bible study group under the umbrella of Calvary Chapel. In 1977, John Wimber, a former jazz musician and manager of the Righteous Brothers (a duo that became famous soon after Wimber's departure for their hit song "You've Lost that Lovin' Feeling") started a similar Calvary Chapel group in Yorba Linda, California. In 1982, the founder of Calvary Chapel, Chuck Smith, criticized Gulliksen's and Wimber's emphasis on the public exercise of the gifts of the Holy Spirit and encouraged them to form a separate movement. The leadership of the new movement soon passed to Wimber, who incorporated the Association of Vineyard Churches in 1985.[21]

The Vineyard movement began as an association of churches with the same "spiritual DNA," rather than as a traditional denomination. Wimber taught that ten essential emphases constitute the Vineyard's "genetic code": accurate Bible teaching, contemporary worship, gifts of the Holy Spirit in operation, active small groups, ministry to the poor, physical healing, church planting and world missions, unity with the whole body of Christ, evangelistic outreach, and equipping the saints for ministry. Wimber did not grow up attending church, but as his wife Carol described it, John was a "beer-guzzling, drug-abusing pop musician who was converted at the age of 29 while chain-smoking his way through a Quaker-led Bible study." Even after his conversion—in the heart of countercultural southern California of the 1970s—Wimber never developed any great respect for denominational religion, which he perceived as routinized and culturally irrelevant. Rejecting hierarchical assumptions of church leadership, Wimber famously taught that every lay Christian gets to "do the stuff" of healing, and everyone "gets to play." Nevertheless, reflecting Wimber's introduction to Christianity through the Calvinist-influenced Calvary Chapel, the Vineyard maintained a strong emphasis on God's sovereignty in healing.[22]

In considering the gifts of the Holy Spirit enumerated in 1 Corinthians, Wimber picked up on the *word of knowledge*. The Bible offers little instruction concerning the content or mode of transmission of such words. Wimber interpreted words of knowledge as divinely revealed information that most often concern health problems that God wants to heal at a particular moment. According to Wimber, people might receive words of knowledge by hearing them, seeing them, thinking them, dreaming them, finding themselves saying them, or, most commonly, feeling them as a sympathetic pain in their own bodies. In this model, prayer for healing consists most basically of blessing what God is already doing and asking for "more."[23]

During the 1970s and 1980s, the Vineyard both drew inspiration from global sources and exerted a significant international influence. Wimber borrowed many of his ideas on the relationship between "signs and wonders" and church growth from two-thirds-world students at Fuller Theological Seminary School of World Missions in southern California, where Wimber was an adjunct instructor. The Signs and Wonders movement over which Wimber exercised leadership emphasized that spiritual gifts such as healing and prophecy overcome resistance to the gospel, producing revivals and church growth. Wimber insisted that he began to preach about the "kingdom of God" as being displayed through "power evangelism" before he had any personal experience with divine healing—which began to be reported in his services only ten months later. During the 1980s, the Vineyard influenced thousands of Catholic, Anglican, evangelical, and mainline churches worldwide through international "equipping seminars," as well as through Wimber's numerous books, especially *Power Evangelism* (1986) and *Power Healing* (1987). At the time of Wimber's death in 1997, there were five hundred Vineyard churches in the United States and two hundred fifty in other countries; by 2011, the number of Vineyard churches worldwide exceeded fifteen hundred, two thirds of which were outside the United States.[24]

As of 2011, the Vineyard still calls itself a movement, but it no longer shies away from being classed alongside other denominations. As the sociologist Max Weber predicted and as has seemed largely borne out, with institutionalization comes the routinization of charisma. During Wimber's lifetime, the Vineyard's characteristic teaching that the kingdom of God is both "already" and "not yet" spawned an atmosphere of eager anticipation of seeing apparently divine healings for the first time. Over time, the emphasis shifted from pressing in for breakthroughs toward explaining why there are not more successes. This change in emphasis is in striking contrast to movements that grew out of the Vineyard via the Toronto Blessing and borrowed even more substantially from the global South. These outgrowth movements came to reject the Calvinist "blueprint model" (that everything that happens must by definition reflect God's will) for a "warfare model" of a clash between kingdoms in which humans (alongside angels and demons) actively participate. Randy Clark emphasizes *sovereign healings* as one among many categories of healing available, and words of knowledge as a tool for building other people's faith to receive healing rather than as an almost-complete list of healings available at the time. Although some Vineyard churches have continued to participate in ANGA-affiliated networks, others have backed away. It is telling that when Clark resigned from pastoring a Vineyard church in St. Louis, Missouri in 2001 to focus on developing an international ministry network, his former congregation breathed a sigh of relief and turned their attention to domestic concerns. When Clark returned to St. Louis to hold a School of Healing and Impartation in 2006, few of his former congregants could be found in the audience. Indeed, by the early 2000s, Vineyard USA had developed its own identity distinct from a broader international movement.[25]

Even as Vineyard USA has increasingly looked inward, the global context of the revivals that burst forth at the Toronto Airport Vineyard cannot be overemphasized. Toronto itself is one of the most multicultural cities in the world; one hundred forty linguistic groups and two hundred distinct ethnic origins are represented, and members of many different local cultural communities visited the Toronto Blessing. Despite Arnott's and Clark's expressed surprise at the scope of what took place in 1994, both had already been using their global ties to seek what they understood to be manifestations of the Holy Spirit. In 1993, John and Carol Arnott had visited Argentina in order to receive prayer for impartation of a "fresh anointing" of the Holy Spirit from the Argentinian revivalist Claudio Freidzon. News had spread to North America that Freidzon's stadium-size meetings were characterized by people falling down, laughing uncontrollably, crying with joy, and acting as if inebriated. Freidzon had in turn avowedly received the new anointing through prayers from the Palestinian Canadian American healing televangelist Benny Hinn, who traces his anointing back to the American healing evangelist Kathryn Kuhlman—who in turn points back to the Canadian American healing evangelist Aimee Semple McPherson (1890–1944), who gestures back toward the American healing evangelist Maria Woodworth-Etter (1844–1924), whose meetings were known even in the nineteenth century for people falling down and experiencing trances, visions, prophecies, and healing. It was also in 1993 that Clark attended meetings in Tulsa, Oklahoma led by Rodney Howard-Browne, a South African missionary to the

United States. Howard-Browne was a self-described "Holy Ghost bartender" who serves the "new wine" of the Holy Spirit and invites people "to drink"—shocking imagery for pentecostals and evangelicals who had been raised on the teaching that Christianity enjoins teetotalism. Howard-Browne's meetings were characterized by people falling down, laughing, and experiencing "drunkenness in the Holy Spirit." When Clark returned home, similar phenomena occurred at the St. Louis Vineyard, and again at a regional Vineyard meeting, reports of which formed the immediate backdrop to Arnott's invitation to Clark to visit his church.[26]

Given that the Toronto Blessing emerged from preexisting global pentecostal connections, it is not surprising that its leaders envisioned the event as a catalyst for global revival. In the autobiography he titled *Lighting Fires,* Clark claims that God "may have lit a fire in Toronto, but I quickly realized that the Lord intended to set the world ablaze, using Toronto as a torch to ignite other flames." According to Clark, "there's a connection between revival, real revival and missions." Prior to visiting Toronto in 1994, Clark had never traveled outside the United States. By 1995, he had begun accepting international preaching invitations that would take him and hundreds of North Americans he influenced to preach salvation and healing in partnership with churches of every major denomination on every continent. Clark has preached in venues ranging from simple churches in the United States and overseas with fewer than a hundred members, to a U.S. arena packed for a Benny Hinn healing campaign, all the way up to open-air events in India that attract crowds numbering over one hundred thousand people.[27]

The Apostolic Network of Global Awakening

As international travel became an increasing focus for Clark, he resigned as pastor of the St. Louis Vineyard and moved to Mechanicsburg, Pennsylvania to develop ANGA. Clark avers that God has called him specifically to be a "Fire Lighter, Vision Caster, and Bridge Builder." Rather than planting churches or forming a new denomination, he sees his role as "fire lighter" as one of "imparting" the presence and

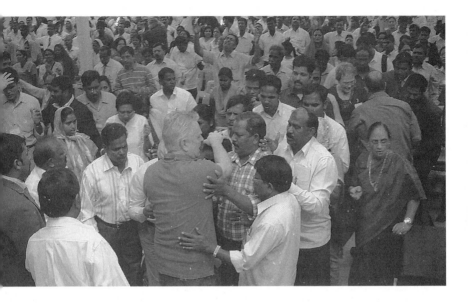

Figure 1.1. Randy Clark praying for impartation of spiritual gifts at a pastors' conference, Bangalore, Karnataka, India, 2010. Courtesy Global Awakening.

gifts of the Holy Spirit, especially to leaders of churches of all denominations (figure 1.1). Clark notes with satisfaction, "I've preached in Catholic churches, Lutheran churches, Pentecostal churches," and to Southern Baptists, Presbyterians, Greek Orthodox, Anglicans, Word of Faith, New Apostolic, and Methodists, "all over the world." The "vision" Clark casts is "power evangelism"—a term he borrows from Wimber—to expand the kingdom of God by preaching the gospel while demonstrating the kingdom with healing from sickness and deliverance from *demons* (evil spiritual beings believed to cause mental, spiritual, and physical problems, including sickness). The "bridges" Clark seeks to build are relationships that connect "apostolic leaders and other strong leaders" around the world, both with ANGA and with each other. An online directory lists 226 churches and ministries, most of them in North America, that belong to ANGA. The Pennsylvania headquarters hosts various thematic conferences; a one- to two-year

Global School of Supernatural Ministry; a Healing Center that combines the Spokane, Washington–based International Association of Healing Rooms (IAHR) model with the Restoring the Foundations program birthed at TACF; and the administrative office for an online bookstore that sells a variety of books, training manuals, pamphlets, and DVDs. Clark and affiliates also itinerate across North America and the world to offer four-day Schools of Healing and Impartation, as well as international evangelistic campaigns in which "little ole me"s— or ordinary church members—are the prayer ministry team.[28]

The Apostolic Network of Global Awakening is one of a number of transnational, cross-cultural, relational, and institutional networks whose divine healing practices are contributing to the global expansion of Christianity. Global Awakening is not so high profile—or so wealthy—as some pentecostal television ministries. Televangelists such as Benny Hinn (who, for instance, attracted 7 million people to a campaign in India in 2005) or the Igreja Universal do Reino de Deus (the Universal Church of the Kingdom of God, a Brazilian church known for its public displays of healing and exorcism, which claims to have planted over five thousand churches in 176 countries) might be more familiar. Global Awakening—like many of its network affiliates, such as Iris Ministries in Mozambique—has steered away from prosperity teachings that emphasize that Christians can become wealthy by sowing money into the kingdom of God via contributions to the speaker's ministry, even though such teachings are effective in raising funds.[29]

When GA appeals for funds (which the group does not seem to do so often, lengthily, or obtrusively as do some other observed ministries), it is often to pay for transportation for the poor to attend campaigns. Many of those who attend GA rallies outside the United States are bused in from impoverished areas on the urban outskirts. An oft-screened video advertisement shows Clark asking an Indian pastor why he sent so few of his people to a convention—and the answer that it was because GA had sent only one truck. The appeal is for wealthy conference attendees to look beyond their own needs to enable others from around the world to attend meetings where they too can presumably experience the power of God. In addition to taking up offerings during North American conferences, GA follows the common para-church model of recruiting so-called partners who make a monthly financial commitment of at least twenty-five dollars, in return for which they receive symbolic benefits, such as preferential conference seating. Iris Ministries has eschewed asking for financial support or instituting a financial partnership program (avowedly trusting God to provide resources without such pleas), although IM leaders do allow network allies such as GA to engage in fundraising on IM's behalf. In addition, Heidi and Rolland Baker speak at North American and European conferences, thereby cultivating sympathy for their work in Mozambique.[30]

Few organizations have approached ANGA's activism in networking leaders and members of diverse Christian traditions worldwide. Clark seeks to bring diverse "streams" of the church together. Healing "streams come together to make a major healing river of God. My purpose," says Clark, "is not to put any stream down, but to say here is the stream, here is the teaching, here are the strengths and the weaknesses. This weakness can be handled by this stream over there that is strong in that area. We need all streams flowing together." Because GA uses conferences and training materials to equip pastors and the laity to return to their *own* churches with new resources rather than seceding to form a new denomination, it is difficult to quantify the organization's influence. Yet there is reason to believe that this influence is substantial and that the activities of ANGA are representative of a large number of similar transnational healing networks—such as those brokered by Mensa Otabil, Reinhard Bonnke, David Yonggi Cho, Sérgio Von Helder, Mahesh Chavda, David Hogan, Dennis Balcombe, and Leif Hetland—several of which overlap with ANGA's own networks to greater or lesser degrees.[31]

The Revival Alliance

The overlapping networks that grew out of the Toronto Blessing reflect a shift away from the denominational organization of Christianity toward more fluid relational and institutional networks that embrace a global Christian identity. Global Awakening's core relational network is termed the Revival Alliance. It consists of Randy and DeAnne Clark (Mechanicsburg, Pennsylvania); John and Carol Arnott (Toronto, Ontario); Ché and Sue Ahn (Korean and Filipina Americans based in Pasadena, California); Georgian and Winnie Banov (Georgian was born in Bulgaria, but their headquarters is in Valrico, Florida); Bill and Bennie Johnson (Redding, California); and Rolland and Heidi Baker (born in the United States but based in Pemba, Cabo Delgado, Mozambique). Members of the Revival Alliance frequently speak at each other's conferences, as well as inviting speakers with whom they have looser ties, such as the Kenyan-born Indian American Mahesh Chavda. The nondenominational conference circuit prominently includes GA's annual Voice of the Apostles conference, a forum for regularly rearticulating a common vision and a relational gathering point for ANGA members. The conference attracted nearly five thousand attendees in 2011.[32]

Each member of the Revival Alliance constitutes the axis of its own relational network, which partially overlaps with that of ANGA. John and Carol Arnott developed a vision for TACF as an international hub for some of the churches and ministries that caught "fire" in Toronto in 1994. This was accomplished, first, by establishing eleven campuses of TACF around the Toronto area, and by planting churches (each of which bears the name Catch the Fire!) in Raleigh, North Carolina; London, England; Oslo, Norway; Reykjavik, Iceland; and Montréal, Canada. In 2009, TACF was renamed Catch the Fire Toronto! in order to reflect the more-than-local reach of the church. (One might ask whether this move marks a key moment in the transformation of a relational network into a denomination, and whether this will inevitably lead to the routinization of charisma.) John and Carol Arnott also provide "apostolic leadership" for Partners in Harvest (PIH), an international "fellowship of churches," and "family of churches, a network of people." Partners in Harvest serves many of the same functions as a denomination, but seeks to avoid the institutionalizing tendencies of formal denominational structures. According to a 2009 declaration of purpose, PIH offers a "primary relational affiliation and covering" for two hundred churches in the "western" world and seven thousand churches in developing nations (most or all of which, it seems, entered via Iris Ministries). The association avowedly differs from a denominational hierarchy in that affiliated churches remain "autonomous, self-governed entities" that are "bound together" not by a "top-down, controlling, pyramid structure" but by "our common DNA. This DNA is foundational for our mission and values. It links us together in a profound relationship built on love, respect, honor, and a desire to bless each other." Friends in Harvest (FIH) is a "secondary level of association," intended to cross denominational lines and to unite churches and ministries "whose primary accountability structure is denominational in nature, yet who desire to relate with others flowing in revival."[33]

Making a similar transition from denominational to relational connections, Bill Johnson, a fifth-generation Assemblies of God pastor, withdrew Bethel Church in Redding, California from the Assemblies denomination in 2006 after becoming increasingly aligned with Toronto-inspired networks. In an open letter explaining this decision, Johnson insisted that the withdrawal was "not a reaction to conflict but a response to a call . . . to create a network that helps other networks thrive—to be one of many ongoing catalysts in this continuing revival." Johnson says of Revival Alliance relationships that "there's a sense of family. . . . I don't really care who belongs to whom. I love partnerships and friendships." Johnson first met Clark through mutual friends who encouraged Johnson to attend a conference at Clark's church in St. Louis, Missouri in 1997, after which Clark agreed to visit Redding. Johnson looks back to the impartation of spiritual gifts received through that visit as a watershed that "really turned it up a notch as far as the realm of miracles . . . It went from a miracle happening every week to daily; it just was a dramatic increase for the whole church and myself included." Since that time Johnson and Clark have developed a "really close friendship . . . We're together maybe half a dozen times a year. It's probably my strongest relationship in ministry outside of our own church." This kind of relational connection, in Johnson's view, matters more than organizations or denominational ties.[34]

As of 2011, Johnson spends an estimated one hundred eighty days each year traveling to speak at ANGA-related conferences and evangelistic healing rallies across the United States and around the world. Bethel Church also attracts many short- and long-term visitors through its three-year School of Supernatural Ministry, School of Worship, Healing Rooms Ministry, and Transformation Center—which focuses on "inner," or emotional, healing and deliverance using the "sozo" model of restoring concepts of God wounded by unhealthy parental relationships. Bethel International is the church arm that focuses on equipping and networking national leaders in Brazil, Mexico, Nicaragua, Croatia, Kenya, and Norway. This work includes sponsoring Schools of Supernatural Ministry and Missions Training, and establishing children's homes and reaching into migrant-worker camps. In Brazil, for example, Bethel's school has "raised up a leadership team of young Brazilian revivalists" whose goal is to "transform and disciple all nations," going out from Brazil as missionaries, and "building bridges from Brazil to other nations." Bethel also aligns itself with ministries that have their own network orbits, as in Kenya, where Bethel works alongside Heroes of the Nation, a nonprofit organization that has children's homes in five African nations—not only providing food and shelter, but also "raising a generation of revivalists."[35]

Other Revival Alliance members similarly emphasize both networking and fostering revival in national churches and working in very poor communities. Ché Ahn attended a Toronto-influenced Vineyard conference in Anaheim, California in 1994, began laughing uncontrollably, and experienced healing from depression. Ahn then traveled to TAV and received further healing. John Arnott visited Ahn's church, which soon became known as "the Toronto of southern California." As of 2011, the Ahns are pastors of the multiethnic HROCK Church in Pasadena, California. One outreach of HROCK is Harvest International Ministry (HIM), which works with the world's poor. The HIM network connects sixty-five hundred churches and ministries in forty countries, supporting local groups as they establish churches and children's homes. The Banovs founded the group Global Celebration, through which they oversee a fellowship of thirty-five churches in Bulgaria and travel worldwide to host evangelistic meetings and outreach events, especially targeting the widely despised gypsies of eastern Europe, and very poor communities in southeast Africa and Central America. All of the Banovs' non-U.S. events include "Love Feasts" during which they feed local people their favorite foods.[36]

It is not uncommon, and certainly not looked down on, for ministries to forge explicit ties with multiple network hubs. Rolland and Heidi Baker, the founders of Iris Ministries, are core members of ANGA's Revival Alliance. They also call themselves "Partners in Harvest Iris," thereby affirming a relational connection to Toronto. Heidi Baker denies that the PIH link positions IM merely as a subsidiary of the PIH network. According to Baker, IM has "so many churches, and it's our DNA." In other words, there is something distinctive about IM-network churches that is not equivalent to what characterizes PIH churches. "But," Baker continues, IM has also adopted the PIH label because "we love them so much, so we linked. It's like a loose link, but it's really a family link." Baker appreciates that "Toronto has modeled a resting place for the Holy Spirit. . . . That's why Toronto has so much impact on missions, because they've taught missionaries that they're allowed to rest. They're allowed to press into God's presence and still be missionaries. That's the huge difference between Toronto and old-time missions. . . . There's a rhythm: to rest and to run to the heartbeat of God." The Bakers selected the name "Ministerio Arco-Iris" for their own network because the phrase means "rainbow ministry" in Portuguese, and they believe that the "Son" shines through the various gifts he gives his people to produce a "beautiful result." The IM network connects over ten thousand churches in Mozambique and twenty-four other countries (prominently including India). Network members provide homes and food for more than ten thousand orphaned children (figure 1.2).[37]

The network model is organized along the lines of family relationships. Thus, there are implicit, and to an extent explicit, lines of authority. Indeed, it was through this same model of oversight that the Association of Vineyard Churches disfellowshipped TAV in 1995. Nevertheless, within a few years the Arnotts rose to the position of apostolic leaders in their own revival-oriented network, PIH. Members of ANGA's Revival Alliance, including the Arnotts, submit themselves to mutual accountability to each other and exert apostolic oversight of affiliated churches and ministries. The purpose of accountability, according to Bill Johnson, is not limited to helping each other avoid sin but also has the more positive connotation of calling each other

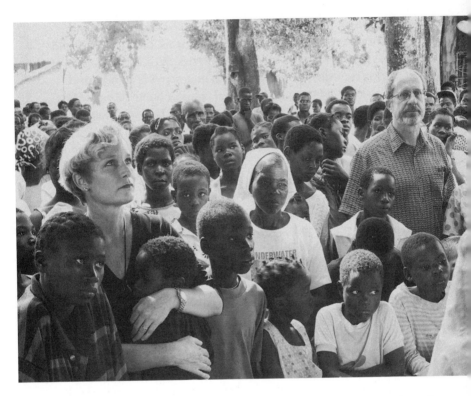

Figure 1.2. Heidi and Rolland Baker in Dondo, Sofala, Mozambique, 2001. Courtesy Patrick J. Endres.

toward divine "destiny." This model of accountability depends on its members' expressing commitment to relationships, because there are few official channels for disciplinary action.[38]

The "Lakeland Outpouring" that began in April 2008 provides an instructive example of how network accountability functions. Revivals at the small Assemblies of God Ignited Church in Lakeland, Florida captured international attention through nightly broadcasts via the Internet and the satellite station GOD TV. Within days, the Lakeland revival was attracting thousands of pilgrims from across the United States and dozens of other countries, many of them seeking and claiming to experience physical healing. So many visitors converged on the small host church that the meeting organizers were constantly scrambling to seek a series of new venues—including an eight-thousand-seat convention center, a baseball stadium, and a ten-thousand-seat tent erected on the grounds of a local airport cum campground. Members of the Revival Alliance (John Arnott, Ché Ahn, and Bill Johnson, plus another prominent pentecostal leader, C. Peter Wagner) visited the Lakeland stage, publicly ordaining and extending a "spiritual covering" over the principal revivalist—the thirty-two-year-old Canadian Todd Bentley, an unconventional, tattoo-covered evangelist who freely admitted to being a former drug addict and convicted criminal and who, even after his radical conversion, has continued to sport spiked jewelry and ride Harley-Davidson motorcycles.[39]

By August, the Lakeland revivals halted as Bentley withdrew from nightly ministry. It was significant that pilgrims had not been attracted to a place where the Holy Spirit seemed to be moving as at Toronto but to a single revivalist and his apparent "healing anointing." Shortly thereafter, it was announced that Bentley was divorcing his wife and marrying a ministry intern who was the nanny of his three young children—and that he had been asked by the board of his own organization, Fresh Fire Ministries, in Abbotsford, British Columbia, to withdraw from public ministry. Members of the Revival Alliance expressed a commitment to Bentley's emotional and spiritual "healing and restoration," jointly issuing a public statement in October 2008. The report insisted that "while there must be no toleration or whitewashing of sin . . . the quickness to condemn and abandon a fallen comrade has caused us as much concern as has the actual sin of our friend." In an interview conducted one week after the issuance of this report, Bill Johnson sounded a less confident tone than that of the public statement, citing a history during which Bentley had never embraced a genuine accountability relationship but had called only in times of crisis. Bentley had indeed phoned Johnson during the Lakeland scandal and had traveled to Redding, California to spend three days with Johnson. But Johnson questioned the impact of these meetings. For Johnson's part, "I will confront, but I am not heavy-handed in trying to rake him over the coals or punish him. . . . In one sense, yes, we have a relationship but in a practical sense we have to have time together." Despite Johnson's assessment of the weakness of his accountability relationship with Bentley, Johnson nevertheless agreed to join a team of three, which included the prominent pentecostal leaders Jack Deere and Rick Joyner, to "help give oversight to get him healed up." Bentley relocated to the headquarters of Joyner's Morningstar Ministries in Pineville, North Carolina, and Joyner sponsored Bentley's rerelease into public ministry in October 2010. In August 2011, Johnson issued a public statement to "recommend" Bentley's ministry as an example of "grace" and "restoration."[40]

Cultural Flows from the Global South to Global Awakening

The relational network model embraced by the Revival Alliance and other ANGA affiliates implies a high value on building bridges across national and even continental borders. Pablo Deiros, pastor of the large Del Centro Evangelical Baptist Church in Argentina, admitted to first meeting Clark with "some reservations" because the Toronto Blessing had stirred up controversies in Argentina that "created a lot of trouble for me." After spending several hours getting to know Clark, Deiros decided that he was "an honest servant of God" and agreed to minister with him on various occasions, commenting in 1998: "How much I have learned from him!" Clark also borrowed much from Latin American revivalists such as Deiros. Indeed, it was because of reports of revivals in Argentina, Colombia, and Brazil that predated Toronto that Clark traveled to Latin America to observe the revivals firsthand. Clark wanted to find out why evangelistic events seemed more effective in Latin America than in North America—reportedly attracting sixty thousand people to a typical campaign with retention rates for new converts of 85 to 90 percent, in contrast to the 6 percent average retention for smaller rallies in the United States.[41]

Clark has since sought to combine Billy Graham's interdenominational networking and follow-up through local churches with the supernaturalist approaches of the Latin Americans. Clark emulates the Argentinian Omar Cabrera's strategies of evangelizing through healing conventions, asking God to send healing angels, explaining words of knowledge, and asking people to begin waving their arms in the air for others to see once they feel 80 percent better. Clark borrows from the Argentinian evangelist Carlos Annacondia and his Director of Deliverance Ministry, Pablo Bottari, in praying en masse against demonic oppression followed by one-on-one ministry in a designated deliverance tent to bring individuals *liberación* from demons. The view that demons are behind many diseases leads into the idea that *deliverance ministry* is often a prerequisite to the effectiveness of prayers for healing. Clark's *Ministry Training Manual* (2002), which is used by churches worldwide and has been translated into eight languages with several more translations under way, takes its section on deliverance directly from Bottari's book *Libres en Cristo,* which has been translated from Spanish into English as *Free in Christ* (2000). Heidi Baker, for example, says that the models taught by Clark—who was borrowing from Bottari—"on praying deliverance and forgiveness have really helped us here in Mozambique." Thus, teachings flowed from Argentina to Mozambique via the United States. Cabrera, Annacondia, Bottari, and the Brazilian worship bands Casa de Davi (House of David) and Nova Geração (New Generation) have also conducted campaigns, cultivated friendships with North American ministry leaders, and marketed their books, CDs, and DVDs in the United States and Canada.[42]

Clark became particularly interested in Brazil—spending fifty to sixty days there annually over a ten-year period—after hearing what he understood to be a prophetic word from God: that there would be a revival in Brazil twelve times greater than the one in Toronto, just as Argentina and Brazil's Iguaçu Falls are twelve times larger than Niagara Falls, and that a missionary movement would go from Brazil to Mozambique, in both of which Portuguese is spoken. An added advantage, in Heidi Baker's view, is that Brazilians' "standard of living is not so high that it's such a culture shock" to move to Mozambique. When preaching about salvation and healing in Brazil, Clark often draws his sermon illustrations from Mozambique "with the intention of building a bridge between that country to this new country." Global Awakening works closely with networks of local Pentecostal, Baptist, and New Apostolic movement churches and ministries, such as Casa de Davi and Nova Geração in Brazil and IM in Mozambique, seeking to build international bridges among the groups in its global network.[43]

International Ministry Trips and Global Community Building

Hundreds of North Americans each year participate in a GA international ministry trip; the most popular destination is Brazil. Traveling with GA can be viewed within the overlapping frameworks of short-term missions, Christian tourism, and religious pilgrimage. A Brazil trip is moderately expensive: $2,500 for two weeks, including transportation, the best hotels, and buffet breakfasts and meat-heavy lunches. By contrast, the $3,500 Mozambique trip fee does not include lodging or meals; IM provides these at no charge but accepts donations to defray expenses. Participants sleep in hostel-style bunk rooms under mosquito nets, share quarter-star, co-ed bathrooms and showers, often go without running water or electricity, and are offered the same rice and beans served to the base's resident children and pastors in training. It is notable, however, that a number of the North Americans who traveled to Mozambique with GA in 2009 seemed unable to cope with these living conditions for even two weeks; most supplemented their diets with meats and desserts brought from home, and several visited a nearby hotel to dine and shower. Although the modal age of Mozambique trekkers is a bit younger than the age of those bound for Brazil, most GA travelers are middle-class empty-nesters or retirees with time and money on their hands, who want more than a tourist experience. Sometimes trip attendees "raise support" by asking family, friends, and church giving committees for donations, but most attendees pay their own way from saved earnings. Although many trip members have disposable income, for some the decision to travel with GA involves financial sacrifice—which may seem particularly worthwhile if one has a personal need for healing. Many people on a given trip have traveled with GA before and are already acquainted with others from previous trips. Small church groups sometimes travel together, but more often individuals and couples come on their own, expecting and generally finding an immediate sense of community with others influenced by the same conference speakers and books.[44]

The leading reason people give for traveling with GA is that they are tired of listening to other people's stories of the miraculous and want stories of their own. Many—including leaders such as Clark and Baker—point back to at least one time in their lives when they experienced God's love for them in a particularly intense way through healing. Such an experience whetted their appetites to experience more of the love of God and to express greater love for God and for other people, including those from other cultures. Most team members, whether pastors or laity, also feel dissatisfied with their local church and want to participate in a community of like-minded believers and to receive personal attention from dynamic leaders.

Participants always refer to GA network leaders such as Randy Clark and Heidi Baker by their first names, without titles; many insist that they decided to go on a trip because Randy extended a personal invitation to travel with him—although Clark would likely not remember most of these individuals since he typically extends a hundred such invitations at a single conference. The accessibility of leaders such as Clark constitutes a draw for pentecostals who cannot attract similar notice from higher-profile figures such as the televangelist Benny Hinn. Hinn also leads international trips but keeps his distance from attendees who might at most hope to stand within a few feet of "Pastor Benny." On a GA trip, it is possible to sit next to "Randy" at breakfast. Hinn, moreover, cultivates an aura of his own distinctive anointing, whereas Clark insists that, in the words of one his book's titles, *God Can Use Little Ole Me*—which refers to Clark and to every team member, whom Clark encourages to pray for the sick and to expect to see miracles through their own prayers. Clark also assures people that they are not on their own in working up enough faith for their own or another's healing; he and other team members are available to pray repeatedly.[45]

The pace of most GA trips is intense. On a typical day in Brazil, the team rises in time to eat breakfast and travel by bus for up to an hour before a 9:00 A.M. meeting. The service breaks up by 1:00 P.M., after which the team eats lunch at a local restaurant—the last formal meal of the day. During the afternoon, there might be an hour or two back at the hotel, but on some days this time is spent visiting an orphanage or rehabilitation center. Then, it is time to get back on the bus to go to the evening meeting—which might last from 6:00 P.M. until after midnight, when light snacks are provided by local churches. Bedtime is typically after 1:00 A.M., followed by an early start the next day. Rooming groups—GA assigns two team members per hotel room— take turns praying for one-hour shifts throughout the night. During a two-week trip, the team is given at least one afternoon to buy souvenirs and visit a single tourist site; during a trip to Rio de Janeiro in 2007, the trip coordinator pointed out the famous tourist beaches outside the bus window, noting that there was not time to stop. The intensity of the trip is part of the appeal. This type of travel is a pilgrimage experience in which participants enter into a liminal, transformative zone distinct from their everyday routines. Although an expression of globalization, the trip provides a rare opportunity to escape the constant sensory input, work and family obligations, and communication demands of life in a globalized world. Long airplane and bus rides, hours spent singing and praying every day, the difficulty and expense of calling home or accessing the Internet, and trip policies against watching television—all create an atmosphere in which the sacred is expected to intrude into the mundane world at every moment.[46]

Although volunteering as short-term missionaries, trip participants expect to get as much as they give. This shift from older philosophies of Christian missions (which is also observable among nonpentecostals) can be read as reversing patterns of colonialism and cultural imperialism by exhibiting greater sensitivity to the weaknesses of North American Christianity and the strengths of other cultures. Conversely, North American missionaries can be understood as products of engrained patterns of imperialistic thought that reinforce rather than resisting problematic aspects of globalization. Short-term pentecostal missionaries feel compelled to travel to other countries less by their desire to pray for the sick—who can be found in abundance at home— than by their desire to benefit from cultural others' experiences of pain and its relief. At its best, the practice of divine healing constitutes a strategy of resistance against oppressive social structures by recognizing the bodily reality of poor people and affirming the worth of female, nonwhite bodies, about which it appears that God cares enough to heal and empower as conduits for transferring healing to others. It is also the case that local churches and holistic ministries, such as IM in Mozambique, do often provide long-term relief and development aid. Yet at the conclusion of mass rallies such as those commonly held in Brazil, short-term visitors quickly leave without making any commitment to the individuals for whom they prayed and without working to transform the political, economic, and social structures that contribute to ongoing suffering by limiting access to nutrition and basic health care. Indeed, participation in GA international trips seems to confirm the prior assumption of some North American pentecostals that the problems confronting the developing world are so severe that miracles offer the only viable solution. After returning home, North American pentecostals may be even less likely to engage in political or social activism that addresses the systemic material causes of global health crises. These pentecostals may even be confirmed in self-satisfied complacency, since they have done their part by replacing an annual vacation in the Bahamas with a ministry trip to Brazil.[47]

North American GA team members and Christians in host countries such as Brazil and Mozambique nevertheless share many values, beliefs, and practices in common, and they often identify as members of a single church universal. During their first day after arriving in Brazil in September 2007, a team of sixty North Americans stepped off their tour bus and filtered into the pews of a large, unfinished concrete church building in Rio, from which they could view dilapidated housing through cut-outs in the walls that served as windows. Within fifteen minutes, the visitors had joined in with the local congregation as all participated in a common culture of singing songs to God—in Portuguese, with English translations projected overhead for the visitors' benefit.[48]

Linguistic differences are viewed as superficial barriers to communication within the church universal. Because God—as well as angels and demons—presumably understands prayers in every language, participants expect that healing can take place even when communication is imperfect. Glossolalia is seen as a universal language that reaches God directly. Brazilian churches do attempt to provide translators, but their abilities vary, and often there are more North Americans than translators (figure 1.3). Global Awakening provides team members with a CD of Portuguese phrases commonly used in praying for healing and urges memorization. Yet most team members observed arrive without having learned much, if any, Portuguese. They simply plan to rely on the provided translators, a stance that might be criticized as reflecting North American cultural arrogance. Disregard

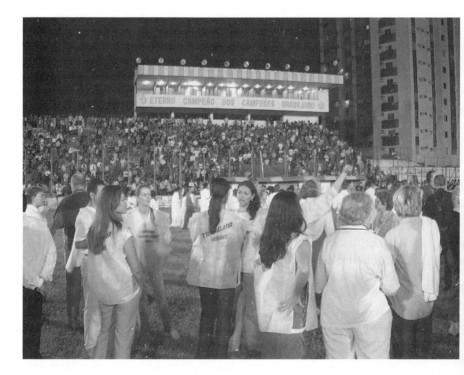

Figure 1.3. Brazilian translators assisting Global Awakening team at a stadium campaign in Belém, Pará, Brazil, 2004. Photograph in author's collection.

for the cultural respect displayed by learning someone else's language extends to most visible GA preachers—with the significant exceptions of Baker, who is fluent in Portuguese and conversant in several local Mozambican languages, and Clark, who uses as much Portuguese as he can while preaching and even when conversing with English-speaking Brazilian pastors. Other ANGA network preachers—some after as many as twenty trips to Brazil—continue to speak exclusively in English, even when repeating such a common refrain as "Praise God," which could easily be rendered as "Glória ao Deus." Nor have most GA team members done any background research on Brazilian churches. Yet at least some assume, condescendingly and inaccurately, that Brazilians know very little about Christian practice—as, for instance, when I observed the U.S. leader of a joint intercessory-prayer meeting in Rio instructing Brazilian coleaders and participants in how to conduct intercessory prayer. There are almost always, in the larger meetings, a few Brazilians fluent in both Portuguese and English who can prevent such major miscommunications as giving public testimony to a healing that obviously has not occurred. It seems probable, however, that team members working with less-proficient translators do make unsubstantiated claims, especially because those requesting prayer might not want to disappoint the person praying.[49]

Rather than obscuring cultural differences, the ideal of a global Christian community puts value on using differences to correct weaknesses in each cultural expression of Christianity. One reason Brazilian churches invite GA to visit—much as North American churches invite international visitors—is that they want an outsider's perspective. Sometimes this leads to sharp criticisms, as when Clark directed a pointed sermon at pastors in the equatorial town of Imperatriz, Maranhão in northeastern Brazil. Clark urged those gathered to set aside their translations of old American hymns in favor of new Portuguese songs created in the Brazilian revivals, and to shed their climate-inappropriate, dark, two-piece suits and ties, which they had modeled after the clothes of U.S. missionaries. Clark also urged the pastors to stop sitting onstage—joking that these were bad seats that gave them a view of the back of the preacher's head—and follow GA's democratized model of having leaders mix with the congregation.[50]

Cross-cultural criticism goes in both directions. Brazilian leaders of Casa de Davi called on a U.S. team visiting the group's headquarters in Londrina, Paraná, Brazil to repent of national sins, which the Brazilians believed had caused 9/11 and Hurricane Katrina. Writing a chapter for a book edited by Clark and marketed in the United States, the Argentinian Pablo Deiros argued that the need for deliverance ministry is greater in North America than in Latin America, and he estimated that 80 percent of U.S. church members are demonized although most do not realize it. When Pablo Bottari speaks in the United States, he criticizes practices accepted in North American churches that he sees as dangerous dabbling with the occult.[51]

The Twin Engines of Supernaturalism and Democratization

North Americans take from cross-cultural interactions with pentecostals from the global South an expectation that God performs miracles and that suprahuman agents, such as angels and demons, help or hinder healing. These views push against a North American "faith plus holiness equals healing" formula carrying the implied accusation that those not healed must lack faith or holiness. It is significant, however, that North American pentecostals often borrow this supernaturalism—out of context—from pentecostals in Latin America and elsewhere. Most economically and politically marginalized Latin American pentecostals are poignantly aware of the material context for their experiences of bodily suffering. Although they call on supernatural aid, many also engage in political and social activism and pursue entrepreneurial economic activities, because they assume the existence of a dynamic interaction between the material and spiritual worlds. North American appropriators are more likely to rely solely on spiritual rather than material solutions—at least when contemplating the seemingly overwhelming needs of the developing world. At the same time, GA exports healing models—including those originating in Latin America but repackaged in democratized forms—to Latin American and African churches that had previously defined healing and deliverance as the special province of gifted evangelists or pastors.[52]

Global Awakening team members are most likely to express discomfort not with supernatural healing claims—however implausible these may sound to outsiders—but rather with apparent demonic manifestations, which sometimes involve unseemly bodily expressions, such as vomiting, biting, screaming, clawing, or writhing, that sit uneasily with North American middle-class sensibilities of decorum. Although Clark emulates Latin American evangelists in commanding demons to leave from the platform, he admittedly does not like to teach on deliverance or handle one-on-one deliverance himself. Every GA team member is expected to pray for healing, but only those who feel comfortable with deliverance are asked to place an identifying mark, such as an orange sticker, on their name badges so that other team members can find them if the need arises. Deliverance is also a sensitive issue in many Brazilian churches, whose pastors may either emulate or react against the highly dramatized exorcism tactics (for instance, publicly provoking the spirits of African-Brazilian religions such as Candomblé) employed by the influential Universal Church of the Kingdom of God. Although most participants in GA conferences agree about the basics of divine healing, impassioned disagreements arise—among North American team members, between North Americans and Brazilians, and among Brazilians—over how deliverance should be performed.[53]

As North Americans gain a heightened expectation of the supernatural, they disseminate a democratized model for how divine healing should be practiced. Global Awakening's contribution is less theological—because Brazilian churches already commonly embrace a theology that God heals miraculously—than practical, teaching and showing by example that God will heal through the prayers of ordinary church members (figure 1.4). Whenever Clark travels to Brazil, he takes with him a team of sixty to one hundred eighty self-described homemakers, businesspeople, physicians, retirees, and teenagers whose prayers for healing are represented as being as effective as Clark's. One reason that Brazilian churches invite Clark—and invite him to return

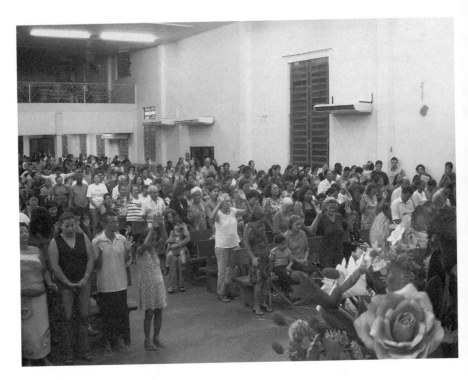

Figure 1.4. Foursquare Gospel Church service, Belém, Pará, Brazil, 2004. Photograph in author's collection.

repeatedly—is that he does not emphasize his own unique gifts so much as his goal of equipping local churches to continue praying for healing after the conclusion of a campaign. A large proportion—by one estimate, 86.4 percent—of Brazilian Christians attest to having received divine healing, but a much smaller proportion—an estimated 11.4 percent—claim to have been used by God to heal others. In contrast, a survey of U.S. Pentecostals found that 70 percent claimed healing from a physical illness and 67 percent claimed to have been used as "instruments of divine healing." A survey of visitors to the Toronto Blessing found that 34 percent of respondents reported a subsequent increase in being used by God to physically heal others.[54]

Global Awakening typically offers morning training sessions as well as evening healing services. In addition to teaching, team members model how to pray for healing—particularly mentoring young translators, who by the end of a weeklong convention are beginning to pray on their own. Global Awakening uses some training materials developed in North America, including a five-step healing model and instructions on how to receive words of knowledge, materials introduced by John Wimber in the 1970s. North American–authored prayer models are coupled with training materials developed by Latin Americans, such as a ten-step deliverance model created by Pablo Bottari in the 1980s. During a typical morning training in Rio, Clark's associate Rodney Hogue, in the characteristic drawl of a Southern Baptist from Texas that his interpreter had trouble translating, taught on deliverance. He emphasized the need to "close doors" to demonic activity by forgiving others, breaking soul ties established by sex outside of marriage, and renouncing occult involvement; the premise was that once demons no longer have a "legal right" to oppress a person, they must obey commands to depart that are issued in the name and authority of Jesus of Nazareth (even when commands are given in a soft-spoken, undramatic manner). Hogue taught Bottari's deliverance model filtered through several layers of linguistic mediation, the formula having been translated from Spanish to English to Portuguese. Some teachings—particularly on controversial topics such as deliverance— seem to be more acceptable to Brazilians when re-presented with the stamp of North American approval, rather than being communicated more directly by other Latin Americans.[55]

As clearly as teaching, modeling, and imitation play roles in how GA transmits healing practices, Clark's central theological contribution is the concept of *impartation*. Pointing to biblical precedents such as the apostle Paul's encouragement to his disciple Timothy not to forget the gift given to him through the laying on of hands and prayer, Clark envisions healing as more contagious than disease, and the anointing, or oil-like spread, of the Holy Spirit as a tangible, transferable power, or love energy, that is caught rather than taught and imparted to others through human touch. The emphasis on impartation encourages the democratization of healing practices, because anyone can become anointed by receiving impartation—and, indeed, new leaders within ANGA networks can emerge from just one dramatic impartation experience. But the emphasis also singles out certain leaders, such as Clark, as particularly anointed. Regardless of Clark's repeated insistence that people can be healed through the prayers of any team member—and that often the greatest miracles occur through someone else's prayers—there is always what insiders refer to as a long "Randy line" of those who will settle for prayer from no one else.[56]

Every international trip begins with an impartation service for the GA team, during which Clark lays hands on each person. One team member, George, a university-employed biomedical researcher who recounts that he was divinely healed of a brain tumor (see chapter 4), described the impartation experience: "Randy prayed for me to impart gifts of healing, and it was really powerful. My right hand was shaking for a long time after that. Then I had some other person pray over me, and it was powerful. . . . Later, I saw Randy standing by himself and asked for a second prayer of impartation, so he did. My hand was still shaking, so he just said something like 'I bless the power in that right hand.'" George went on to explain his apparent greediness for prayer: "I want as much anointing as I can carry, because there are many people who need healing. . . . The crusade that night was to be the most powerful yet for me." Among those he believed healed through his prayers after he received impartation were two blind, orphaned brothers, aged seven and ten. An impartation service for Brazilians is always included in a multiday conference; GA team members who have received impartation help to pray for Brazilians.[57]

Healing Practices and Global Revivalism

On a steamy, 90-degree evening in 2007 in Imperatriz, Maranhão, Brazil, the Miracle Healing Crusade sponsored by twenty local churches and featuring Randy Clark and his GA team attracted ten thousand attendees, 5 percent of the town's population. The night before, a marching band waving a welcome banner lettered in English had greeted Clark and the seventy other North Americans who had volunteered to travel with him at their own expense. As the campaign began, Clark called a young Brazilian woman up to the platform to sing. Sylvia—a local television news anchor—electrified the audience with a popular Brazilian song, "Poderoso," or "Powerful [God]." Many of those present knew Sylvia and the story she retold that evening. Two years before, she had come to a GA convention in Imperatriz. Doctors had sent her home to die from cancer of the thorax. Sylvia had arrived at the 2005 rally weighing a mere 80 pounds, too weak to stand, and coughing up blood. Clark and some of his team had spent an hour praying for Sylvia as she claimed to feel the power and love of God coursing through her body. By the end of the prayer, Sylvia believed herself miraculously healed and felt strong enough to stand up to testify of her healing and to sing a song of praise to God. During the past two years, Sylvia had remained symptom-free, soon regaining a healthy weight and returning to her broadcasting job.[58]

After Sylvia sang and gave her testimony at the 2007 campaign, Clark announced that the power and love of God were present to heal that night, just as God had healed Sylvia two years before. Clark called up members of his team to deliver words of knowledge: pain in the right knee, kidney failure, lower back pain. Clark prayed over the entire congregation using a mixture of English, which an interpreter translated, and brief Portuguese phrases he had memorized. Clark began by welcoming the Holy Spirit and asking God to send angels to assist with the healings. He commanded each of the problems mentioned in the words of knowledge to be healed in Jesus's name and took authority over all sicknesses, pains, and demons present, commanding them to leave in Jesus's name. Clark then asked the audience to test their bodies to see what they were able to do now that they could not do before and to find out whether their pains had disappeared. He asked those whose conditions were at least 80 percent improved to wave their arms so that others could have their faith encouraged. Scores of arms began to wave around the auditorium, and people filed up to the stage to testify to their healings. Clark gave an altar call, telling those who were not Christians but who had just witnessed the power and love of God that they now had an obligation to respond by placing their trust in Jesus and renouncing all other gods and spirits. Dozens streamed forward to pray, after which they were greeted by local pastors, who counseled them as new believers.

Clark then released his team to pray one on one with those who still needed healing. Lines formed behind each team member, as people eager for prayer came forward. With the help of Brazilian translators—mostly young adults who had learned English in school—team members conducted brief interviews: "What is your name? Why do you want prayer? Are you a Christian? What was going on in your life when the pain began? Is there anyone you need to forgive? Have you ever been involved in the occult?" Team members led those who needed healing through short prayers to forgive those who had wronged them and to renounce participation in "occult" practices. Then they prayed briefly for healing: "In the name of Jesus, demons, leave now. Be healed in Jesus's name. Check your body. A little better? Let's keep praying. Check again. No pain left? Praise God!" Around midnight, Clark called his team back to the buses, promising more prayer at tomorrow night's service.

Prayer for healing and evangelism typically go hand in hand at GA conferences. In Imperatriz, Clark gave an altar call for salvation from sin following Sylvia's testimony of physical healing. Team members also evangelize as they pray for healing. Oblivious to scholars' explanations of healing claims as attributable to misdiagnosis or the placebo effect, believers relate intense subjective experiences of God's expressing love through healing. Pentecostals envision salvation in material as well as spiritual terms, providing health for both body and soul.[59]

During a typical campaign interaction, a young man named Carlos requested prayer because he had pain caused by a lump on his foot. Carlos watched as several people in line before him claimed to experience healing. When Carlos's turn came, team member George, introduced above, asked Carlos whether he was a Christian. When Carlos said no, George told him that Jesus wanted to heal the whole person, not just his foot, and asked him whether he wanted to experience the love of God by becoming a Christian. George clarified that this would mean renouncing all other gods and spirits and trusting in Jesus only. Carlos said that he wanted to do this, so George, with the help of his translator, led Carlos through a prayer to accept Jesus as his only savior. Then George commanded the spirits of infirmity to leave Carlos and commanded healing to his body in Jesus's name. Carlos soon reported that all pain was gone, and those around him attested to seeing the lump that had been on his foot disappear. One of the local pastors then took over to counsel Carlos as a new Christian.[60]

North Americans who participate in GA's international ministry trips believe that healing should be equally available at home, while confessing a higher expectation of seeing miracles in places such as Brazil, Mozambique, or India, where faith in the supernatural seems more common and where there is less opportunity to rely on doctors instead of God. Global Awakening leaders urge team members to use the faith boost gained from an international trip to pray more expectantly once they return home. Global Awakening also conducts healing schools and sells books, CDs, and DVDs in the United States and Canada that attempt to demonstrate the accessibility of miracles— especially in marketplace spaces sacralized by the performance of healing rituals. The idea is that Christians should be on the lookout at stores such as Walmart for fellow shoppers who complain of pain or have an obvious sickness or disability, offering to pray for their healing. In 2009, GA began production of videotaped North American marketplace healing practices designed for broadcast on nonreligious networks as reality TV. The premise is that North American Christianity will be revitalized once people experience, not just read or hear about, the power and love of God.[61]

Notably absent in the valorization of marketplace healings is any sustained critique of economic injustices. Healing advocates do envision their performances as counteracting selfish consumerism. Yet this same discourse can be read as contributing to the very commercial processes that offers of free prayer purportedly destabilize. By harmonizing prayer and commerce, sacralizing rituals seductively transform highly suspect consumer-oriented spaces into sites of religiously legitimate activities. There is nothing here to subvert white, patriarchal, capitalistic, U.S.-dominated policies that subsidize multinational corporations by paying inadequate wages to two-thirds-world workers in substandard working conditions. The practice of marketplace healings implies an acceptance of existing economic conditions as a given, rather than subjecting them to critical scrutiny. By marketing healing prayer—especially as North Americans borrow inspiration from pentecostals in the two-thirds world—to supplement rather than criticize marketplace practices, North American pentecostals often make opaque their own complicity in oppressive economic relationships. At the same time, pentecostal networks also play a role in meeting practical physical needs for food, shelter, and basic medical care among the world's poor by deploying natural as well as supernatural means.[62]

Conclusion

As of 2011, seventeen years after the genesis of the Toronto Blessing, the revivalist waves set in motion by this event have surged through the fluid, partially overlapping pentecostal networks bridged by ANGA, reaching across the boundaries of geography, denomination, ethnicity, language, and social class. As pentecostals from the global South and from North America engage in shared network activities and participate in multidirectional cultural flows, they sustain and deepen their sense of membership in a global community for which healing prayer is a defining ritual. In some instances, the globalization of healing practices obscures or intensifies economic and political inequities, but cases can also be cited in which very poor people directly or indirectly experience tangible benefits. North Americans may not expect to see many miracles at home, but they do expect miracles in such countries as Brazil or Mozambique. Lay Brazilians or Mozambicans may expect miracles to occur, but perhaps not through their own prayers. Participation in globalized healing networks fuels the twin engines of supernaturalism and democratization, which together forcefully propel the growth of pentecostalism.

A central activity in ANGA conferences and international ministry trips is prayer for healing. The following chapters examine social constructions and empirical effects of healing prayer from a series of complementary vantages, beginning with controversies over prospective clinical trials of prayer and retrospective evaluation of before-and-after medical records; looking in turn at perceptions and measurements of healing; using longitudinal follow-up to assess any effects of prayer practices over time; and offering a theoretical model to interpret outcomes of praying for healing.

CHAPTER 2

Why Are Biomedical Tests of Prayer Controversial?

✦

For the last five hundred years, since the beginnings of what scholars term *modernity*, Europeans and North Americans have hotly debated these questions: Can and should the effects of prayer for healing be tested empirically? If so, what methods and standards of evaluation should be employed? There is indeed a fascinating history of great reversals concerning where cultural groups have positioned themselves on these questions. Nor is this subject a matter of merely antiquarian interest. Debates over empirical investigations of prayer are raging with particular intensity at the present cultural moment. What motivated Christians' opposition to empirical studies in the nineteenth century seems to have been fear that God would not respond to tests with results favoring his existence and intervention. As a handful of biomedical scientists, some of whom were also Christians, began to employ their accustomed methods of study to prayer and found evidence suggestive of an effect, other members of the scientific community became alarmed about the potential implications of these positive results for the meaningfulness and authority of what they understood as real science.

This chapter traces a history of the controversies surrounding biomedical studies of prayer for healing in the modern world. The chapter argues that despite problems in past practice and intrinsic to the endeavor, studies of intercessory prayer have the potential to provide insight into any empirical effects of praying for healing—especially if researchers shift attention from "distant" to "proximal" prayer studies.

Regardless of the prevalence and widely assumed efficacy of prayer for healing, its clinical effects are poorly understood, in part because of serious limitations in how prayer has been studied. Of particular concern are findings like those of a well-publicized study of heart patients, which reported that patients who knew they were the objects of intercessory prayer did worse rather than better. If prayer could have negative effects, however indirect, then the frequency with which it is practiced should generate public concern. If, on the contrary, prayer is on balance therapeutically beneficial, researchers may be able to learn something about when, how, and why praying for healing makes a difference. Even in the industrialized world, where biomedical science is the most sophisticated, convenient, and affordable, many illnesses still baffle medical doctors, and people continue to suffer lifelong, debilitating conditions and to die of disease. If one turns to the developing world, even basic medical care remains unavailable or inaccessibly expensive for as much as 80 percent of the population. Given the magnitude of global health problems, arguments that a priori deny the legitimacy of studying how religious practices such as prayer might affect health are intellectually and ethically problematic.[1]

From the Council of Trent to the Lourdes Medical Bureau

Although today often framed as a struggle between "science" and "religion," disputes over the efficacy of prayer for healing arose in a quite different cultural context—as a controversy during the sixteenth century between Catholics and Protestants, with the former group successfully appealing to scientists as willing allies. The Roman Catholic Church demanded that Protestant dissidents produce miracles as *proof* that God approved their novel doctrines. Protestants, notably John Calvin (1509–1564) and Martin Luther (1483–1546), rebutted that they did not need miracles because theirs was no new doctrine but simply the gospel of Christianity. In Luther's words, "Now that the apostles have preached the Word and have given their writings, and nothing more than what they have written remains to be revealed, no new and special revelation or miracle is necessary." To explain the absence of an experience of miracles, Calvin developed the doctrine of *cessationism* to argue that miracles had ceased with the end of the biblical era because they were no longer needed to confirm the gospel; thus, "the gift of healing disappeared with the other miraculous powers which the Lord was pleased to give for a time." God might still heal in response to prayer, but such healings were not miraculous, and most healing should be expected through medical means. By claiming ongoing miraculous healings, Calvin argued, the Catholic hierarchy perpetuated superstition.[2]

In response to Protestant charges, the Counter-Reformation Council of Trent (1545–1563) established more stringent guidelines for evaluating miracle claims presented in proceedings for the canonization of saints. Ninety-five percent of purported miracles—dating from medieval times through the end of the twentieth century—involved healings of physical illnesses, for most of which medical doctors provided testimony. The Tridentine guidelines were predicated on a skeptical approach to claims and a demand for evidence, prominently including that presented by physicians, with the goal of finding scientific explanations for asserted miracles. In the seventeenth century, Paolo Zacchia (1584–1659), a lawyer and chief physician for the Papal States, articulated a set of requirements that, although more fully elaborated over time, set the terms for subsequent adjudication of claims brought before the church. For healings to be considered miraculous, the diagnosis had to be unquestionable; the prognosis incurable; the recovery instantaneous, complete, and permanent; and with no suggestion that nature or medical treatment could be responsible. At the most frequented Catholic healing shrine, Lourdes, France, established in 1858, the church in 1883 established a medical bureau that includes non-Catholic doctors. This bureau has strictly applied a modified version of Zacchia's standards, accepting just sixty-seven out of more than seven thousand investigated claims as medically inexplicable. By contrast, Protestants—ironically, given their critiques of alleged unreasoning Catholic superstition—have been more leery of the medical gaze.[3]

The Prayer-Gauge Controversy

The question of whether prayer should be tested empirically was first asked publicly in close to its current form during the 1870s, at a moment when European and American scientific and religious communities were undergoing changes that prompted them to seek proofs of particular kinds. Mid-nineteenth-century Protestants continued to discount Catholic miracle claims, whether or not validated by medical procedures such as those employed at Lourdes. Yet many of these same Protestants came to envision bold, specific prayer requests as what the historian John Corrigan calls "a sign and measure of faith," or proof that Christians were doing their part in a contractual relationship with God. In this model, prayer was primarily petitionary, and—to quote directly from prayer manuals of the period—directed explicitly at the goal of obtaining "for the petitioner the blessings which he needs," or, in short, "getting things from God." The best prayers were not self-interested, but "intercessional, on behalf of others." Nineteenth-century Americans felt ambivalent about praying for healing because of widespread church teachings that God sent sickness to discipline his children and aid their spiritual sanctification. The official service for the Visitation of the Sick in *The Book of Common Prayer* of the Church of England, introduced in 1549 and still in print today, prescribes that the minister say to the sick person:

> Whatsoever your sickness is, know you certainly that it is God's visitation. And for what cause soever this sickness is sent unto you: whether it be to try your patience for the example of others and that your faith may be found in the day of the Lord laudable, glorious, and honourable, to the increase of glory and endless felicity; or else it be sent unto you to correct and amend in you whatsoever doth offend the eyes of your heavenly Father; know you certainly, that if you truly repent you of your sins, and bear your sickness patiently, trusting in God's mercy, for his dear Son Jesus Christ's sake, and render unto him humble thanks for his fatherly visitation, submitting yourself wholly unto his will, it shall turn to your profit, and help you forward in the right way that leadeth unto

> everlasting life. / Take therefore in good part the chastisement
> of the Lord.

Notwithstanding such exhortations, most people, understandably, wanted healing more than they wanted sickness. A growing number of Protestants believed, and publicly claimed, that prayer produced tangible, this-worldly results, prominently including physical healing. Effectual prayer seemed to Protestants, who enthusiastically embraced the Scottish Common Sense Realist strain of the Enlightenment and especially the inductive methods of Francis Bacon (1561–1626), to provide empirical evidence of the truth of Christianity.[4]

Meanwhile, the position that came to be called scientific naturalism was emerging, newly bolstered by Charles Darwin's plausible account, in *The Origin of Species* (1859), of how life evolved without presupposing the necessity of divine intervention. In the seventeenth century, René Descartes (1596–1650) had proposed a dualistic model of the material world as distinct from "mind" or "spirit." In the eighteenth century, David Hume (1711–1776) had reasoned that "miracles" are invalidated by the known regularity of the material world of nature. In the nineteenth century, a "new Humean argument" emerged that miracles are, rather, invalidated by the unknowability of nature, because human knowledge seems too limited to prove that any event has violated natural law. Immanuel Kant (1724–1804) argued that human knowledge is limited to that which is observable in the phenomenal world, whereas the noumenal, or that which is real, is outside the realm of verification. Thomas Huxley (1825–1895) coined the phrase *scientific naturalism* in 1892 to describe an empirical approach to gathering knowledge about the material world that rejected supernatural explanations of phenomena. Naturalism can refer to a purely methodological commitment to naturalistic explanations. But Huxley had in mind something more: a philosophical commitment to materialism, tantamount to agnosticism or atheism. The idea of conducting a scientific experiment to study the empirical effects of prayer was first proposed by scientific naturalists—and ardently opposed by Protestant clergy. After months of intense public controversy, the issue largely faded from public interest until a century later, reemerging with the sides in the debate strangely reversed—but this gets ahead of the story.[5]

In what became known as the "prayer-gauge controversy," the religiously skeptical physicist John Tyndall (1820–1893) issued a challenge to Christians who claimed that prayer made a difference in the natural world. Precipitating this challenge, in 1871 the prince of Wales became seriously ill with typhoid fever. The British Crown requested national prayers for healing, and when the prince recovered the prayers were credited. Tyndall questioned the presumed causal connection in a letter mailed to the London *Contemporary Review* in June 1872 titled "Prayer for the Sick: Hints towards a Serious Attempt to Estimate Its Value." Tyndall—avowedly at the suggestion of a well-known British surgeon, Sir Henry Thompson—proposed a test of the efficacy of prayer. One ward of a hospital, containing patients whose diseases and mortality rates were best understood, should become the object of special prayers for a three- to five-year period, after which mortality rates would be compared with those of patients with similar conditions in a regular hospital ward. No one ever took Tyndall up on his challenge, which, however, generated a firestorm of public controversy in British and American newspapers and books. Proponents of the test assumed that scientific methods both could and should arbitrate all truth claims. By claiming that prayer "produces the precise effects caused by physical energy in the ordinary course of things," Tyndall averred, religion had stepped onto the ground of science and should therefore be tested by the rules of science. The notion that prayer could influence a presumably closed natural system was profoundly disturbing to Tyndall because it challenged a fundamental premise of modern scientific inquiry, that the universe is governed by regular, predictable natural laws.[6]

Despite the enthusiasm of some Protestants for declaring publicly the efficacy of intercessory prayer, they recoiled at Tyndall's challenge. Protestant respondents worried that prayer could not get a fair trial by scientists on their terrain, in a hospital setting with doctors adjudicating the results. More than objecting to the terms of the challenge, Protestant critics rejected the very idea of subjecting prayer to a scientific test. On the one hand, Protestants affirmed that because God created the world using natural laws, scientific investigation should provide evidence of divine activity. On the other hand, they denied the appropriateness of testing whether God answers prayers in a naturalistically consistent way. They argued, first, that the challenge reflected a misunderstanding of the personal nature of God, which in their view, implied that divine power is inherently untestable by methods used to measure impersonal natural forces. The challenge, moreover, reflected a misunderstanding of the nature of prayer, which, the Protestants insisted, is no more binding on God than a child's requests of a parent. By this reasoning, it seemed unlikely that God would answer prayers offered as part of a study since such prayer would not be motivated by genuine concern for the sick but by the mere desire to test prayer and reduce it to a scientifically measurable force. This last worry, indeed, constituted the core Protestant fear: a test was being proposed that they did not think prayer could pass.[7]

Following this logic, some Protestants backed away from claiming effects of prayers for healing, whether or not as part of a study. Writing in 1892, twenty years after the prayer-gauge challenge, the editor of the widely circulated U.S. *Methodist Christian Advocate,* James Monroe Buckley, frankly worried that claiming that prayer results in healing "seriously diminishes the influence of Christianity by subjecting it to a test which it cannot endure. It diverts attention from the moral and spiritual transformation which Christianity professes to work, a transformation which wherever made manifests its divinity, so that none who behold it need any other proof that it is of God." Buckley avoided the danger of failure by redefining "proof" in nonfalsifiable terms, as unquantifiable moral and spiritual changes, rather than as verifiable answers to prayer.[8]

In the meantime, however, scientific naturalists were unwilling to allow their challenge simply to be sidestepped. Because no Christians expressed willingness to participate in a prospective study, in August 1872, two months after Tyndall issued his challenge, Francis Galton, a cousin of Charles Darwin, published in the British *Fortnightly Review* his own retrospective study of the past effects of intercessory prayer, titled "Statistical Inquiries into the Efficacy of Prayer." Galton, who referred to prayer as a "perfectly appropriate and legitimate subject of scientific inquiry," reasoned that because the Church of England admonished parishioners to pray for the British sovereign as well as for clergy and missionaries, those who had been the recipients of so much prayer should, if prayer exerted a beneficial effect, have higher life expectancies than the general population. Galton found the reverse to be true and concluded that the experiment disproved the efficacy of prayer.[9]

Prior to the prayer-gauge debate, Catholics and Protestants principally argued with each other—with additional divisions among various Protestants—over the relationship between prayer and healing. The cultural battle lines began to shift as scientific naturalists issued challenges with implications for all of Christian prayer.[10]

Pentecostal Prayer Studies

By the early twentieth century, biomedical science had developed into a self-confident profession with an unsurpassed degree of cultural authority. Given the apparent objectivity of science in determining medical truth about illness and healing, more marginal cultural movements had to appeal to the language and methods of science in order to claim legitimacy. As the historian David Lindberg has aptly observed, "'Science' and 'scientific' are often simply employed as general terms of approval—epithets that we attach to whatever we wish to applaud." The very fact of the increasing availability of scientific means of measuring the effects of medical alternatives such as prayer seemed logically to require that the results be measured—but how to go about taking such measurements remained highly contested. From Tyndall and Galton's victories through the first half of the twentieth century, debates over the efficacy of prayer for healing shifted from large-scale trials back toward earlier efforts to confirm or deny that particular cases of healing might be attributable to prayer.[11]

The influential early Pentecostal John G. Lake (1870–1935) provides a revealing case study of nonscientists appropriating apparently scientific language and methods in an attempt to validate prayer. In many respects, Lake fitted the stereotype of an "antimedical" Pentecostal. Blaming medical doctors and cessationist theologians for permitting the deaths of eight of his fifteen siblings, Lake renounced all medical assistance to trust God alone for healing. Lake, three of his siblings, and his wife all apparently recovered from illnesses after learning the prayer-only model practiced by the controversial Scottish-born, Australian-raised divine healing advocate John Alexander Dowie (1847–1907), at his Chicago Healing Home. Having repudiated medical science for the pragmatic reason that divine healing seemed more effective, Lake spent the rest of his life trying to demonstrate that divine healing was itself a science, the results of which could be verified empirically.[12]

Lake theorized that "pneumatology" was a "science of Spirit," by which one could uncover the "laws of the [Holy] Spirit, a discerning of the modus operandi of the Spirit's working." Lake argued that even Jesus had used "scientific" methods to heal the sick, and taught his followers to employ at least four scientific means: the prayer of faith, the prayer of agreement, the anointing of the elders, and the laying on of hands. Despite his rejection of the naturalistic assumptions underlying medical science, Lake developed an enduring interest in scientific investigation while taking medical courses at Northwestern University. Like many of his contemporaries fascinated by the recent invention of the dynamo, or electrical generator, Lake described prayer as a dynamo that attracted the Holy Spirit—which Lake envisioned as a "tangible substance," much like electricity, which was powerful enough to control every "form of materiality." According to Lake, when people prayed, the Holy Spirit physically took possession of the human body, producing chemical interactions that affected every cell—for instance, causing "waves of heat" to pass through a person's body, or "dematerializing" a tumor in a kind of supernatural "surgical operation." The Holy Spirit could literally "impregnate" any "material substance," which explained the healing properties of handkerchiefs that had, since New Testament times, been prayed over and sent to the sick. Since Jesus's followers did not possess the same degree of the Holy Spirit's anointing as did Jesus himself, it sometimes took repeated prayers to obtain healing.[13]

Like other irregular healers of his era, Lake adopted the title "doctor," although he lacked medical credentials, or even a college diploma.

As a self-styled doctor, Lake operated a Divine Healing Institute, popularly known as Healing Rooms, in Spokane, Washington, from 1914 to 1920. Lake viewed the Spokane healing rooms as a kind of laboratory for finding out not only "that God healed," but also "*how* God healed." Challenging doctors to make scientific examinations the "test of the truth of the message," Lake orchestrated a series of experiments to demonstrate the interconnectedness of the supernatural and material realms. He claimed to have convinced faculty at Northwestern to attach instruments to his head that registered "vibrations of the brain" and to take microscopic x-rays as Lake invited the Holy Spirit to flow through his body. The scientists reportedly observed readings that exceeded their instrument's measurement capabilities. Lake then asked the doctors to connect a monitoring device to a man hospitalized for an inflamed bone while Lake prayed for healing; the doctors, according to Lake, saw "every cell" respond to his prayers. On another occasion, Lake allegedly placed live bubonic plague cells in his hand under a microscope, challenging doctors to watch the cells die on contact as the Holy Spirit surged through his body. As a further empirical test, Lake sent healing-rooms clientele to a nearby x-ray lab before and after prayer in order to chart the progress of healing. Although Lake renounced the naturalistic paradigm that formed the foundation of modern medicine, he constructed an alternative science of healing in which supernatural forces acted in measurable ways to affect the material world.[14]

Lake attracted a great deal of notice from other Pentecostals during his own lifetime and became a hero for subsequent generations—who today still widely boast that Lake "documented" (reflecting a privileging of scientific-sounding language) one hundred thousand healings, mostly from incurable conditions, although no documentation apart from Lake's own estimate seems to exist. Cal Pierce, a retired real estate developer, re-opened the Spokane Healing Rooms in their original location in 1999 and established an International Association of Healing Rooms (IAHR), which had, within a decade, networked more than two thousand healing rooms (not counting numerous unaffiliated but similarly inspired healing rooms) in almost every state and more than forty countries. Today's healing rooms explicitly affirm conventional medical science and few of them have shown much interest in empirical tests of prayer or even in collecting medical documentation of avowed divine healing. Healing-rooms staff occasionally claim that medical doctors refer their hopeless cases to them. Christian medical doctors sometimes volunteer to pray with local healing-rooms teams. For the most part, however, Lake and the later healing-rooms movement have never made it onto the radar of nonsectarian medical practitioners or media outlets. As a result, little public controversy has surrounded their dramatic claims—which include healings of virtually every type of condition from headaches to cancers.[15]

Psychosomatic Prayer Studies

Since Tyndall and Galton, mainstream biomedical research on prayer and other religious rituals has focused on psychosomatic, or mind-body, effects for which naturalistic causal explanations are readily available. The psychology of religion developed as a subfield of the emerging discipline of psychology in the late nineteenth century, at a time when allied fields were all professionalizing and developing laboratory-research programs affiliated with major universities. Early psychotherapists such as Sigmund Freud (1856–1939) evaluated religion negatively as a form of psychopathology. Accordingly, scientists looked less at the alleged benefits of prayer than for ways that religious beliefs could cause physical harm. In a widely heralded article on "'Voodoo' Death," published in the *American Anthropologist* in 1942, Walter Cannon (1871–1945), a professor and the chairman of the Department of Physiology at Harvard Medical School, looked for psychobiological mechanisms through which beliefs in "voodoo" rituals or "witchcraft" curses can cause death in so-called primitive societies. Cannon traced physiological pathways by which negative emotions such as fear and anger produce nerve impulses that arouse secretions in the adrenal glands, which in turn cause the liver to release sugar into the bloodstream, and push blood into the heart, lungs, central nervous system, and limbs. Cannon concluded that a "persistent and profound emotional state" causes excessive activation of the sympathico-adrenal system, which "may induce a disastrous fall of blood pressure, ending in death."

For Cannon, religious beliefs could be bad for one's health for identifiable physiological reasons.[16]

If negative emotions such as stress, anxiety, depression, unforgiveness, and fear could be physically harmful, it seemed equally plausible to some scientists that positive emotions such as joy, peace, love, hope, forgiveness, and religious ecstasy might indirectly cause physical benefits. Researchers in an emerging field of psychosomatic medicine, of which the Swiss psychiatrist Adolf Meyer (1866–1950) was a key architect, sought positive therapeutic uses for observed mind-body connections.[17]

A prospective clinical trial—the first prospective trial of prayer on record—conducted in 1957 evaluated the psychotherapeutic value of praying for one's own healing. Envisioning prayer as a potential adjunct to conventional psychotherapy, the study differentiated subjects who prayed with versus without receiving directions from their therapist on how to pray. Forty-five subjects were divided into three groups of fifteen, not randomly, but on the basis of their therapeutic preferences. The group that received regular psychotherapy without prayer improved on average 65 percent in psychological measures. The "Random Pray-er" group—those who prayed as they were accustomed to doing to overcome their problems—did not improve. The "Prayer Therapy" group—those who followed a prescribed course of group and individual prayer assignments designed according to psychotherapeutic assumptions about beneficial types of prayer—on average improved 72 percent in psychological measures. Fascinating as an early example of efforts to integrate psychotherapy and prayer as well as to conduct empirical research on the efficacy of prayer, the 1957 trial did not immediately inspire many similar studies.[18]

From the 1940s to the 1980s, researchers did publish a number of studies on the therapeutic effects of suggestion and hypnosis. Some authors suggested that prayer might work by inadvertently hypnotizing recipients. The American psychiatrist Jerome Frank, in his now classic book *Persuasion and Healing* (1961), interpreted prayer and psychotherapy as essentially similar: both used the power of suggestion to stimulate the body's natural capacity for healing. Frank came to the interesting conclusion that the "evidence that an occasional cure of advanced organic disease does occur at Lourdes is as strong as that for any other phenomenon accepted as true." Frank accepted the empirical "fact" of religious healing, but explained it naturalistically in terms of poorly understood mind-body connections.[19]

Other twentieth-century scientists objected to the premise of using empirical methods to investigate the effects of prayer. A textbook on the *Psychology of Religion* published in 1984 dismissed the possibility of worthwhile empirical study: "If a deity can meaningfully answer a believer's prayer, and if prayer is to remain a spiritual rather than a magical exercise, then surely that same deity would make sure that all empirical studies of the efficacy of prayer will turn out inconclusive! The evidence of the effectiveness of prayers, as they touch events in the material world, remains outside the domain of science. The faithful who want to believe can believe, and the skeptic who chooses not to believe could not be convinced." The textbook sounds a theological note in asserting that any real deity would oppose scientific investigation in order to "protect" faith. Implicitly, religion that claims empirical effects is not real religion, but "magic." The textbook sidelines religion to the "spiritual" realm, while attributing to science exclusive authority to determine what is real in the "material" world.[20]

Much as nineteenth-century Protestants resisted studying prayer because they feared that studies would not show an effect, the worry expressed by the 1984 psychology textbook seems to be that studies of the efficacy of prayer might *not* turn out inconclusive but would appear to provide evidence for the existence of a deity who acts in measurable ways in the material world. The textbook goes on to enumerate the explicitly "safer," psychological benefits of prayer, which serves the "same functions as psychotherapy." The text explains the efficacy of "faith healing": "In most cases of illness the primary factor, or an important secondary one, is the restoration of a balanced state of mind. That is what faith can do, and it does not (scientifically speaking) matter whether the faith is placed in God, a shaman, a sugar pill, or tinged alcohol on a wart." The textbook asserts that—scientifically speaking— the efficacy of prayer is reducible to a placebo effect. The textbook thereby invokes science simultaneously to delegitimize the empirical study of prayer and as the standard by which religious claims about healing should ultimately be measured—and dismissed.[21]

Since the mid-twentieth century, there have been a spate of publications attributing the efficacy of prayer to the "placebo effect"—which is critically characterized by the anthropologist Thomas Csordas as a "black-box" mechanism or rhetorical device often used to label instead of explaining poorly understood effects of suggestion and expectations on physical health. Despite the popularity of the placebo concept, a highly regarded Cochrane systematic review concludes that properly controlled trials have failed to show any major health benefits from placebos, except in some cases modest reductions in patient-reported symptoms such as pain.[22]

Over the past several decades, researchers have become increasingly interested in identifying precise physiological and psychosocial mechanisms by which prayer may benefit health. Harvard Medical School's Herbert Benson hypothesized the existence of a "relaxation response"—a phrase that became the title of his 1975 bestselling book—to account for cases in which prayer exerts positive effects—for example, by lowering heart and breathing rate. In the developing field of psychoimmunology, the biochemist Candace Pert investigated how emotional states alter chemicals in the body; for instance, endorphins (mood-elevating substances released by the brain) and other neurotransmitters (chemical messengers) act on the endocrine and immune systems. Other researchers have focused on cardiovascular pathways by which, for example, negative emotions can stretch the arterial walls, creating sites for plaque deposits and increasing arterial pressure and heart rate. Larry Dossey, a medical doctor, has provocatively suggested that one day physicians who do not prescribe prayer may be subject to malpractice suits. Dossey is not a traditional supernaturalist; rather, appealing to the "new physics," he envisions "mind" as infinite and nonlocal, allowing one intellect to connect with another to exert a therapeutic influence. As researchers focused on local rather than nonlocal operations of the mind, it became popular after 2000 to use MRIs to look for structures in the brain that were activated during prayer and meditation. Whether negatively or positively evaluating the effects of religion, psychosomatic approaches to studying prayer have diminished the apparent need for supernaturalist hypotheses of how prayer works by positing naturalistic mechanisms by which prayer can affect health.[23]

In a complementary line of research, investigators have examined psychosocial mechanisms by which prayer and other religious practices can benefit health. Studies point to religious proscriptions against use of alcohol, tobacco, and caffeine; participation in social support networks; and the role of beliefs and rituals in creating positive emotional states, such as freedom from anxiety about the future. Doctor Harold G. Koenig, the codirector of Duke University's Center for Spirituality, Theology and Health, has developed an international reputation for his many publications showing a generally positive correlation between high degrees of religious practice and spirituality and better health and longevity. The psychologist Kenneth Pargament has likewise shaped a field of research on the potential efficacy of religious practices, such as prayer, as strategies for coping with illness.[24]

At an Impasse: From the Prayer-Gauge Controversy to Distant Intercessory Prayer Studies

As was the case during the late nineteenth century, at the turn of the twenty-first century, modern science sets the standards for evaluating the risks and benefits of intercessory prayer. In contrast to research on the psychosomatic and psychosocial effects of prayer, since the 1980s scientific researchers have published scores of prospective, randomized, controlled studies of the effects of distant intercessory prayer. Because psychosomatic and psychosocial explanations do not obviously account for distant prayer claims, such studies have generated a strong public backlash in the scientific community and news media.

The recent propensity to study distant prayer—as well as widespread opposition to such studies—reflects both popular interest in spiritual healing and general respect for medical science and is therefore extraordinarily revealing for a number of reasons. First, it is illuminating to compare the early twenty-first century situation with the prayer-gauge controversy of one hundred years ago. During the 1870s, scientific naturalists such as Tyndall and Galton insisted on using scientific methods to investigate the empirical effects of prayer. Christian clergy publicly refused to test prayer in this way, and no prospective trial was attempted for most of a century. In today's cultural context, the roles have been dramatically reversed, and it is scientific naturalists who most often object to studying prayer—for reasons that are as much theological as scientific. Some, though not all, of the researchers who have undertaken prayer studies are themselves known or assumed to be Christians or adherents of other theistic religions such as Judaism or Islam. The religious commitments of those studying prayer have generated concern among other researchers that purportedly scientific studies illicitly serve hidden religious agendas. At the same time, other Christian spokespersons have continued to denounce the idea of testing prayer—even while insisting that claims of spiritual healing could be accepted only if substantiated by the very type of study that they claim on principle should not be attempted. A closer look at several of the biomedical studies that have generated the most public debate—those by Byrd, Harris, Cha, Benson, and a Cochrane Review—will help to flesh out the issues at stake.[25]

In 1988, the cardiologist Randolph C. Byrd and colleagues attracted a great deal of largely favorable, and some aggressively negative, public notice by publishing, in the peer-reviewed *Southern Medical Journal,* the results of a prospective, randomized, double-blinded, controlled study—the gold standard of rigorous scientific research methods—that found positive therapeutic effects from distant intercessory prayer "to the Judeo-Christian God." Conducted in the coronary care unit of the San Francisco General Medical Center over a ten-month period in 1982–1983, the study compared the outcomes of 201 patients in a control group with those of 192 patients in an experimental group that received prayer from "born again" Protestant and Catholic Christians active in "daily devotional prayer" and "fellowship with a local church"; both Protestant and Catholic intercessors were recruited. Byrd matched patients and intercessors from the same denominations, providing intercessors with the patient's first name, condition, and diagnosis. Intercessors were instructed to pray "for a rapid recovery and for prevention of complications and death, in addition to other areas of prayer they believed to be beneficial to patients." The study found that

"the prayer group had less congestive heart failure, required less di-
uretic and antibiotic therapy, had fewer episodes of pneumonia, had
fewer cardiac arrests, and were less frequently intubated and venti-
lated." Byrd acknowledged limits to his study's methods, for instance
the impossibility of ensuring that members of the control group did
not pray for themselves or receive prayer from intercessors not enrolled in the study. Although critics picked up on such methodological limitations and challenged Byrd's decision to enroll only "born
again" Christians as intercessors, many readers evaluated the overall
study design as scientifically sound. This study inspired numerous
other researchers to follow the same basic design in trying to replicate
the results.[26]

Anticipating controversy, the *Southern Medical Journal* published a
favorable commentary as a preface to Byrd's article and a second, simultaneously published study demonstrating positive effects of religion in the recovery of burn patients. The commentary, "Religion and
Healing," was written by Dr. William Wilson, professor emeritus of
psychiatry at Duke Medical Center. Wilson began by acknowledging
that "there is no doubt that the following two articles published in this
issue are likely to arouse strong passions and considerable prejudice in
some readers who believe that religion is not worthy of scientific consideration . . . [or is] not relevant to medicine." In Wilson's view, the
articles were important because they highlighted a "problem that increasingly faces science in its search for truth. That problem is the
challenge of the theory of quantum mechanics to our cosmology. It
has changed our mechanistic view of the universe." Calling the questions Byrd raised "quite valid ones for scientific inquiry," Wilson emphasized the potential clinical value of such studies in helping to
"enlarge our therapeutic armamentarium." Wilson concluded by calling for "more research on the role of religion in healing."[27]

Not every reader of the journal issue agreed with Wilson's conclusion. In a subsequent issue, the *Southern Medical Journal* published
a sharply critical letter to the editor. The author, Dr. Steven Kreisman,
was a North Carolina emergency-room physician who worried that
"medicine's greatest accomplishments since the Age of Enlightenment
were made possible by the fundamental characteristics of that age: a

respect for reason." Medicine had advanced precisely by restricting its purview to understanding scientific laws, which "permit no miracles and which are intelligible without reference to the supernatural." In implying that prayer works by invoking supernatural aid, Byrd's and Wilson's articles, and indeed "the July 1988 *Southern Medical Journal,*" had done a "disservice to the science of medicine and, therefore, to mankind in general." Kreisman pejoratively referred to Byrd's "'scientific' study" by placing the word *scientific* in quotation marks; he thereby questioned the scientific merits of the study, although he did not present any substantive critiques of the study design or methods. Kreisman did not specifically target the burn-patient study for criticism—likely because it restricted its analysis to the role of religion as a coping mechanism without claiming it had direct effects on health. Kreisman concluded that "by trying to undermine reason and by giving credence to faith as a valid epistemology, [Wilson's and Byrd's] articles are an attempt to return medicine to the Dark Ages, and to reduce physicians to the same status as witch doctors and faith healers." Kreisman appended a warning that "if the *Southern Medical Journal* is to be taken as a legitimate medical publication, it must explicitly state it will no longer publish articles of this kind." Kreisman not only indicted the study authors as unscientific but also questioned the medical legitimacy of a journal that would allow their publication.[28]

Kriesman was correct, perhaps even prophetic, in observing the receptivity of the *Southern Medical Journal* to publishing research on prayer. In addition to publishing Byrd's research in 1988, the *SMJ* would provide a home for a study of Christian prayer by Dale Matthews in 2000 (discussed below) and my research group's article in 2010. Indeed, I submitted our article to the *SMJ* because it had previously published related research. One may conjecture that the journal's location in Birmingham, Alabama, which is in the southern "Bible Belt," has attracted editors and readers interested in studies of Christian prayer. It should also be noted, however, that the vast majority of articles published by the *SMJ* since 1988 have had nothing to do with the subject of spirituality and health.

An editor's note responded to Kreisman's criticism of Byrd by reaffirming the publication decision. Byrd's article had been "subjected to the usual peer-review process and judged to report properly designed and executed scientific investigation, with a recommendation for publication." The editor explicitly "reject[ed] the thesis" of Kreisman's conclusion regarding the Dark Ages and "decline[d] to categorically deny publication to any work fulfilling the *Journal*'s established criteria." The editorial note concluded by implying that the editor took the more reasonable position, because the journal's open policy "includes Dr. Kreisman's negative response, which I welcome, since it indicates that the *Journal* is stimulating thought and debate, a primary function of any scientific publication." Thus, the editor rebutted the charge of scientific illegitimacy by defining the role of a scientific publication as encouraging open debate regardless of the religious presuppositions of the participants as long as the methods are sound according to scientific standards.[29]

Following publication of Byrd's study, the highly prestigious *Archives of Internal Medicine* published a replication study by William S. Harris and colleagues in 1999. Similar to Byrd, Harris conducted a prospective, randomized, double-blind, parallel-group controlled trial of the effects of intercessory prayer on 990 consecutively admitted coronary patients. Half the patients received prayer from intercessors who believed in a "personal God who hears and answers prayers made on behalf of the sick," and half did not. The group that received prayer exhibited better outcomes than the control group. Although comparable to Byrd's study in methods and results, Harris's paper generated a great deal more public criticism from other scientists—in part because it was published in a higher-impact medical journal and in a cultural climate that during the intervening decade had become more hostile to the concept of using scientific methods to study Christian prayer.[30]

The *Archives of Internal Medicine* received so many scathing response letters that the editors published an entire section of rebuttals from physicians in a subsequent issue of the journal. These responses questioned the study's methods. For instance, the letter writers objected to the sponsoring hospital's decision to waive the requirement of informed consent for prayer (a decision discussed by Harris in the original article), but their more fundamental question concerned the legitimacy of conducting a scientific study of intercessory prayer. One of a number of critics, Dr. Prakesh Pande, discounted the possibility of implementing a randomized study of intercessory prayer—because God is presumably omniscient. Pande forwarded a theological argument in which he quoted the biblical injunction against putting "God to the test," from which he concluded that he "failed to see" any reason for "further randomized studies" of prayer. Doctors Richard Sloan and Emilia Bagiella similarly concluded that "religion does not need medical science to validate its rituals" and urged an end to similar research for the theological reason that it "trivializes" religion. Dr. Donald Sandweiss characterized the idea of studying prayer as "pseudoscientific mischief." A letter coauthored by Mitchel Galishoff and nine other physicians suggested—again invoking a theological frame of reference—that "perhaps the real conclusion is that God's grace is greater than our skills and immeasurable by our tools." Such criticisms apparently protect religion from blasphemous tests and trivialization; in effect, the refusal to study the effects of commonly employed religious healing practices dismisses without investigating such measures as irrelevant to the empirical world. Harris nowhere invoked theological reasoning or drew theological conclusions; his article's conclusion disavows that the study had "proven that God answers prayer or that God even exists. It was intercessory prayer, not the existence of God, that was tested here." Yet Harris's critics drew scientific conclusions about the lack of merits of his research—and all similar research—on the basis of theological premises of their own.[31]

It should perhaps not be surprising that theological and scientific arguments intertwine in debates over prayer studies. The practice of praying for healing, after all, involves an appeal for divine or supraempirical action in the natural world. Religious ideas—and Protestant, Catholic, and Jewish traditions in particular—have shaped the development of American cultural institutions, including the educational and medical systems. Even doctors and researchers who have rejected religious truth claims or supernatural theologies still draw on a cultural repertoire to which religion has contributed concepts and vocabulary. It is also the case that battles among scientists over a variety of research questions can become acrimonious and degenerate into ad hominem exchanges (and for that matter, the same holds for religious adherents debating theology). In this sense, controversy over the legitimacy of using empirical methods to study prayer is by no means unique.

It can nevertheless seem jarring when theological arguments appear in journals that ordinarily restrict their purview to empirical questions. The *Archives of Internal Medicine*—which it is worth emphasizing is one of *the* leading medical journals—published in 2001 an article by the psychologist John Chibnall and colleagues titled "Experiments on Distant Intercessory Prayer: God, Science, and the Lesson of Massah"—a title that explicitly refers to a story in the Bible. Chibnall argues that "the very idea of testing distant prayer scientifically [is] fundamentally unsound" because there is no obvious naturalistic causal mechanism. Chibnall accuses the authors of prayer studies of "attempting to validate God through scientific methods." First charging prayer researchers with a lack of scientific objectivity, the article proceeds to offer theological arguments against the study of prayer: "In the major religious traditions, prayer that tests for a response from God in the way the intercessor requires would not be considered prayer at all because it requires no faith, leaves God no options, and is presumptuous regarding God's wisdom and plan. Where is faith if science can validate the power of prayer?" Chibnall resorts to theological arguments to support the assertion that studying prayer is inherently unscientific.[32]

The critical backlash elicited by Harris's study and the more general concerns voiced by Chibnall were tame compared with the controversy generated after Dr. Kwang Yul Cha and colleagues at Columbia University published in the peer-reviewed *Journal of Reproductive Medicine* in 2001 a study that found a large positive effect on in vitro fertilization from distant intercessory prayer. Korean women who received prayer from Christian intercessors in Australia, Canada, and the United States conceived at twice the rate (50 percent) as women in the control group (26 percent). The results of the study were so unequivocally positive that critics averred that "if true, [it] was a landmark study," since it appeared "to show astonishing results." Consequently, the study became the subject of an unusually high degree of public scrutiny. A *New York Times* story provoked the U.S. Department of Health and Human Services to conduct a formal investigation (with the cooperation of Columbia University) of whether the authors were ethically and legally culpable for failing to secure informed consent from subjects who did not know that intercessors were praying for them. The investigating committee concluded that no "further involvement" on its part was needed once Columbia's Institutional Review Board offered to conduct an "educational in-service" for the Obstetrics and Gynecology Department.[33]

The uneventful end of official investigations did not stop the most outspoken critic of the Cha study, Bruce L. Flamm, a clinical professor of obstetrics and gynecology at the University of California, Irvine, from publishing a response article titled "'Miracle' Study: Flawed and Fraud" (2004). Despite the title of Flamm's response, the study's authors did not claim that their results should be viewed as "miraculous." Flamm faulted the study for its complexity, charging that the "study protocol was so convoluted and confusing that it cannot be taken seriously." More to the point, Flamm argued that the results themselves provided grounds for suspicion: "The first lesson this paper teaches us is that we should be highly suspicious of studies that appear to show astonishing results. Of course, every once in a while someone will discover something that is truly astonishing! Nevertheless, such results wave a red flag indicating extreme caution should be taken as the study is reviewed." Beyond advocating caution, Flamm went the further step of charging the authors with fraud—without presenting evidence to back this accusation beyond the remarkable nature of the results. He asked rhetorically, "Is it more likely that this study is flawed or fraudulent or that the authors have demonstrated the existence of a supernatural phenomena and thus have made perhaps the most important discovery in history? But worse than flaws, . . . one must consider the sad possibility that the Columbia prayer study may never have been conducted at all." This is an extraordinary charge, given that it was presented without any supporting evidence.[34]

Flamm continued, moreover, to shift the discussion into an asserted conflict between "religion" and "science." According to Flamm, "it is one thing to tell an audience at a tent revival that prayers yield miracle cures but quite another thing to make the same claim in a scientific journal. By doing so, faith healers cross the line into the domain of science, a domain where superstitious and supernatural claims are not taken seriously." This is a fascinating claim reminiscent of an argument made a century earlier by Tyndall that religion was illegitimately crossing over into the domain of science by claiming effects for prayer. But it is notable that Tyndall had drawn the opposite conclusion—that such claims necessitated rather than delegitimized scientific inquiry into the empirical effects of prayer. An obvious difference is that Tyndall was confident that scientific inquiry would yield results invalidating the effectiveness of prayer, whereas Flamm was responding to a randomized, double-blind, prospective study that apparently demonstrated prayer to be a highly effective therapeutic measure.[35]

Cha responded to Flamm's charges by suing him for defamation. Cha lost the court case, lost an appeal, and lost a further appeal to the California Supreme Court, which awarded Flamm approximately $100,000 for legal costs in 2010. Meanwhile, Cha's reputation was tarnished by separate allegations that he had plagiarized a different article in 2005. In addition, one of Cha's coauthors, Daniel Wirth, a lawyer without a medical degree, attracted initial mistrust because he had a record of publishing articles in parapsychology journals that are widely regarded as pseudoscientific. Wirth, as it happens, made his critics' job considerably easier by committing unrelated financial fraud that subsequently led to his imprisonment.[36]

The in vitro paper's third and final coauthor, Rogerio Lobo, the chairman of the Obstetrics and Gynecology Department at Columbia University, reacted to the public controversy that followed the paper's publication by withdrawing his name from the study—three years after the fact of publication. Lobo explained that his role had been relatively minor since he had only helped with the write-up subsequent to data collection, contradicting a Columbia University press release that had described him as the principle investigator. The *Journal of Reproductive Medicine* also backed down in the face of the groundswell of criticism, removing the online version of the article from its website, first temporarily and then permanently. The controversy, and particularly Lobo's withdrawal, also led the authors of a 2009 Cochrane Review of studies on intercessory prayer to exclude the Cha study from its analysis. Cochrane Reviews are regularly updated, systematic reviews that summarize and interpret the cumulative results of medical research. These reviews are widely accepted as the best single source of reliable evidence about the positive and negative effects of health-care interventions. To safeguard review quality, the Cochrane Library provides an online system for users to submit feedback should they find gaps or problems in the published reviews. Review authors regularly update their reviews, taking this feedback into account; published criticisms and responses can be read by subscribers as a part of the reviews. In excluding the Cha study, the Cochrane Review authors acknowledged that "we may have been incorrect in doing this and still do not have proof that the study was bogus." The incident illustrates just how charged debates over prayer research can become.[37]

The Cochrane Review did include a study by Herbert Benson, then the director of Harvard Medical School's Mind/Body Medical Institute—the same Benson who popularized the psychosomatic mechanism of a "relaxation response." In an apparent effort to replicate Byrd's and Harris's findings, Benson and colleagues published in the *American Heart Journal* a prospective, randomized controlled "Study of the Therapeutic Effects of Intercessory Prayer (STEP)" on coronary artery bypass graft (CABG) patients. This large-scale, multicenter trial included nearly eighteen hundred subjects at six U.S. hospitals. One group of subjects received intercessory prayer after being told that they might or might not receive prayer; one group did not receive prayer after being told that they might or might not receive prayer; the third group received prayer after being informed that they would receive prayer. Intercessors were given the first name and the initial of the last name of each subject and instructed to pray "for a successful surgery with a quick, healthy recovery and no complications." Instead of replicating Byrd's and Harris's results, the study's findings seemed to present an important challenge to the earlier studies by concluding that "intercessory prayer itself had no effect on complication-free recovery from CABG, but certainty of receiving intercessory prayer was associated with a higher incidence of complications." This was the first widely publicized study of intercessory prayer that suggested that prayer might actually be bad for one's health. The study did not imply that the prayers themselves were harmful or beneficial; rather, it suggested that the knowledge that one has become the subject of intercession may induce stress and fear about the seriousness of one's condition. These negative emotions can have adverse effects on coronary and overall health. Despite Benson's negative findings, critics objected that his study still seemed to assume that prayer is generally benign.[38]

What critics did not emphasize was a significant methodological difference between Benson's study and those of Byrd and Harris. Many of the intercessors selected by Benson would not have qualified under either Byrd's or Harris's protocols because they would not be widely recognized either as "born again" Christians or as believers in a "personal God who hears and answers prayer." Avowedly because no other religious groups would agree to participate in the study as it was designed—a fact that in itself points to a gap between Benson's idea of prayer and that of many religious practitioners—Benson's sole representative of Protestant prayer was Silent Unity of Lee's Summit, Missouri (although the study did also employ Catholic intercessors). Silent Unity is the prayer ministry of Unity, a "new religious movement" (NRM) that traces its origins to the late nineteenth-century New Thought movement. Unity's cofounder Myrtle Fillmore taught, "We do not promise to say a prayer of words and have the saying work a miracle in another individual. Our work is to call attention to the true way of living and to inspire others to want to live in that true way." Similarly, May Rowland, Silent Unity's director from 1916 to 1971, explicitly described "prayers of supplication or petition" as "useless." Rather, those in need of healing should learn to say "affirmative prayers containing 'I Am statements of Truth,'" describing the situation as it should be. As of 2011, many Unity practitioners continue to understand prayer not as supplication to a personal deity outside the self but as an exercise of the divine and human power of mind. Every time a prayer request is received, a Silent Unity worker not only prays but also sends a personal response letter—in order to instruct the person submitting the request how to think and pray "affirmatively." Thus, by employing intercessors who may practice a form of prayer that diverges from traditional Christian constructions of prayer, Benson's study sacrifices construct validity.[39]

In contrast to Unity, pentecostal Christians are more likely to envision prayer in relational terms. Conceiving of themselves as being in a relationship with a personal deity, many pentecostals do pray for their own healing and also request distant intercessory prayer from fellow believers. But—and this is a crucial point—many pentecostals consider *proximal* intercessory prayer (PIP)—a term I coined to refer to in-person, direct-contact prayer, frequently involving touch, by one or more persons on behalf of another—to be especially efficacious. Many pentecostals (as well as other Christians) model PIP on New Testament accounts of Jesus and his disciples laying hands on the sick. Pentecostals may conceptualize the Holy Spirit's *anointing*, sometimes represented by oil, as a tangible, transferable substance, or love energy. Anointing for healing presumably can be communicated through human touch, because physical bodies function as conduits of spiritual power. Comparing anointing with electricity or radiation therapy, certain pentecostals believe that efficacy correlates with frequency and length of exposure, types—including theological correctness—of prayers, "faith" and anointing levels of those receiving and offering prayer, and even the anointing level of the physical location in which prayers are offered. Some persons, moreover, are considered more anointed than others, or as "specialists" in praying for particular conditions. The Charismatic Catholic Francis MacNutt (b. 1926) reputedly specializes in arthritis, whereas Heidi Baker claims to specialize in hearing and to a lesser degree vision—but only in certain places, especially in Cabo Delgado Province of Mozambique.[40]

Prayer studies that have widely inclusive criteria for admission of intercessors fail to differentiate among intercessors who are reputed to have more or less anointing, or to believe different things about prayer and to practice it in divergent ways. Many pentecostals hold that someone who prays for healing "if it be thy will" (expressing theological uncertainty about God's will for healing) will likely get worse results than someone who prays with confidence that healing *is* God's will for today. Studies that have been criticized for overly narrow inclusion criteria—for instance, those that include any "born again" Christian or anyone who believes in a "personal God who hears and answer prayer"—may actually be too broad to capture significant differences in practices across individual intercessors. Even the most reputedly "anointed" intercessors acknowledge that their own results vary, somewhat unpredictably, from one occasion to another. For example, the Vineyard founder John Wimber noted that on some nights everyone seemed to get healed, but on other nights no one did. Wimber denied that he had more "faith" or "holiness" on some nights and claimed not to know what accounted for the difference—except for noting that God is sovereign and has the prerogative to heal when and where and what he wants.[41]

Francis MacNutt has suggested that there is inevitably a gap between the anointing levels of intercessors and that of Jesus of Nazareth. Thus, "there can be more or less power, more or less authority in me, since I am not God, but only share in his life, . . . I want to grow closer in union with Jesus Christ, so that more of his life, his wisdom, his authority and his healing power will work through me to heal others. But this, too, is a process and takes time." An advocate of *soaking prayer*, or praying personally for extended periods of time for a single person, MacNutt has argued that duration and frequency of prayer (which he compares in this regard with radiation therapy) matter greatly to the potency of healing power communicated, and that more serious conditions generally require lengthier prayer. Yet prayer studies rarely specify the duration of prayers administered. MacNutt, a former Dominican priest, has also emphasized the efficacy of sacramental approaches to healing—use of material means through which divine grace is communicated—such as laying on of hands, anointing with oil, or eating the Eucharist, all of which depend on physical contact and ritual actions on the part of both intercessors and recipients.[42]

The inappropriateness of most previously implemented study designs to *this* kind of prayer is readily apparent. For example, efforts to study "blinded" prayer obscure the presumed role of "faith" on the part of those receiving and offering prayer. A person receiving prayer cannot respond with faith without knowing that someone is praying. Pentecostal healing evangelists often note that their level of faith corresponds to the level of personal connection and even physical presence that they have established with the prayer recipient. For example, Randy Clark frequently admits publicly that he does not have enough

faith to pray at a distance. During one of Heidi Baker's visits to a pentecostal conference in Cleveland, Ohio in 2009, she learned that another
missionary from Mozambique was on a respirator in the Cleveland
Clinic. On a tight schedule between speaking at one conference and
catching a flight to an engagement in another city, Baker could have
interceded at a distance. Instead, she and her chauffeur, a local pastor,
braved downtown traffic on a morning when President Barack Obama
happened to be visiting the Cleveland Clinic. Baker reportedly got
through police blockades to the clinic and prayed for the woman—who
recovered from her ailment—and made it to the airport just in time for
her flight. Despite this level of emphasis on proximal prayer—even by
pentecostals such as Clark and Baker who are widely reputed to be
particularly "anointed"—most prayer studies provide intercessors with
minimal information about the patients for whom they are supposed
to pray, typically a first name and a condition requiring prayer.[43]

It is understandable and appropriate that scientific researchers have
been cautious about the masking of theology as scientific reasoning.
However, it is also clear from the above discussion that theological assumptions *do* inform the arguments of those who have opposed prayer
studies as well as motivating certain researchers to conduct such studies. The problem, this chapter argues, is not that theological analysis
has been employed by either side, but that it has been used for argu-
mentative purposes—whether to imply a supernatural causal mechanism or to delegitimize empirical study—rather than as an analytic
tool. Indeed, lack of theological understanding by researchers designing prayer studies and conducting meta-analyses has meant that even
if intercessory prayer, as it is most often practiced contextually, "works,"
most study designs would likely not be able to find existing empirical
effects, because they do not isolate the prayer phenomena that practitioners claim to be effective. To phrase this as a problem of science,
most distant-prayer studies have been designed in such a way as to
lack construct validity. Thus, it is scarcely surprising—even assuming
for a moment the efficacy of intercessory prayer—that many studies
have failed to find an effect.

In an effort to draw some more general conclusions from the multi-
tude of studies of distant healing that have been published in recent

years, scholars have published several systematic reviews of the literature. A foundational—and problematic—assumption of such review
articles is that all "prayer" is everywhere and always the same, a kind
of uniform energy that either does or does not work. Review articles
have treated together distant intercessory prayer and other forms of
"distant" or "energy" healing such as Therapeutic Touch and external
qigong that posit a different healing mechanism (such as *prana, qi* versus
Holy Spirit, Jesus) that may engender correspondingly different levels
of anticipated efficacy, as well as involving different practices. To sim-
plify, practitioners of Therapeutic Touch and qigong, for instance,
seek therapeutic benefits by redirecting impersonal, universal life-force
energy. Despite the political correctness in a pluralistic society of including representatives of different religious and spiritual healing traditions in the same study, failing to distinguish among types of "distant
healing" is a major methodological problem that makes it impossible
to isolate a single phenomenon for study. There is an inadequate evidential basis for generalizing findings from studies of one class of healing
technique to another, yet researchers persist in making such generaliza-
tions. The resultant literature yields uncertainty as to whether prayer or
distant healing are therapeutically beneficial, neutral, or detrimental.[44]

Of particular interest is "Intercessory Prayer for the Alleviation of
Ill Health," a Cochrane Review by Leanne Roberts and colleagues first
published in 2000 and updated in 2007 and 2009. The Roberts review
merits extended discussion because it illumines several of the key
issues at stake in controversies over distant prayer studies. Typical of
Cochrane Reviews, the Roberts review included only *randomized,
controlled trials* (RCTs), and certain studies—such as the controversial Cha article discussed above—were excluded. All together the 2009
review includes ten studies with a total of over seven thousand participants. The review includes Benson's study, as well as a 2001 study by
Mitchell Krucoff and colleagues that encompasses not only Unity, but
also Jewish and Buddhist prayer.[45]

On the basis of this collection of widely divergent studies, Roberts
concluded that "the studies that have been done, reported and included
in this review do not show an effect of intercessory prayer. However,
because this review highlighted no clear effects does not mean that

intercessory prayer does not work. The limitations in trial design and reporting are enough to hide a real beneficial effect and we found no data to contraindicate the use of prayer for seriously ill people." Roberts also concluded, however, that "we are not convinced that further trials of this intervention should be undertaken and would prefer to see any resources available for such a trial used to investigate other questions in health care." The review elaborated that "the evidence presented so far is interesting enough to support further study. However, if resources were available for such a trial, we would probably use them elsewhere. There are many other treatments that are in urgent need of evaluation and that are likely to be more suited to investigation in a randomised trial." Although discouraging rather than advocating further studies of intercessory prayer, the authors' language was not strong enough for critics of the review because it opened a glimmer of hope for legitimizing further research.[46]

One set of critics, Karsten Juhl Jørgensen and colleagues, picked up on the suggestion that "available studies merit additional research" and, having expressed disappointment at learning that the review had not been intended as a "joke," accused Roberts of presenting a "scientifically unsound mixture of theological and scientific arguments." This is a noteworthy reaction, given how generally unencouraging the review was of future intercessory prayer studies. What concerned Jørgensen, as it did Chibnall cited above, was that prayer studies have no "credible mechanism." In the absence of an easily identifiable naturalistic mechanism, "a statistically significant result is less convincing in a trial of prayer or homoeopathy than in a trial of a new non-steroidal, anti-inflammatory drug that has a similar molecular structure as existing drugs with a documented effect and that has been effective in animal studies." Thus, the authors asserted that "most researchers" would consider randomized trials of prayer "futile," because "any observed effect would more likely be due to the play of chance, bias or fraud, than to divine intervention." The invocation of divine intervention, a category absent in Roberts's language, shifted the discussion from a debate over empirical effects—the explicit grounds for dispute— to a perceived conflict between religion and science. Jørgensen frankly worried that "if we were to accept the authors' theological reasoning, all scientific research would become meaningless." Roberts responded to this theological critique by shifting the discussion back onto the terrain of science: "We have proceeded on the basis that empirical claims are made for prayer and that these can be empirically tested."[47]

Another of the Cochrane Review's critics, the Australian Dr. Chris Jackson, requested an "overhaul" of the report, in which the authors—in order to discourage "a lot of pseudoscience being done in this area"—should include "an argument against further IP [intercessory prayer] studies being performed" and argue that "scientific study of prayer ought to be limited to its social effects ideally using qualitative methodologies." Jackson's offer of qualitative research on social effects as a kind of consolation prize implies that although prayer may serve social functions, it cannot credibly be posited to exert "real" empirical effects. Jackson objected to quantitative research of any kind precisely because it may convey scientific legitimacy.[48]

Roberts's response to Jackson's critique effectively isolates what is at stake in this kind of criticism. The first potential reason for delegitimizing future prayer studies is that the "scientific results show IP to have been disqualified or confirmed with a very high degree of certainty. The results are by no means conclusive enough for us to urge such a course on this basis." The second possible rationale for exclusion is that it is "inherently flawed to use randomised controlled trials (RCTs) to investigate this subject." Roberts and colleagues devoted the rest of their response to exploring the implications of this latter rationale, concluding that "we cannot agree with Dr. Jackson that studies of this kind should be ruled out, simply because this cannot be recommended without making assumptions of a philosophical and theological nature, whether theistic or atheistic." Such assumptions "cannot be a reason for a journal to rule out a meta-analysis." The review's authors revealed that, "as it happens, the theological-philosophical convictions of at least one of the authors involved in our review disposes them against the use of RCTs for investigating IP. He or she holds that this must be put to one side and wishes to examine the empirical evidence as empirical evidence." The Cochrane Review's authors stood by their original position in the 2009 report, concluding that one cannot "rule out further RCTs for IP on *a priori* grounds separate from 'theological' assumptions as to the properties of the God in which one does or does not believe. One could not urge for these studies to be discontinued on *a priori* grounds without bringing theological ideology into science. IP may be studied by empirical means until such time the empirical findings themselves suggest an end to the studies." This exchange cuts to the heart of many of today's debates over distant intercessory prayer studies—which arise from theological-philosophical concerns about the implications of prayer studies, rather than disputes over the empirical evidence itself.[49]

A final question raised by these charged debates over published prayer studies is the effect of deeply held convictions on the peer-review process itself. It seems plausible—and unpublished anecdotal evidence suggests that the possibility is more than theoretical—that reviewers who have staked out strong positions against the concept of studying intercessory prayer might have difficulty objectively refereeing such studies on their merits. It took five years for Byrd to publish the results of his research and three years for Benson to publish the results of his study. Although there is no clear evidence as to what accounted for these particular delays, one might wonder whether these authors encountered publication setbacks because of reviewer bias, or similarly whether the authors of other well-conducted studies have been unable to publish their results in peer-reviewed journals for ideological reasons.

New Directions: Proximal Intercessory Prayer Studies

Despite the implicit agendas that a close reading of criticisms of prayer studies reveals, these criticisms do point to substantial problems with the methods that have heretofore been employed in studying any effects of intercessory prayer. Research methods developed in other fields of biomedical research have dictated the methods employed in prayer studies—as well as determining the types of prayer considered or excluded—rather than study designs growing out of the particular nature of the phenomena under consideration. Researchers have attempted to conduct randomized, controlled trials of distant intercessory prayer modeled after studies of experimental drugs largely because RCTs are considered the gold standard of rigorous scientific research.

Distant intercessory prayer, conducted in laboratory settings rather than in contexts where prayer would naturally occur, has been targeted because it is easiest to control for certain potential confounds. Chief among these are *placebo effects*—improvements that occur for psychosomatic reasons because subjects believe they are receiving a therapeutic intervention, regardless of whether that intervention has any intrinsic therapeutic value. Another potential confound, *empathy effects*, are similar to placebo effects in that the concern and attention expressed by a medical or religious healer may itself produce therapeutic benefits; hence, the above-cited Cochrane Review included only studies in which intercessors had no relationship to the patients for whom they provided prayer. Similarly, *Hawthorne effects*, named after the factory where they were first observed, are short-term improvements resulting from the motivational effect of attention paid to subjects during a study regardless of the nature of the experimental intervention. *Hold-back effects* are the tendency of those who are being evaluated before and after an intervention unconsciously to perform worse at first in order to demonstrate an improvement later. *Demand effects* are the other side of the coin: subjects may perform better during posttests in order to meet the presumed expectation of those conducting the study. *Practice effects* are the tendency of subjects to perform tasks better when they have more experience, which can be gained during the course of a study.[50]

Distant-prayer studies present the advantage of avoiding all these potential confounds—because subjects do not know whether or not they are receiving study-related prayer and are not asked to perform any tasks before or after prayer interventions. Yet the Cochrane Review makes an important point—that distant intercessory prayer may not be especially well "suited to investigation in a randomised trial." There are inherent methodological challenges to using RCTs to study the empirical effects of distant intercessory prayer, such as the difficulty of establishing appropriate control groups. There is, for instance, no way to prevent patients (or their families and friends) in a control group from also praying. Accepting the premise that RCTs may not be the best way to study distant intercessory prayer does not—as the Co-chrane authors also note—necessarily lead to the conclusion that researchers must abandon as "futile" all controlled research on the empirical effects of prayer.[51]

Despite the emphasis on distant intercessory prayer in the litera-ture, Dale Matthews and colleagues, in a prospective, controlled study of the effects of intercessory prayer on patients with rheumatoid ar-thritis published in the *Southern Medical Journal* in 2000, found no significant effect for patients receiving distant intercessory prayer. The authors did, however, find that patients experienced statistically sig-nificant improvements in symptoms with direct-contact, or what may be called proximal, intercessory prayer, compared with patients who received medical treatment alone. Subjects in an experimental group each received a total of six hours of in-person prayer, and an addi-tional six hours of group instruction in the theology of healing prayer, over a three-day period. Although acknowledging possible confounds of Hawthorne and placebo effects, Matthews's study design, compared with the above-discussed studies, better corresponds to how interces-sory prayer is practiced contextually. This is not surprising given that one of the study coauthors, Francis MacNutt, is a well-known Catho-lic Charismatic healing practitioner. If anything, study participants may have received an "overdose" of prayer, if the goal was to simulate natural prayer settings where it is uncommon, at least among western-ers, to devote anywhere close to six hours in three days praying for someone's healing even when practicing "soaking prayer." At religious healing conferences, it is more typical for prayer sessions to last some-where between one minute and an hour total, with a median of per-haps five to ten minutes. In healing rooms settings (such as those affili-ated with the IAHR), prayer sessions may last from a mode of twenty minutes up to two hours, but rarely longer.[52]

More unfortunately, the condition isolated for study by Matthews, rheumatoid arthritis, is relatively susceptible to psychosomatic improve-ments. The study reported that improvements in swollen and tender joints and reduction in pain and functional disability were not accom-panied by a parallel reduction in serum inflammatory markers, sug-gesting that "clinical improvement might be attributable more to alteration of patients' perceptions regarding their illness than to changes in inflammatory pathways affecting their joints." The study did not clarify whether improvements resulted from the prayer itself, or from attention, touch, social support, counseling, and exchanges of forgiveness offered, all of which have been shown to have therapeutic effects. The potential role of these psychosocial effects is nontrivial, especially given the long duration and high intensity of interactions (twelve hours over three days) both among subjects and between subjects and intercessors during the study—perhaps reflecting the most positive personal attention and group interaction the subjects had experienced in a long time.[53]

Despite its clear limitations, the Matthews study illumines a major gap between most research on intercessory prayer and how intercessory prayer tends to be practiced—a crucial problem if the goal of researchers is to evaluate the empirical effects of a commonly employed health-related practice. Studies of proximal, as opposed to distant, intercessory prayer may help to overcome the current state of impasse and chart a route toward a better understanding of what happens when people pray for healing.

Conclusion

The idea of testing the empirical effects of prayer has generated both interest and controversy since the beginnings of modern science. The availability of clinical methods that *could* be applied to prayer for healing has led certain people to conclude that such tests *should* be performed, while causing others to question the appropriateness of mixing biomedical techniques with religious concepts. Practitioners of science and religion have at various times been found on both sides of this debate. The arguments employed by all parties provide insight into competing constructions of religion, science, prayer, and healing in the modern world. As will soon become apparent, controversies over prospective clinical studies of prayer have a parallel in similarly contentious efforts to test healing prayer through retrospective evaluation of medical records.

CHAPTER 3

Are Healing Claims Documented?

✦

In 1953, the British Medical Association, in response to a request from the Archbishops' Commission on Divine Healing formed by the Church of England, established a committee to conduct a retrospective investigation of medical evidence for divine healing through prayer. The committee proceeded by distributing a questionnaire to British physicians asking them to provide medical documentation of any spiritual healings with which they were familiar. Seventy physicians responded to the survey by describing anomalous recoveries that they attributed to divine intervention. The committee dismissed most of the cases as psychosomatic improvements in "functional" rather than "organic" conditions. In such cases, although "patients suffering from psychogenic disorders may be 'cured' by various methods of spiritual healing, just as they are by methods of suggestion and other forms of psychological treatment employed by doctors, we can find no evidence that organic diseases are cured solely by such means." The committee discounted cases of apparent cures of organic disease as attributable to "wrong diagnosis, wrong prognosis, remission, or possibly of spontaneous cure . . . due to chance." The committee concluded that they found no medical evidence of divine healing through prayer.[1]

The investigative committee report is important not only for its conclusion but also for how it was reached. The committee's judgment contradicted the assessments of most of the physicians on whose data the report relied—none of whom, according to samples printed in an appendix, seems to have offered psychosomatic explanations for cases presented. The committee rejected the medical opinions of surveyed physicians because "the majority of the doctors who replied [to the questionnaire] believed in prayer and so were naturally prejudiced in its favour." The committee instead "drew to a considerable extent on the cumulative experience of its members." Adopting theological arguments similar to those used by opponents of clinical studies of prayer, the committee affirmed that "the essential object of spiritual ministrations must always be the reception of spiritual grace, and not necessarily physical improvement," because there are "many other ways" besides cure "in which Divine love and mercy may reach out to those in need." The report urged that rather than "demand" physical healing, patients should use prayer primarily to help them "accept the limitation and course of the illness and glorify God through it," and gain a "willingness to accept Divine will." Reasoning from personal experience and theological convictions, the medical committee argued not only that prayer does not result in real cures but also that prayer should not be used to seek physical healing.[2]

The committee justified its negative verdict on the medical value of prayer on the basis that the physicians surveyed had failed to provide sufficient medical documentation. The "alleged claims were not supported by detailed case histories and full pathological reports." The committee was quite likely accurate in this assessment. It is rare for patients or physicians to present "detailed," "full" medical documentation that reveals an apparently inexplicable postprayer change in condition. Yet even if the cases of healing dismissed by the British Medical Association had resulted from prayer, the kinds of documentation required by the investigative committee might not have existed because of the nature of medical record keeping. Documentation will not exist if a patient did not visit a doctor and undergo laboratory tests both before and after a religious healing experience. Many people pray for healing before going to their doctor. Once a problem has been resolved, patients may see no reason to return to their physicians. Medical progress notes are in any case typically brief and oriented toward tracking specific markers of disease or health in order to provide effective treatment. What seems most relevant at the time of treatment may differ substantially from what later investigators might consider important in determining causation. Few of those who seek medical care, let alone their doctors, are concerned with keeping comprehensive records in anticipation of one day experiencing a religious healing for which they must provide documentation. Yet the absence of medical evidence is sometimes, as in the case of the British Medical Association investigation, treated as positive evidence of the absence of real cure.[3]

Claims of healing through prayer often raise questions about whether a patient was sick in the first place or healed in the second. In cultures in which the biomedical profession is respected—if not always liked—it seems obvious to many that doctors are best qualified to arbitrate assertions of illness and healing by providing medical documentation. The term *medical documentation* can refer simply to the system of record keeping used by healthcare professionals. Often, however, what people mean in reference to healing prayer is "biomedical proof" that someone was "really" diseased and is "really" cured—and that modern medicine cannot account for the recovery.[4]

Parallel to the history of controversies over clinical studies of prayer is a complex history of how scientists and religious practitioners have constructed medical documentation as evidence for or against the healing power of prayer. Efforts to provide medical evidence for miraculous healing date back to the sixteenth-century Catholic Church, which by the nineteenth century had famously formed a medical bureau to investigate claims of healing at the shrine of Lourdes. In the first half of the twentieth century, a maturing medical profession used the general absence or ambiguity of medical records from before and after prayer as grounds for bolstering biomedical authority and dismissing religious healing claims. By the 1990s, the turn toward "evidence-based medicine" by a self-confident medical community diminished interest in explaining anomalous cases in favor of large-scale, prospective trials of predictable effects.[5]

European and North American Christians, and particularly pentecostals who make divine healing testimonies a core of their identity, have expressed an intriguing ambivalence toward the value of medical documentation. Early denominational Pentecostals, concerned that medicine might conflict with faith, sometimes avoided medical treatment and sometimes used modern forms of evidence, such as x-rays and photographs, to argue that prayer is superior to medicine. From the 1960s to early 1990s, Charismatic Christians sought to shed anti-medical stereotypes and actively cultivate support from Christian medical doctors in using medical documentation to validate divine healing claims. Since the 1990s, pentecostals have largely backed away from their earlier interest in medical documentation. Embracing a *postmodern* cultural identity that esteems science and spiritual experience, pentecostals may seek to "prove" healing by pointing to the "evidence" of sensory experience, such as feelings of heat, sensations akin to electricity, or diminished pain, as well as visionary experiences. Postmodern pentecostals generally welcome medical treatment, yet may consider medical documentation of religious healing to be superfluous and even dangerous to faith.[6]

The answer to the question posed by this chapter—Are healing claims documented?—is generally "no," or at least not in such a way as would persuade those not already inclined to believe in prayer's healing power that anything supernatural has transpired. This chapter explores the history of debates over the uses, limits, and meanings of medical documentation, assessing the reasons scientists and religious practitioners have at times pursued or avoided documentation efforts. I argue that there are inherent constraints on what medical records can prove or disprove about healing prayer. Yet when complemented by other perspectives, medical records do provide one revealing lens through which to examine healing claims.

Wielding Medical Records against Healing Claims

Much as scientific naturalists first had the idea of testing the efficacy of prayer through clinical studies, those skeptical of religious healing made the first systematic efforts to collect medical documentation—in order to show that healings either did not occur or could be explained naturalistically. One of the earliest large-scale investigations was conducted in 1923 in Vancouver, British Columbia. The Vancouver General Ministerial Association formed a committee composed of eight physicians, three university professors, a lawyer, and eleven Protestant ministers to investigate claims made during a healing campaign of the itinerant Pentecostal healing evangelist Charles Price (1887–1947) that had attracted more than ten thousand attendees nightly to a Vancouver arena. The investigative committee could scarcely be described as neutral; most members were friends who shared a common antipathy to the Price campaign, and several of them had already publicly opposed Price.[7]

After spending six months collecting evidence from 350 people whom Price had anointed with oil and prayed would be healed, the committee concluded that only 5 of the individuals had been cured, all of them of merely "functional" ailments, although 38 others had exhibited improvement due to an "improved mental and spiritual outlook." More disturbing, within six months, 39 had died and 5 had gone insane; in addition, 4 family members of those who had sought prayer also succumbed to insanity. A minority report issued by two dissenting members of the committee challenged the objectivity of the study, noting that the committee had investigated only a small percentage of the 6,000 people anointed and had not collected a representative sample, since many of those approached had refused to appear before the committee because they mistrusted its impartiality. Indeed, after the pro-Price Baptist Ministerial Association passed a resolution refusing to cooperate with the investigation on account of the committee's biased composition, the committee recruited subjects by advertising for volunteers in the newspapers.[8]

The committee's procedures raised questions about its objectivity in interpreting the medical evidence. For example, the committee dismissed as "functional" the dramatic claim of healing from clubfoot—accompanied by a shortened leg and curvature of the spine—of one Ruby Dimmick without interviewing her, her father, or her own doctor, who had concluded that the recovery was "miraculous." The committee based its conclusion largely on a certificate of examination from the Toronto Orthopedic Hospital indicating that at the time of admission Dimmick had been free of "organic disease." The committee interpreted this certificate as indicating that medical specialists had "pronounced her deformity to be of a functional nature," and thus susceptible to "auto-suggestion." In so doing, the committee ignored the context of the hospital certificate. As a facility that specialized in treatment of "deformities," the hospital had required that Dimmick be free of infectious disease as a condition of admission. Thus, the certificate said nothing of the nature of her disability, which had indeed been deemed severe enough to warrant admission. The committee likewise summarily dismissed claims of healings from tuberculosis and cancer on the grounds that the original diagnoses must have been mistaken.[9]

The investigative committee offered the modern, scientific "evidence" of x-rays and photographs as apparently transparent windows onto reality in order to make its position appear objective and irrefutable. As one anti-Price newspaper promoted the committee's apparently fact-based approach: "No attention will be paid to the statements of those treated. Only actual conditions as shown by the several examinations will be used in arriving at a decision." A published report of the committee's findings presented, for instance, an x-ray of congenitally dislocated hip sockets to discount one individual's claim of experiencing healing from difficulty walking. Diagrammed arrows and captions educated viewers on how to interpret the duplicated film—as indicating that no structural change in the hip joints had occurred (figure 3.1). The examiners dismissed the testimony of several nearby observers who reported hearing this person's joints snap into place at the moment of healing. The report rebutted that "congenital dislocations do not 'snap' into place when reduced, as the socket is undeveloped and the head of the bone does not fit." Everyone had to admit that the subject could walk better after the "healing," but the committee attributed this obvious improvement to an inconsequential improvement in "muscle function," rather than "real" structural change.[10]

Supporters of Price responded to criticisms by also publishing photographs—of healthy-looking patients with their discarded medical paraphernalia as "proof" that those testifying to healing now enjoyed restored health (figure 3.2). As the historian James Opp aptly summarized, "the embedded 'truth' of photography proved to be malleable in the hands of both critics and proponents of faith healing." Drawing radically different conclusions, both sides recognized the presumed authority of modern, medical "evidence" in adjudicating claims of illness and healing.[11]

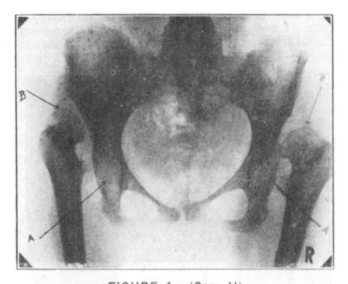

FIGURE 1.—(Case H).
Double Congenital Dislocation Hips. "A" indicates position of hip-sockets. "B" indicates position of heads of hip-
bones which are out of the sockets.

Figure 3.1. "Double Congenital Dislocation Hips." Published in *Report on a Faith-Healing Campaign held by Rev. C. S. Price in Vancouver, B.C., May 1923*, 9. Courtesy The United Church of Canada, BC, Conference Archives.

Displaying Medical Records to Support Healing Claims

During the first half of the twentieth century, those wishing to discredit divine-healing claims most often took the initiative in soliciting medical documentation. By the 1960s, Christian participants in the era's Charismatic renewals increasingly sought out medical documentation of their own accord. In an effort to enter the cultural mainstream, Charismatic leaders such as Kathryn Kuhlman and Oral Roberts repudiated the antimedical positions adopted by many earlier denominational Pentecostals and aggressively recruited medical allies. Roberts primarily took the tack of seeking to demonstrate the complementarity of divine and medical healing, best symbolized by his building of the City of Faith Medical and Research Center in Tulsa, Oklahoma (opened

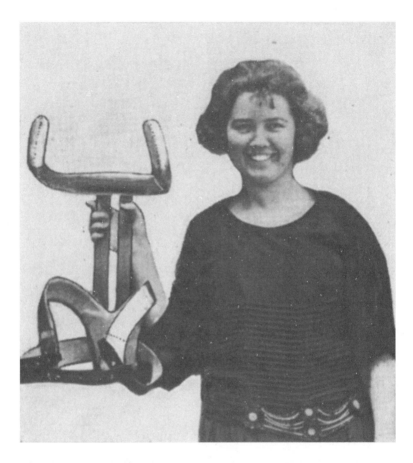

Figure 3.2. Edna Lang holding her now-discarded back brace after experiencing healing in a Charles Price campaign. Published in the Pentecostal periodical *Golden Grain* (September 1926): 33. Courtesy Flower Pentecostal Heritage Center.

in 1981 but closed in 1989 as a financial failure), where, he claimed, the "healing streams of prayer and medicine must merge."[12]

Like Roberts, Kuhlman affirmed that God often works through doctors and medicine to heal. But she also insisted that God has the "power to heal instantly without the material tools of scientific medicine." Kuhlman apparently got the idea of collecting medical records to bolster the credibility of healings reported during her "miracle services" after the nonsectarian *Redbook* magazine commissioned an avowedly skeptical reporter, Emily Gardiner Neal, to write an article on Kuhlman in 1950, titled "Can Faith in God Heal the Sick?" Like other naturalistically oriented investigators, Neal collected medical and x-ray records and workmen's compensation reports as well as testimonial letters from those claiming or witnessing anomalous healings. Unlike previous investigators, Neal and *Redbook*'s editors—who wrote a foreword to Neal's article endorsing her findings—became convinced by what they saw that people really did experience healing in Kuhlman's services. Neal was sufficiently impressed that she converted from agnosticism to Christianity and embarked on her own career as a lay Episcopal minister of healing.[13]

Kuhlman in turn became convinced that medical documentation could be a potent apologetic device for persuading skeptics of divine healing claims. Kuhlman began a lifelong campaign to document healing through prayer in order "to offer proof of the power of God." She solicited help from Neal as a ghostwriter and from a panel of supportive physicians who evaluated submitted medical records. Kuhlman published a collection of twenty case reports, each of which was backed by before-and-after medical records, under the title *I Believe in Miracles* (1962). Emulating criteria established by the Lourdes Medical Bureau, Kuhlman published only cases for which the following criteria could be shown: First, the disease or injury had been medically diagnosed as resulting from an organic or structural problem, involving more than the unexplained failure of a body part to function. Second, the healing had to have occurred rapidly, involving changes that could not easily be explained as psychosomatic. Third, the patient's primary physician had to verify the healing. Fourth, the healing had to have occurred long enough in the past that it could not readily be diagnosed as remission. *I Believe in Miracles* became a bestseller, prompting Kuhlman to write two sequels—*God Can Do It Again* (1969) and *Nothing is Impossible with God* (1974)—which together contained an additional forty healing narratives, each of them backed by medical evidence.[14]

The book trilogy presented recoveries from a range of diseases and disabilities, with disproportionate emphasis given to serious conditions with clear diagnoses. Twelve individuals reported dramatic recoveries from cancer that their doctors had diagnosed as terminal. Several reported the disappearance of unwanted growths such as goiters; others insisted on the reappearance of decayed bones and tissues. For instance, James McCutcheon's doctor reportedly exclaimed, "This is truly a miracle," when x-rays showed that a piece of bone had mysteriously grown over a broken hip that five operations had failed to restore. Injured by molten iron in an industrial accident, George Orr, a World War I veteran, had been blind in his right eye for over twenty-one years when he claimed to regain his sight during a miracle service. The same doctor who had diagnosed his disability attested that Orr's left eye, which had deteriorated from the strain of overuse, was perfectly restored and that his right eye was 85 percent functional. Seventeen years later, an investigator interviewed Orr and reported that he still enjoyed good vision. Three other individuals unexpectedly recovered from paralysis secondary to injury or disease; five experienced the discontinuance of symptoms of multiple sclerosis. Five attested to instantaneous deliverance from drug or alcohol addiction. Other ailments apparently healed included emphysema, asthma, arthritis, heart conditions, diabetes, myasthenia gravis, stroke, and curvature of the spine.[15]

Kuhlman particularly sought out cases for which psychosomatic explanations seemed inadequate. For this reason, she included seven testimonials of the healing of infants or young children of such maladies as congenital bone deformities, epilepsy, blood diseases, eczema, and hydrocephalus. One such healing reportedly came to a four-month old baby who had been born with a dislocated hip. The baby was the daughter of Richard Owellen, M.D., Ph.D., a cancer researcher, professor, and staff doctor at Johns Hopkins University. After watching his baby's leg straighten, Dr. Owellen announced: "I had often wondered if many of the healings I had seen weren't psychosomatic. . . . But a four-month-old baby doesn't know enough to have a psychosomatic healing." Owellen deployed his medical qualifications, knowledge of psychosomatic medicine, and former avowed skepticism to bolster the credibility of his personal experience.[16]

Many readers walked away from Kuhlman's publications persuaded. A 1970 *Time* magazine article concluded that "miraculous cures seem to occur" and termed Kuhlman a "veritable one-woman shrine of Lourdes." Not everyone was similarly impressed, but it was notable that those on both sides of the debate over Kuhlmlan's miracle services undertook the strategy of collecting medical evidence either to discredit or to confirm claims of healing through prayer. Kuhlman's most vocal medical critic, William A. Nolen, M.D., wrote a widely heralded exposé, *Healing: A Doctor in Search of a Miracle* (1974). Nolen was a small-town surgeon who often wrote for the popular press. After attending a Kuhlman service in Minneapolis in 1973, Nolen interviewed twenty-three people who believed themselves healed and reported on five presumably typical cases: multiple sclerosis, migraine headaches, bursitis, acne, and varicose veins. All five narrators affirmed that they were still healed, but Nolen explained each case as psychosomatic or trivial rather than miraculous. Nolen also followed up with five cancer patients who initially claimed healing but later found they were mistaken; two of them died shortly thereafter.[17]

In response to Nolen, another medical doctor, H. Richard Casdorph, M.D., Ph.D., F.A.C.P. (born c. 1929), published a collection of ten medically documented case reports of healings during Kuhlman services, under the title *The Miracles* (1976). Casdorph is a research scientist who received training in cardiovascular diseases at the Mayo Clinic, served on the faculty of the UCLA Medical School and the University of California Medical School, Irvine, and has produced more than eighty articles and presentations on heart disease. In endorsing Kuhlman, he published before-and-after photographs of x-rays, laboratory films, and medical reports of ten individuals, whose real names and other identifying information he provided—noting that Nolen had not provided similar means of authentication. Casdorph selected diseases that were both more serious than the healing claims Nolen highlighted and, in most cases, more difficult to class as psychosomatic: bone cancer, kidney cancer, two cancerous brain tumors, two instances of rheumatoid and/or osteoarthritis, osteoporosis, multiple sclerosis, a massive gastrointestinal hemorrhage, and heart disease.[18]

Casdorph's critics did not substantively challenge his findings, although they did question the representativeness of the phenomena he recorded and attacked his credibility on the basis of his unrelated research interest in chelation therapy, an alternative treatment for heart disease. One religious critic without medical credentials of his own summarily dismissed Casdorph's book, marveling that "perhaps the most striking feature of the entire book is not the nature of the cases described but the fact that there are only ten of them" (the same number of cases reported by Nolen). Nolen and Casdorph publicly debated on the *Mike Douglas Show* in 1975, bringing with them one of Casdorph's case studies—the teenager Lisa Larios, whose testimony of being healed from terminal bone cancer at age twelve had earlier appeared in *Nothing is Impossible with God*. Neither Nolen nor Casdorph changed opinions as a result of their debate, but the televised encounter suggests widespread and growing interest in evaluating claims of healing through prayer using medical evidence.[19]

In emulation of Kuhlman and Casdorph, the prominent healing televangelist Benny Hinn published a volume of ten healing narratives, *Lord, I Need a Miracle* (1993), for which a physician, Donald Colbert, M.D., wrote a foreword. Colbert attested to having personally reviewed the medical files for each subject included in the volume. For example, David Lane had been diagnosed with adenocarcinoma of the rectum by rectal biopsy; a colorectal surgeon had told Lane that he had thirty days to live without surgery or three months with surgery. Lane elected not to undergo surgery, radiation, or chemotherapy, or to take any other medicine, but he did attend a Benny Hinn miracle service. Nine months later, when Lane went to a doctor for an appendectomy, this doctor wrote in his medical report: "free of metastatic carcinoma . . . no evidence of malignancy." Other conditions reported as healed in the volume include chemical hypersensitivity, a cerebral pseudotumor causing blindness, metastasized bladder cancer, lupus, Hodgkin's disease, thoracic outlet syndrome, pulmonary vascular hypertension, coronary artery disease, and congenital severe hearing impairment.[20]

Although medical technology has improved the means available for medically documenting—or challenging—healing claims since the 1970s or even the 1990s, relatively few comparable documentation efforts have been undertaken by either supporters or detractors of claims of healing through prayer. It seems noteworthy that pentecostal leaders born outside North America have initiated most post-1990s documentation efforts, perhaps because they do not share the same social experiences that led many North American pentecostals to back away from documentation. The pentecostal healing evangelist Mahesh Chavda—an Indian born in Kenya who migrated to the United States (and is loosely affiliated with ANGA)—included limited documentation in his book *Only Love Can Make a Miracle* (2002): before-and-after photographs of a Pakistani woman whom Chavda claims had been healed of blindness (figure 3.3), and a notification of death for a six-year-old boy from Zaire (now the Democratic Republic of Congo) whom Chavda insists was raised from the dead (figure 3.4). Similarly, the German pentecostal Reinhard Bonnke, who has spent most of his evangelistic career in Africa, included medical documentation in his video *Raised from the Dead* (2003). The film narrates the story of a Nigerian man, Daniel Ekechukwu, who claims to have been resuscitated during a Bonnke crusade after spending three days in a mortuary. The film includes interviews with the man and his family, friends, and the examining physician, Dr. Josse Annebunwa, who displays the patient's death notice for the camera while describing the signs observed that led him to order removal to the mortuary. There were no respiratory movements, no breath sounds, no heart sounds, no pulse, and the pupils appeared fixed and dilated (figure 3.5).[21]

The most systematic early twenty-first-century documentation efforts appear to have been undertaken by the Korea-based World Christian Doctors Network (WCDN), founded in 2004 by a group of Christian medical doctors in Korea. The WCDN has hosted annual international conferences in the United States, Norway, Ukraine, Italy, and Australia, attracting several hundred Christian and some non-Christian physicians to each conference. WCDN conferences consist of PowerPoint presentations of cases, which include patient histories and diagnoses, illustrated by before-and-after medical records—including x-rays, CT and MRI films; endoscopic, microscopic, retinal,

A   **B**

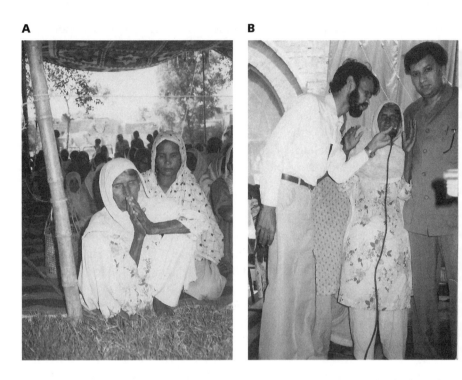

Figure 3.3a–b. Sixty-year-old Pakistani woman reportedly born blind. (a) Photograph taken by Mahesh Chavda during an evangelistic campaign in Pakistan. (b) Photograph of this same woman later testifying to healing. She reported seeing a brilliant flash of light followed by the restoration of her vision after Chavda said, "Now, Lord Jesus, show these people that the message of the gospel is true." Reprinted with permission from Mahesh Chavda, *Only Love Can Make a Miracle* (Charlotte, NC: Mahesh Chavda, 1990), Courtesy Chavda Ministries International.

and ultrasonographic photographs; and doctors' opinions—much like what physicians might present at regular medical conferences. The key difference is that the case reports are explicitly designed to demonstrate that the healings in question are so remarkable that divine attribution is plausible. Cases presented include conductive hearing loss, distortion of visual field by Harada disease, gastric cancer, metastasized breast cancer, spina bifida, sterility, pulmonary tuberculosis, herniated discs, and intracerebral bleeding.[22]

A

C.S.S.P.
C. A. D. Z.
As. Ebeyl No 10 Q. Mikon'o
Zone de KIMBANSEKE
———

Kinshasa 22/06/1985

N/Réf. :

V/Réf. :

Objet : Transfert de Malade
KATshinyi Mikaikai.

Cit. Médecin.
Je vous envoie l. enfant : KATshinyi. sexe. masc à
Age. 6 ans.
Reçu à 9h.00 du Matin au dispensaire avec
- Hyperthermie. T. 40°C T. A. 7/5
- Conseil : Respiration : néant
Battement cardiaque - rien : néant
ne réagit pas à l. injection
Concl. Δ. Paludisme
- déshydratation

N.B. DéCéDé †

Voir hôpital Mama yemo pour un certificat
de décès

Assist. Médical Resp.
IWANGA. SAIBUM

[signature]

B

C.S.S.P.
C. A. D. Z.
As. Ebeyl No 10 Q. Mikon'o
Zone de KIMBANSEKE
———

Kinshasa June 12, 1985

N/Réf. :

V/Réf. :

Objet : Transfer of Patient
Katshinyi Manikai

Dear Doctor,

I am sending to you this child, Katshinyi. - Sex: masculine.

Age: 6 years

Received at 4:00 O'clock in the morning with
- hyperthermia T 104°F B.P. 7/5
- Breathing : none
- Beating of heart: none
- no response to injection
- Malaria
- Dehydration
Note: DECEASED

See Mama Yemo hospital for death certificate

Medical Assistant in Charge
Iwanga Embum

[signature]

Figure 3.4. Death notice for Katshinyi Manikai, Mikondo Clinic, Kinshasa, Zaire, June 12, 1985. (a) Copy of certificate written in French. (b) English translation. Reprinted with permission from Mahesh Chavda, *Only Love Can Make a Miracle* (Charlotte, NC: Mahesh Chavda, 1990), Courtesy Chavda Ministries International.

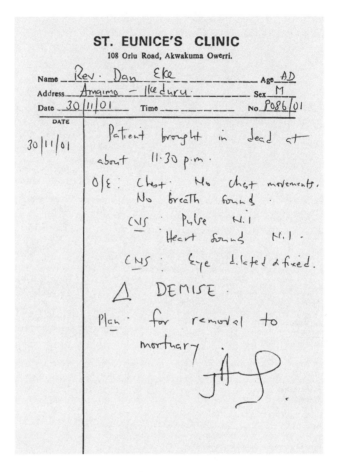

Figure 3.5. Death notice for Daniel Ekechukwu, St. Eunice's Clinic, Akwakuma Owerri, Imo, Nigeria, November 30, 2001. Courtesy E-R Productions, LLC.

Figure 3.6 is the case of Jenny, a woman diagnosed with profound hearing loss whose records indicate improved, though still severely impaired, hearing after prayer. Pure-tone average (PTA) tests conducted in 2004 measured a threshold of 120 dBHL in the right ear and 112 dBHL in the left ear; brainstem evoked response audiometry (BERA) tests done the following day showed no response to sounds in

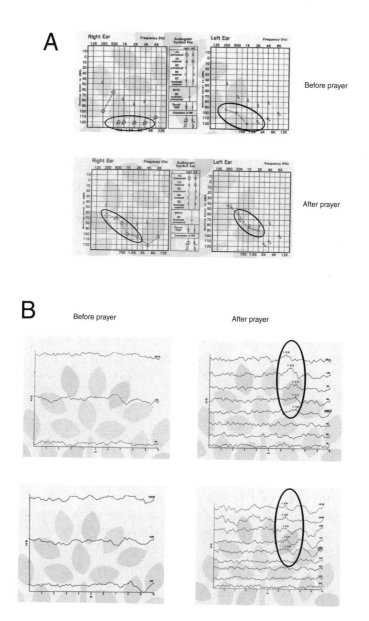

Figure 3.6a–b. Audiology records for Jenny. (a) Comparison of PTA printouts taken three and a half months apart in 2004, showing initial readings of 120 dBHL in the right ear and 112 dBHL in the left ear and subsequent readings of 92 dBHL in the right ear and 78 dBHL in the left ear. (b) Comparison of BERA printouts taken three and a half months apart in 2004 initially showing no response for either ear and subsequently recording a response for both ears at 90 dBHL. Courtesy Brian S. Yeo, M.D.

either ear. Jenny received prayer two months later and at the time testified to being able to hear a loud voice, which she could not hear before prayer. A PTA test conducted three and a half months after the first test measured a threshold of 92 dBHL in the right ear and 78 dBHL in the left ear; consistent with the PTA results, a BERA test that same day found a response to sounds in each ear at 90 dBHL. These test results are consistent with Jenny's claim that she could hear loud sounds after receiving prayer. It is, however, possible that a coincidental ear infection or blockage of wax, which subsequently cleared, accounts for the apparent improvement.[23]

The WCDN is associated with the Manmin Central Church, pastored by Rev. Dr. Jaerock Lee, in Seoul, Korea. This church has been the target of heresy charges, although it has proven difficult to investigate whether there is any evidential basis for such charges. Apart from its own conferences and website, the WCDN's medical claims have not received public scientific scrutiny, because the group has not yet published any of its quite extensive case reports in peer-reviewed journals. The WCDN has given me copies of medical records for a number of cases like Jenny's.[24]

In recent years, the secular media have appeared more interested than many North American pentecostals in medical corroboration of claims of healing through prayer. Indeed, a 2011 online primer on reporting on religion addressed to journalists writing about religious healing claims advises: "Seek verification. If someone says their cancer was healed by a preacher, ask for medical confirmation from before and after the alleged healing." In many instances, reporters covering religious-healing stories have—although pressing for medical validation—adopted a strikingly unskeptical tone in their reports, which reflects a recent renaissance of popular interest in spiritual healing. For example, Fox News (in Miami and then in New York) did a story on a Christian cardiologist, Dr. Chauncy Crandall, titled "Raised from the Dead," that attracted over a million website hits. Based in Florida, Crandall is chief of the Cardiovascular Transplant Program at the Palm Beach Cardiovascular Clinic and has also helped with Bonnke crusades in Africa and presented cases at WCDN conferences. In 2006, he attracted national U.S. media interest when he declared a man dead after forty minutes of failing to resuscitate him following a heart attack—and then declared that the same man had been miraculously brought back to life. Having "called the code" and on his way out of the emergency room ward, Crandall had avowedly heard God tell him to pray for the man and try the defibrillator one more time—after which his heart began to beat. Fox reported Crandall's—and his patient's—accounts in a matter-of-fact style, in part because the dramatic claim was vouched for by a respected medical professional.[25]

Crandall claims that many of his patients have been healed through prayer, as he describes in his book, *Raising the Dead: A Doctor Encounters the Supernatural* (2010). When I asked Crandall whether he had medical documentation for other claims, he demurred that "documentation is always very difficult since few doctors will ever document a miracle in their hospital notes." Crandall acknowledged, "I have just recently started to document prayer, healing in my notes but insurance comp and other physicians look down on this and in fact I have received letters/requests from physicians to stop this practice." Crandall's statement is telling both because it highlights the relative dearth of medical documentation being presented alongside recent healing claims (compared with the 1970s) and because it suggests that one reason is resistance from naturalistically oriented physicians who consider notations of miracles unscientific. Indeed, there has been a multifaceted cultural transition in the last several decades.[26]

Resisting Medical Documentation as Contrary to Faith

Up until the 1970s, those wishing to discredit spiritual healing claims pointed to an insufficiency of medical documentation. In the 1960s and 1970s, and to a lesser extent through the early 1990s, Charismatics responded by producing voluminous medical records. Since then, neither side, at least in the United States, has seemed so interested in using medical records as evidence in debates over healing. One explanation may be that medical standards for evaluating purported documentation have changed. Thus, medical records that convinced doctors in the 1970s that something more than natural had occurred may not have convinced—or even interested—doctors in the first decade of the twenty-first century. Moreover, the scientific community's attention has shifted toward the standard of evidence-based medicine built on large-scale clinical investigations—including studies of distant intercessory prayer.

Yet it also seems that North American pentecostals themselves have become decreasingly concerned with medical documentation. Many pentecostals have embraced a postmodern epistemology that pairs a high esteem for science with resurgent interest in the evidential value of narrative, individual experience, and physical sensation; this turn stems in part from disillusionment with the demonstrated potential of medical evidence to prove anything to the satisfaction of skeptical audiences. Within this general tendency, Charismatics in the stream of Kuhlman, the Vineyard movement of the 1980s, and the Toronto Blessing of the 1990s, have been relatively more attentive to objective measures compared with classical Pentecostal denominations such as the Assemblies of God—or nonpentecostal evangelicals, who have tended to emphasize faith and faithfulness in trusting God over the presentation of proof to outsiders.[27]

The Vineyard movement marked a transition away from Kuhlman's strategy of collecting medical records back toward an earlier Pentecostal emphasis on personal testimony—but now presented more systematically than in previous eras with the embrace of the new tools of social science. Unlike Kuhlman, John Wimber did not recruit medical doctors as allies. But what he did was to lend support to a social anthropologist, David C. Lewis, to investigate claims of healing at Vineyard conferences. Following a small-scale investigation of a Wimber conference in Sheffield, England that Lewis published as an afterword to Wimber's widely heralded book, *Power Healing*, Lewis conducted a larger-scale study in which he distributed a written survey to 2,470 registrants at a conference in Harrogate, England in 1986. On the basis of quantitative and qualitative analysis of 1,890 completed questionnaires and 100 personal follow-up interviews, Lewis published a book, *Healing: Fiction, Fantasy or Fact?* (1989).[28]

Lewis reported that most Vineyard conference attendees were already in relatively good health, and only a third of them requested prayer for healing of a physical condition. In only 8 percent (68 cases) of the 867 cases of prayer for physical healing—involving a total of 621 people, because some people requested prayer for multiple conditions—did subjects report experiencing total healing. A total of 32 percent (279 cases) reported high degrees of improvement, and another 26 percent (222 cases) reported intermediate degrees of improvement, compared with 42 percent (298 cases) of little or no healing. More than half of those with whom Lewis followed up claimed that they remained healed at the time they were interviewed six to ten months later.[29]

Lewis based his analysis primarily on self-reported degrees and permanence of healing, although he did also seek verification by writing to the subjects' primary care physicians. In several cases, doctors confirmed that patients reported diminished symptoms, or the doctors themselves expressed surprise at the level or rapidity of improvements noted. Lewis concluded that "physical healings did take place," although he had to admit that he found "little documentary medical evidence for claims of healing." Many of those who reported healing did not return to their doctors, and if they did return, further laboratory tests were rarely performed. If objective changes were observable, doctors may have noted surprise, but change in itself, even if unexpected, does not necessarily point to a particular causal mechanism.[30]

Lewis questioned the value of medical evidence in either confirming or discounting perceived healings. To make this point, he cited Dr. David Wilson, Dean of Postgraduate Medical Education at the University of Leeds. Wilson questioned giving "100 percent credence to the 'doctor's diagnosis'" when it means dismissing as irrelevant reductions in patient complaints, for instance, in light of stable x-rays. In Wilson's evaluation, if the "complaint disappears then patient and doctor may be in disagreement because the X-Ray appearance hasn't changed. But surely what matters, what is important, is what the patient feels (or doesn't feel), not the doctor's intellectual concept." Wilson, like Lewis, rejected not the factual content of such medical documentation but its utility in invalidating subjective healing experiences.[31]

Lewis's book was popular among Charismatics in the early 1990s, but—understandably, given its lack of medical support or statistical rigor (much of the book is a stream of anecdotes and descriptive tables rather than quantitative testing of hypotheses)—received virtually no attention from the medical or academic communities. It is possible, moreover, that Lewis's failure to obtain useful medical evidence to confirm healing claims and his conclusion that self-reports are the best standard for evaluating results discouraged subsequent healing ministries from seeking medical documentation. Despite the limitations of Lewis's method, his study does highlight the importance of coupling an examination of medical records with an analysis of how subjects perceive the effects of prayers for healing.

Emulating Wimber's stance toward Lewis, John and Carol Arnott, the pastors of the church at which the Toronto Blessing began, facilitated sociologist Margaret Poloma's study of healing claims at the Toronto services. Poloma's book, *Main Street Mystics* (2003), gained a sizable readership both within the Charismatic movement and among secular scholars. Poloma found in 1995 that 78 percent of participants surveyed had experienced "inner or emotional healing." Of these, 94 percent remained healed two years later. In addition, 22 percent of respondents reported healing of a physical problem. Poloma also observed that as leaders of the Toronto Blessing placed increasing emphasis on healing, over time more people claimed to experience healing. Poloma noted that although Toronto's leaders lacked "resources to pursue medical documentation," they did "often encourage those who claim healings to do so." Nevertheless, it is unclear whether such encouragements generated many results. None were ever published, and my own follow-up with the Arnotts to ask for any collected medical documentation has not yielded a response.[32]

Poloma, collaborating with political scientist John Green, similarly studied healing experiences among classical Pentecostals. A 1999 survey collected responses from 1,827 Assemblies of God adherents from twenty-one congregations across the United States. Of those surveyed, 70 percent reported having experienced divine healing from a physical illness, 85 percent had "witnessed a miraculous healing in the lives of family members and/or friends," and 93 percent had personally experienced "an inner or emotional healing." In an earlier survey, Poloma also found that nearly two-thirds of Pentecostals who attested to healing indicated that the healing came through intercessory prayers from others (including pastors, church members, healing evangelists, family, and friends) rather than by praying for themselves at home alone. (Only 35.5 percent reported the latter.) Those who reported past healing experiences were, moreover, four times more likely than those who did not (80 percent compared with 20 percent) to have responded within the past year to a church altar call for healing prayer. This strong correlation suggests that those who ask for prayer from others are more likely to experience healing, or possibly that those who already have experienced healing through prayer are more likely to seek further prayer when other health problems arise. Poloma also found a strong correlation between belief that healing is available today (rather than having ceased with the apostles) and likelihood of experiencing healing. What Poloma and Green, like Lewis, demonstrated is that Pentecostals and Charismatics *perceive* themselves to be the frequent recipients of divine healing. These researchers did not succeed (Lewis tried; Poloma and Green apparently did not) in using medical evidence to assess whether objective improvements could be confirmed.[33]

If the Vineyard and Toronto movements have become more interested in social scientific than in medical investigations of healing claims, other pentecostals—and especially those coming from classical Pentecostal backgrounds of longstanding resistance to medical science—have more explicitly rejected the proof value of medical evidence. One telling example of this tendency is the ANGA Revival Alliance leader Bill Johnson, pastor of Bethel Church (formerly Assemblies of God) in Redding, California. Johnson employs a full-time staff person, Amy, to collect healing testimonies. The church posts testimonies on the Internet and even sells printed copies in the church bookstore. Yet when I interviewed Amy, she acknowledged that few efforts have been made to collect medical documentation. She said she was "trying to get more," but had found the workload involved in tracking down medical records "nearly impossible" because the ministry receives such an overwhelming volume of testimonies. This explanation suggests that the proliferation of information in an era of globalization works against documentation efforts by making it increasingly difficult to sift through the abundance of healing claims presented.[34]

Johnson has admittedly resisted outside investigations of any medical basis of healing claims. As he explained in an October 2008 interview with Poloma:

> We've had people ask to be able to interview certain people. We allow it in a certain measure. Strangely, a lot of people don't understand, I won't give names of people healed, and I won't give names of doctors. And the reason is because the media is [sic] so cruel. Individuals could handle it well, but once the news gets out it'll become almost public property, and it causes doctors to withdraw because they come under such scrutiny. . . . We work really hard to [protect confidentiality]. I'd rather the word not get out, I'm not interested in promoting what God's doing in Redding, I'm interested in promoting what God's doing in the earth, and if we're a case study for that then that's fine.

Specifically, Johnson fears that medical doctors will not endorse claims of healing through prayer when they come under public scrutiny from the presumably "cruel" media. He would rather the "word not get out" than take the risk that medical investigations might be used to discredit rather than substantiate healing claims. Bethel Church has not responded to my repeated requests for *de-identified* medical records (that is, all names, dates, numbers except years, and addresses are removed, in accordance with the health-care privacy regulations of the Health Insurance Portability and Accountability Act of 1996)—which would not compromise the anonymity of those reporting healing or that of their doctors.[35]

In this October 2008 interview with Poloma, Johnson was likely reacting to several negative, nationally disseminated news articles—from such major media outlets as NBC News, ABC News/*Nightline*, and the Associated Press—on the Lakeland Outpouring of the previous summer. During the revivals, the visiting healing evangelist, the Canadian Todd Bentley, and the pastor of the local Assemblies of God Ignited Church, Stephen Strader, had regularly issued on-the-air challenges to the media to come investigate the nightly stream of dozens of healing testimonies.[36]

When reporters and researchers—including myself—took Bentley and Strader up on the offer and asked for medical documentation, their staff responded by mailing out a thin media binder. The packet contained sixteen brief, undocumented testimonials listing conditions healed, with the names and phone numbers of those reporting healing. An Associated Press reporter noted that Lakeland's staff had asserted that all of these claims had been "vetted by [Bentley's] ministry, with all but three of their stories 'medically verified.' / Yet two phone numbers given out by the ministry were wrong, six people did not return telephone messages and only two of the remainder, when reached by The Associated Press, said they had medical records as proof of their miracle cure. However, one woman would not make her physician available to confirm the findings, and the other's doctor did not return calls despite the patient's authorization." Similarly, a *Nightline* reporter who attempted to follow up with contacts from the media binder concluded that "not a single claim of Bentley's healing powers could be independently verified." I too telephoned the people listed in the binder—and found that the media reports were accurate. Several testimonials provided incorrect contact information; not everyone who could be contacted claimed that permanent healings had occurred; and not even one person contacted produced a single medical record.[37]

My assessment is that none of the major media stories on Lakeland can be fairly described as demonstrating "cruelty." Writers simply reported what was—and what was not—provided to them by Lakeland's leaders, who had after all asked to be investigated. Shortly after the appearance of the national news stories, Strader responded to my e-mail request for de-identified medical records: "Our church has taken a stand that we will provide NO information. The lawsuits and the strife to the families is JUST NOT WORTH IT. . . . You just can't imagine the hardships that the media puts on all of us. . . . It's just overwhelming." It is unclear how provision of the requested *de-identified* medical records (which could not be associated with specific individuals) could result in lawsuits against or strife for involved families. A few weeks later, it became clear that Strader was concerned about media scrutiny for more reasons than the difficulty of meeting their standards of medical proof. News broke that the Outpouring's central figure, Todd Bentley, was leaving his wife and marrying his intern, and—at the urging of his ministry's board and numerous other pentecostal leaders (including Johnson)—taking a leave from public ministry.[38]

Even after scandal ended the Lakeland Outpouring, Strader published a volume of undocumented testimonials, *The Lakeland Outpouring: The Inside Story!* (2008), affirming the genuineness of the revival. The 158-page book includes a four-page chapter on medical verification. In it, Strader reiterated that "we do have a number of healings with good, verifiable reports" that have been reviewed by a "currently licensed and board certified physician" whose identity and specific credentials are not disclosed. Strader cited three cases that this doctor considered "verifiable healings": scoliosis, a liver lesion, and kidney failure. Only in the last instance did Strader quote from the examining doctor's letter—noting an improvement from 25 percent to 75–80 percent renal function with the comment "This God of yours healed you." The unnamed doctor, the "head of the nephrology department of a well-known university medical center," had reportedly been asked by his own university's officials to cease using university letterhead to report on the unusual case.[39]

Strader cited the resistance encountered by the miracle-affirming nephrologist as justification for his refusal to provide more details about the medical documentation claimed. Strader also noted that the physician who reviewed medical records for him had advised against giving out names and contact information for patients or doctors to avoid violating HIPAA (misspelled by Strader as HIPPA) regulations about the protection of personal health information. Strader has, however, at no point commented on a fact that I had previously called to his attention—that HIPAA regulations specifically allow the sharing of de-identified medical records, because no personal information is revealed. Strader's book includes a full-color insert with thirty-seven photographs of Lakeland services, but not one photograph of the alleged medical documentation. This decision is striking for the case of scoliosis described as verified on the basis of before-and-after photographs of the woman's back showing first "severe curvature" and then the "spine very straight." Pentecostals and Charismatics of an earlier era, or those born outside the United States, might have featured such a photograph prominently.[40]

Indeed, Pentecostal resistance to researcher requests for medical documentation predates Lakeland. One major offshoot of Johnson's Bethel Church is the International Association of Healing Rooms, founded by a former Bethel board member, Cal Pierce, in Spokane, Washington in 1999. Like Bethel, the IAHR collects and posts healing testimonies both on location and on the Internet. Acknowledging the authority of medical science, during a videotaped training seminar, Pierce waved a brain CT report in the air—avowedly confirming the disappearance of a steel plate from a Canadian woman's head following prayer. The woman told Pierce that the steel plate had been surgically inserted after her skull was crushed in an automobile accident. Since then, she had suffered migraine headaches and seizures and took debilitating medications; the metal plate consistently set off airport security scanner alarms. The migraines and seizures stopped right after prayer at the healing rooms, leading the woman to ask for a second CT scan at the same hospital where the metal plate had been inserted and an initial CT taken. Pierce read aloud from the second report: " 'Normal brain scan. No evidence of infraction recent or old. The appearance of' the brain, or the 'calvarium [more accurately, skull] is normal.' And the best part is 'there is no metal plate present.' Now that's a testimony. And she went to the airport and passed the test [that is, by not setting off the security scanner alarm]." Reading from an actual medical report gave auditors access to much more specific information than anything provided by leaders of the Lakeland Outpouring. Yet, reflecting ambivalence about the evidential value of medical records and mistrust of how external investigators might use such evidence, IAHR staff members left unanswered my request to see de-identified copies of this woman's first and second CT reports or any other medical records collected by the IAHR; staff members gave only nominal support to my request to distribute written surveys on healing to visitors. After months of repeated follow-up attempts, the IAHR had still produced no completed surveys or medical records.

However, during an interview conducted in October 2011, Cal Pierce did express willingness to provide me with medical documentation.[41]

Interviews with an IAHR staff member, Harvey, whose job it was, when I spoke with him in 2005, to collect and publicize testimonies, provides insight into the basis for the apparent resistance encountered. In Harvey's view, those who already have faith do not need medical records to be convinced that God heals, whereas skeptics who demand medical evidence will not be convinced regardless of the quantity or quality of evidence produced, because they will always be able to find some reason to discount the evidence. Harvey explicitly argued that scientific evidence is inferior to testimonial and biblical evidence because it shows change but does not give an interpretation of why the change occurs, an omission that allows skeptics to "explain away" medical proof. Harvey was interviewed several decades after Kuhlman's systematic medical documentation efforts—which had not succeeded in convincing as many skeptics as pentecostals would have liked, leading to disillusionment with this proof strategy. Visitors to the healing rooms did not, according to Harvey, ask for medical evidence, but they did ask for testimonies of other people's healing experiences. Attempting to convince people who are unwilling to be convinced seemed to Harvey a "waste of time," or worse an opening for the "enemy" to challenge an intellectual basis for faith that depends on x-rays and similar visual evidence.[42]

The argument that empirical research into the medical effects of prayer is a waste of resources has a parallel in a similar argument made by scientists who would prefer to devote available resources to medical trials rather than to clinical studies of the empirical effects of prayer. A key problem for Harvey is that scientific evidence encourages dependence on the sense of sight (associated with the "world") rather than the sense of hearing (associated with faith), because the Bible teaches that "faith cometh by hearing, and hearing by the Word of God"—and the Word is envisioned as inherently aural, even when one uses the sense of sight to read the Bible. Whereas looking for medical evidence breeds doubt, listening to testimonies and the Word's promises of healing "washes away disbelief." Harvey's comments evoke a widely held pentecostal epistemology that assumes a particular hierarchy of the senses—one that privileges hearing above seeing, and in which feeling sensory input rather than seeing is believing. In this framework, healing presumably follows faith, rather than faith following evidence of healing.[43]

In view of this shared framework, it should not be surprising that research efforts at an IAHR affiliate, the Healing Rooms of the Santa Maria Valley, California—which, like Spokane, attracts hundreds of visitors weekly, many of them from long distances away—yielded similarly sparse results. After the organization's director apparently avoided returning my phone calls, e-mails, and postal mail letters, I traveled to Santa Maria and visited unannounced. The staff was very gracious in person and gave as a present multiple videotapes of healing testimonies. Subsequent follow-up yielded several phone numbers of clients reporting healing but a direct refusal to cooperate with survey research or to provide copies of collected medical records (which staff did claim to possess).[44]

The contact information offered by the Santa Maria healing rooms did, however, facilitate a lengthy telephone conversation with a sixty-one-year-old retired police officer, Ralph, who claimed to have been healed of metastasized stomach cancer six years before. Ralph was more than happy to talk on the telephone in order to testify of his healing to a presumably skeptical researcher, but, he demurred, many Christians had encouraged him to seek medical verification of his healing. He had refused all such requests because it seemed to him contrary to faith. In Ralph's words, "I don't want or need a MRI—I live on faith. I've had six years of perfect health. . . . I don't need to test God. They have the law and the prophets. Every lab test would be seen as misdiagnosis to skeptics. . . . I don't need to plead to the doctors 'It's a miracle.' People want to document it, but the skeptics won't stop till they find something to disprove it. . . . Any effort to prove miracles will fail. They'll just dismiss it."   Ralph's statement reflects ambivalence in twenty-first-century pentecostal culture toward the value of medical documentation. Like Kuhlman, many pentecostals today esteem medical documentation as the gold standard of scientific proof. As in the prayer-gauge controversy of the nineteenth century, however, many others worry that skeptics will find some excuse to disprove any evidence presented (partly because of prior experiences of persistent skepticism, even after Charismatics had presented medical evidence). Many pentecostals also retain some degree of the uneasiness that more fully characterized the early Pentecostal era—that medicine and faith may inherently conflict.[45]

In a variation on pentecostal ambivalence toward medical documentation, some evangelical critics of pentecostal healing have taken the position of simultaneously dismissing healing claims for want of medical documentation and also discounting the usefulness of medical evidence to prove anything. The highly respected historian of evangelicalism Martin Marty—who clearly stakes out his personal skepticism toward spiritual healing claims—requires that such claims be supported by medical evidence in order to be taken seriously. Marty asks rhetorically, "Why do not physicians and medical researchers get to measure a leg before and after the Pentecostal prayer that releases God to act to lengthen it? Why are so many verifications of a nebulous, unattributable character?" Marty writes dismissively of claims "that legs were miraculously lengthened by inches or that cancer cells were suddenly transformed to healthy ones" as "extreme" examples of implausibility. At the same time, Marty—like Ralph—rejects the project of seeking to validate faith with science. According to Marty, "an unbelieving generation seeks signs from science and, we are told, these signs will compel faith. / Wanna bet? The Christian circle will not grow an inch because of such 'proof.'" For Marty, alleged scientific proof of the miraculous amounts to an "idol, not testimony"—because idols attempt to represent visually what should be accepted on faith. Marty suggests that the quest for proof itself provides evidence of the absence of faith and implies a dangerous compromise with atheistic science. Such a position—demanding and yet rejecting the proof value of medical evidence—does not seem far removed from that occupied by scientific naturalists who discount the idea of clinically testing the empirical effects of prayer as unscientific, while dismissing religious-healing claims as inherently incredible in the absence of scientific investigation.[46]

What Medical Records Can and Cannot Reveal

Despite the widespread ambivalence I have encountered regarding the proof value of medical documentation, I have tracked down cases of individuals connected with ANGA reporting healing in the 2000s who have produced copies of their before-and-after medical records. Such records typically provide limited information when read alone but constitute one means of inspecting claims that "something" unusual occurred. For example, a signed physician's statement from 2005—written on behalf of a U.S. college student named Joy to explain any absences from class due to migraine headaches—describes Joy as having "vertical heterophoria." This is a visual impairment in which a muscle or nerve weakness causes one eye to turn up or down so that the eyes take pictures from slightly different angles, in Joy's case causing double vision and migraines. This lifelong condition can be largely corrected by prism glasses—and Joy has an optometrist's prescription for such lenses dated 2006. The same optometrist wrote a note dated 2009 stating that she "no longer requires corrective lenses for driving." The medical records do not explain the improvement, but they do confirm its notation by medical professionals (figure 3.7). Interviewed six months later and again two years later in 2011, Joy had not experienced a single migraine or other symptom and continued to see well with both eyes together, despite having discarded her glasses and stopping her antimigraine diet.[47]

Joy offers her own explanation. Shortly before her graduation from college, she began attending mid-week pentecostal services on campus (sponsored by an ANGA affiliate) where she received prayer for healing on several different evenings. One evening,

> we began to pray for my healing. It was a great time of prayer but nothing was really happening. Until they [the worship band] began to play [the song] "Marvelous Light . . . Into marvelous light I'm running, / Out of darkness, out of shame." Well every time the light was mentioned (which happens a lot) God said to me "You get to live in the light, You get to live in the light." Which as you may very well know I can't be in the light when I have a migraine, because it

A

[Redacted] Pediatric Care

[Redacted]

[Redacted]/05

To Whom It May Concern:

[Redacted] is a lovely young woman who has severe, debilitating migraines. They have been well controlled since she received prism glasses. She has vertical heterophoria, which is a medical condition of the eyes caused by muscular imbalance. As long as she has her glasses, she does very well. Other triggers for her migraines are: irregular sleep, irregular meals, stress, and cats.

[Redacted] will occasionally have breakthrough migraines. When she gets a headache, they often last five to seven days. Her symptoms include throbbing pain, vomiting, pallor, and difficulty concentrating. For these headaches, she uses Vicoprofen and goes to sleep. For prophylaxis, she uses Mellatonin in the evenings.

[Redacted]'s migraines may occasionally interfere with her class attendance, but I know she will be a successful college student. She is very stoic and is a dedicated student. She requested that I write a quick note to let you know her migraine history.

If you care for more information, please call anytime.

Sincerely,

[Redacted]

M.D.

B

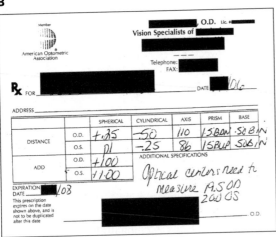

Figure 3.7a–c. Optometry records for Joy. (a) Doctor's letter giving diagnosis of vertical heterophoria, treated by prism glasses, 2005. (b) Optometrist's prescription for prism lenses, 2006. (c) Letter from the same optometrist, who prescribed prism lenses in 2006, indicating that Joy no longer requires corrective lenses for driving, 2009. Courtesy Joy.

C

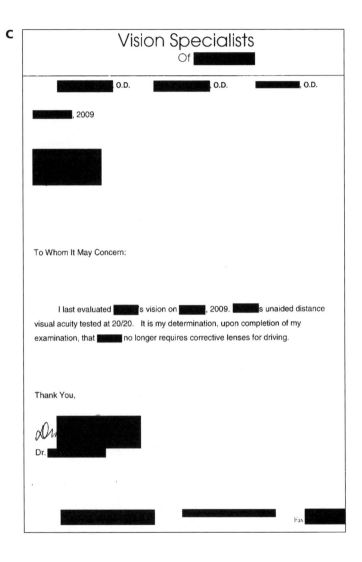

Vision Specialists

Of ▮▮▮▮▮▮

▮▮▮▮▮▮, O.D.   ▮▮▮▮▮▮, O.D.   ▮▮▮▮▮, O.D.

▮▮▮▮, 2009

To Whom It May Concern:

   I last evaluated ▮▮▮▮'s vision on ▮▮▮▮, 2009. ▮▮▮▮'s unaided distance visual acuity tested at 20/20.   It is my determination, upon completion of my examination, that ▮▮▮▮ no longer requires corrective lenses for driving.

Thank You,

Dr. ▮▮▮▮

▮▮▮▮▮▮   ▮▮▮▮▮▮   Fax ▮▮▮▮

hurts too much. But every time darkness is mentioned God says "that is not for you any more, you don't have to live like that anymore." . . . And I am feeling half of my skull being pulled upward (that sounds really weird but that's what happened). Which makes sense . . . kinda . . . since my problem was that my head was slightly lopsided.

> But it didn't hurt just happened. . . . God says to me "Why are you
> wearing those glasses? You don't need them anymore. Take them
> off. . . . I ask to borrow her [the woman praying for Joy] Bible. She
> says yes. And I can read. Normally without my glasses the lines skip
> all over the place and do weird things that are very confusing but
> nothing is happening it is all steady. [The group was] now singing
> "Trading my Sorrows" which goes "I'm trading my sickness / I'm
> trading my pain / I'm laying it down for the joy of the Lord." Which
> is SOOOO true.

Joy's medical records cannot confirm her explanation of the cause of
her healing, but they do indicate an improvement in visual function.[48]

Medical records again tell only part of the story in the case of Art,
who was diagnosed with metastatic melanoma in 1999, when he was
seventy-five years old. During the next twelve months, surgeons removed six secondary tumors in a total of five procedures, and CT
scans revealed that the cancer had spread to the lungs and spinal column. Chemotherapy treatments were suspended because the patient's
hemoglobin levels were too low. Before an attempt to recommence
treatments two weeks later, another CT scan was performed. The report reads, "all clear, no sign of cancer." The treating physician reportedly expressed surprise ("This is unbelievable, I am awed! You have
really made my day. . . . Tell me what you are using, I want to use it for
my other patients.") and agreed not to restart the chemotherapy, instead performing another CT scan three months later. This and three
subsequent CT scans came back clear, and Art continued in good health
when he last communicated with me twelve years later (now age eighty-
seven) in 2011. Read by themselves, Art's medical records are ambiguous in meaning, since he did receive surgery and chemotherapy to
treat his cancer, although the prognosis was poor. Art supplemented
the records with his narrative. He was praying for healing and had
repeatedly received distant and proximal intercessory prayer throughout the year since his diagnosis. Nevertheless, he lost fifteen pounds,
became so weak he had difficulty walking from one chair to another,
and felt cold all the time. But a week after the discontinuation of the
chemotherapy, he was

awakened (*and I mean awakened, I did not just wake up*) on a Thursday morning and saw a figure standing at the foot of the bed dressed in what appeared to be some sort of cassock with a hood that shaded his face so that I could not tell what he looked like. He spoke audibly, aloud, and there is no mistake about that. He spoke only three words, "Nehemiah two two." . . . I don't even remember ever reading that [Bible] verse before and if I had I certainly would never have associated it with healing. As I found the verse my eyes fell on these words, "Why is thy countenance sad seeing that thou art not sick?" I remember saying, "If Jesus says I'm not sick then I'm not sick." Immediately, my complexion changed from pasty white to normal, my body heat returned, my strength returned and my energy was restored.

Art immediately felt well enough to ask his wife to go out to breakfast. Later, his son-in-law noted that the Bible verse quoted had Art's name in it—when read "'thou, ART not sick.' Yes, indeed, how very personal is the lover of our souls." Convinced that God had personally announced his intentions and then healed him, Art self-published his testimony as one of his many subsequent efforts to engage in evangelism and help others experience healing. Like Joy's, Art's medical records are not self-interpreting, but they do provide one window onto healing experiences.[49]

Redefining "Documentation" as Experience

In common with many other pentecostal groups since the 1990s, Global Awakening and Iris Ministries have publicized numerous healing testimonies without seeking systematically to collect before-and-after medical verifications. The reasons have been both logistical and epistemological, and differ somewhat depending on which group one considers. Global Awakening leaders, emulating Wimber and to some degree Kuhlman, covet medical legitimacy but lack the expertise or resources to collect the kinds of portfolios that Kuhlman garnered. Iris leaders care relatively little about their reputation among nonpentecostal medical evaluators. Rolland Baker's standard response to the many people who have asked for documentation of the claim that two hundred fifty people have been raised from the dead through IM is an invitation to come to Mozambique and talk to the families and communities of those resurrected.[50]

Indeed, the Bakers extended permission for an independent filmmaker to do just that. Darren Wilson, a media professor at a small Chicago college filmed an interview with a black South African man, Francis, who claims to have come back to life after having been beaten to death. Interviews with Francis and those who witnessed his surprising recovery constitute one segment of a documentary film of modern miracle claims titled *Finger of God* (2007), in reference to Jesus's claim that his miracles provide evidence that he came from God. The relative popularity of this film (an estimated sixty thousand copies sold, plus many group viewings) in pentecostal circles reflects a growing epistemological emphasis on videographic "documentation"—in preference to medical records, which must be interpreted rather than experienced. As the sociologist Wade Clark Roof has intriguingly argued, the availability of film technologies has heightened the perceived importance of sound and rapidly changing images as offering unique access to reality. In one sense, seeing *is* believing for today's pentecostals as for other postmoderns, but it is a synesthetic blending of sight with sound that can be *experienced,* not just perceived. Indeed, ANGA culture embodies a postmodern blend of esteem for science and quantification with an appreciation of sensory experience and spiritual perception as windows onto truth.[51]

Even if they were more motivated to collect medical documentation, both GA and IM would have a challenging assignment, given the field conditions where their most dramatic healing claims are made. Brazil has a much better medical infrastructure than Mozambique, but even so, many of the poor people who attend GA conferences have at most limited access to medical resources. A sick Brazilian may visit a doctor once, but it is extremely rare for a patient to return to a doctor for "confirmation" of healing if symptoms become manageable or disappear. There tends, moreover, to be relatively little interest in medical verification among many lay Christians in places such as Mozambique and Brazil, where it is common to assume, rather than seeking to prove, a connection between the material and spiritual worlds, and where day-to-day survival is the most pressing concern for most people. Even so, both GA and IM do also regularly conduct conferences in North America and Europe—yet neither group follows Kuhlman's pattern of encouraging attendees to submit before-and-after medical records or requiring medical documentation before endorsing a claim publicly. Nor do GA or IM leaders preach against the use of medicine as contrary to faith; indeed, leaders of both groups avail themselves of modern medical care. Both GA and IM have been exceptionally cooperative with my research inquiries (compared with other groups approached). However, their own top priority is not medical proof targeted at outsiders but the day-to-day work of praying for an endless stream of sick people and building faith among insiders through testimonies—tasks that do not require medical evidence.[52]

Global Awakening staff members have supplied me with contact information for people testifying to healing in their conferences. For example, Patty, then fifty-two years old, was scheduled for surgery in 2010 to repair a dropped bladder and related urinary incontinence. She attended GA's Voice of the Prophets annual conference in Camp Hill, Pennsylvania two months before her planned surgery. While singing worship songs, Patty

> felt a hand pressing into my back and heat going through me. We went back to our seats and Randy came out and was calling out words of knowledge, he called out "A BLADDER WILL BE LIFTED" and no sooner did he say that the power of God hit me so hard I fell backwards and was filled with the joy of the Lord. I could not stop laughing and could not stand up, my friends were holding me up. I could feel a kneading sensation in my lower abdomen, and from that day forward I have had no symptoms. I waited two weeks and called the urologist to cancel the surgery. They would not schedule an appointment for me because I wanted medical confirmation; they said they would just tell the doctor I postponed the surgery. . . . I had to see my gyn. for another matter that he said he would take care of at the same time as my bladder surgery, and I told him I'm not having surgery that the dropped bladder was healed after receiving a word

of knowledge from God and feeling his presence on me. He said let
me examine you!! I was examined by my gynecologist who confirmed that I am healed, there is NO protrusion and NO cystocele
(dropped bladder) my exam was perfectly NORMAL. Praise the
Lord.!!!!!!!!!!!!!! (I have a copy of the progress note stating that I don't
have a dropped bladder anymore, and he wrote "I am healed" after
God experience [sic].) He was in shock, just kept shaking his head,
he said he has NEVER seen this happen before. I told him to get used
to it that he was going to see it happen more and more. He asked if
I told the urologist and I said no they would not let me talk to him,
he said well I'm gonna call and tell him, this is unbelievable.

Figure 3.8 consists of three medical reports, dated 2009 and 2010. The
first two, from Patty's urologist, give the diagnosis of stress urinary
incontinence consistent with sphincteric deficiency, and cystocele, or
dropped bladder, and outlines a plan for surgery. The third note, written by Patty's gynecologist five months after the second urology report,
records Patty's self-reported improvement in symptoms: "USI [Urinary
Stress Incontinence] Better. I got healed. No leaking since God experienced word heard. No USI." The note also records the results of the
gynecologist's pelvic examination: "Normal evaluation. Pelvis normal.
No prolapse. No cystocele. 1. No USI. 2. Endometrial polyp. Schedule
hysteroscopy D & C." Patty had the hysteroscopy procedure done and
reported afterwards that "there was no polyp! only piece of tissue
where it could have been." Patty's relief from urinary incontinence did
not prevent her from having surgery for an endometrial polyp, but the
experience did result in an alleviation of symptoms two months prior
to the scheduled surgery, as well as minimizing the extent of surgical
intervention.[53]

Like Patty, Bethany has collected medical records indicating an
improvement that her health care providers did not expect. Bethany
had been chronically ill for ten years. In 2005, when Bethany was
forty-eight, a neurologist at a university medical center cardiac elec-
trophysiology and autonomic function clinic diagnosed her with "autonomic neuropathy," or autonomic nervous system dysfunction. The
system that normally regulates autonomic functions, such as breath-

ing, blood pressure, heartbeat, digestion, temperature, and other vital functions was not working properly. This caused Bethany a variety of health problems, including poor circulation, difficulty sweating, weakness, irregular heartbeat, intestinal blockages, chronic pain, and a compromised immune system that had made her vulnerable to cancer of the breast and the thymus and frequent infections (documented by more than nine hundred pages of medical records). Medications (an average of ten to fifteen pills, three times a day) provided temporary help in regulating her body's autonomic systems. A 2009 letter from Bethany's neurologist describes the course of her case as consistent with "progressive autonomic neuropathy" and "pure autonomic failure." By December 2009, hospice workers estimated that Bethany had less than six months to live. In 2011, Bethany visited the same neurologist who had been following her case since 2005. The doctor described Bethany as a patient "who previously was suffering from an autonomic neuropathy. On followup today, she tells me that her symptoms have resolved almost completely. I am at a loss to explain why exactly this has occurred, however, the current feeling is that these are autoimmune disorders and there are individuals in whom the immune system will suddenly stop its overactivity and stop attacking parts of itself." The 2011 neurologist's letter describes the resolution of Bethany's health problems but does not identify a particular event that caused her condition to improve after having deteriorated over a four-year period of observation, other than a possible spontaneous remission from a possible autoimmune disorder (figure 3.9).[54]

Bethany believes that she can explain exactly when and why her immune system began to function properly. While hospitalized with a staph infection (methicillin-resistant Staphylococcus aureus, or MRSA) that required surgery, Bethany reported hearing the name "Randy Clark" in her head repeatedly. Bethany did not recall having ever heard the name before, but she made inquiries until she learned about GA, after which she asked friends to take her to a healing school. Clark was unavailable at the time, but one of his associates, Rodney Hogue, prayed for Bethany on April 29, 2010. During the prayer, Bethany avowedly "felt this really warm sensation. It felt like gold hot chocolate was being poured into my body. . . . Then I had the most

A

UROLOGY

████████ MD FACS ████████, MD FACS ████████, DO FACOS ████████, MD

████████, 2009

████████, D.O.
████████████

RE: ████████

Dear Dr. ████:

REVIEWED BY

Mrs. ████ presented today in consultation for stress urinary incontinence. She is a 51-year-old female with the possibility of some neurological issues related to a motor vehicle collision. She has been experiencing worsening of her urinary incontinence. She states that she urinates without warning and there has been significant stress incontinence with horseback riding, trampoline, sneezing, and coughing. She feels as though she urinates with a strong stream and empties well. She denies frequency or urgency. There is a question of possible sensory loss in her lower extremities due to the motor vehicle collision and this may require further evaluation.

Physical exam today reveals a healthy-appearing middle-aged woman. Her abdomen is soft and nontender and her bladder is not distended. Pelvic exam reveals a slight grade 1 to 2 cystocele with significant stress incontinence noted with Valsalva.

Mrs. ████'s gynecologic organs are intact and she has had two vaginal deliveries 18 and 20 years ago. She is presently undergoing menopause.

I discussed the treatment options for Mrs. ████'s stress urinary incontinence and cystocele. She is an excellent candidate for a suburethral sling and possible cystocele repair with mesh. This was discussed with her in detail today. Prior to that, I would like to rule out any neurological pathology with a cystometrogram. I will keep you informed of any findings or plans.

Sincerely,

████████, D.O.

cc: ████████, M.D.
████████, M.D.

████

Phone: ████ • Fax: ████
www.████urology.com

Figure 3.8a–c. Medical records for Patty. (a) Letter from urologist diagnosing stress urinary incontinence and cystocele, 2009. (b) Letter from urologist noting sphincteric deficiency as cause of stress urinary incontinence and outlining surgery plan, 2010. (c) Notes from gynecologist indicating absence of bladder protrusion or cystocele, five months after second urology report. Courtesy Patty.

B

[redacted]

UROLOGY

[redacted], MD FACS [redacted], MD FACS [redacted], DO FACOS [redacted], MD

[redacted], 2010

[redacted], D.O.
[redacted]

RE: [redacted]

Dear Dr. [redacted]:

Mrs. [redacted] presented today in follow-up. She has undergone a cystometrogram revealing a normal bladder contraction and a low pressure voiding pattern consistent with sphincteric deficiency. This in turn is the likely cause of her stress urinary incontinence.

We therefore discussed the cystocele repair and suburethral sling procedure in detail. She definitively desires this procedure and the risks were described in detail today. The risks of injury to adjacent organs, urinary retention, or any other risks associated with this procedure were described.

She has chosen to have this performed in the spring and I will certainly keep you informed of her progress.

Sincerely,

[redacted], D.O.

cc: [redacted], M.D.

[redacted]

REVIEWED BY [redacted] M.D.

C

[redacted] OB-GYN ASSOCIATES, P.C.

[redacted]
Phone: [redacted] | [redacted] Phone: [redacted] | [redacted] Phone: [redacted]

PROGRESS NOTES

Name [redacted] **D.O.B.** [redacted]/57

Allergies

[redacted] 2010 Consultation age 52

11 f SI Better "I got healed"
No leaky since [illegible]
[illegible] " [illegible]

No meds ∅

Pelvic Exam:
(1985)

Pelvic: No [illegible]
Pelvic [illegible]
[illegible]
[illegible]

[illegible]

[illegible]
[illegible]

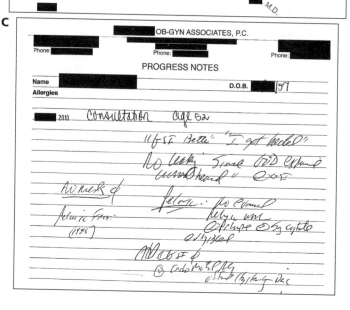

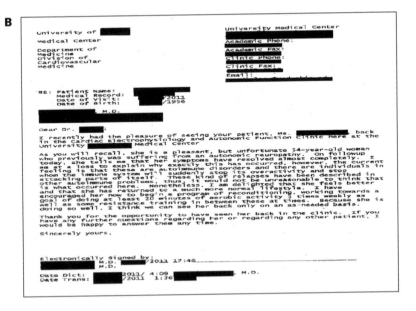

Figure 3.9a–b. Medical records for Bethany. (a) Letter from neurologist noting "progressive autonomic neuropathy" and "pure autonomic failure," 2009. (b) Letter from the same neurologist noting that "symptoms have resolved," 2011. Courtesy Bethany.

startling realization . . . I HAD NO PAIN!!!" She went into the conference lunchroom and ate a meal that included beef stew, salad, white bread, and brownies—foods that previously would have exacerbated her chronic diarrhea—but experienced no ill effects. Bethany had strength to stand during the next conference session, was able to wear a sweater without overheating, sang without becoming dizzy, and the next morning got up by herself and made her own breakfast (none of which she could do before) without taking any further medication. She has since participated in GA international ministry trips and prayed for other people's healing, and she believes that a number of people have been healed through her prayers. As of 2011, Bethany reports that she continues to enjoy excellent health and credits God for her healing.[55]

Similar to Bethany, Daisy has medical records that denote an unexpected improvement of a chronic condition. Daisy suffered from hearing loss in both ears, the result of a hereditary inner-ear problem that went back several generations and had caused her mother to become deaf. Daisy began wearing hearing aids in both ears at age twenty and, over time, her hearing worsened. Hearing tests performed in 1999, when Daisy was forty-one years old, recorded pure-tone thresholds between 41 and 55 dBHL, which is a moderate hearing loss. By 2004 her hearing had deteriorated, as Daisy's recorded thresholds ranged from 55 to 90 dBHL, which is a moderately severe to severe hearing loss. Hearing tests conducted in 2008 showed improved hearing thresholds that ranged from within normal thresholds in the lower frequencies to a moderate hearing loss in the higher frequencies. All tests were performed by a certified audiologist in the same medical office using a sound-insulated testing room, and the 2004 and 2008 tests used the same audiometer (GSI 61) with inserts. Daisy's improved thresholds between the 2004 and 2008 tests do not appear to have resulted from a temporary hearing shift. A hearing screening performed in 2010 indicated "normal" (10 to 20 dBHL) hearing in the speech frequencies in both ears (Figure 3.10).[56]

Daisy explains her improved hearing. On August 27, 2008 (two weeks before her 2008 hearing test), she attended an ANGA-affiliated "prayer summit." While singing worship songs, Daisy "felt my fingers

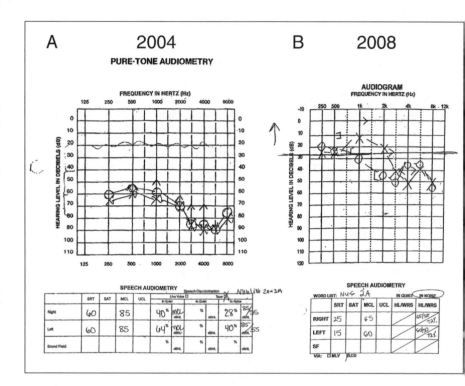

Figure 3.10. Audiology records for Daisy. (a) Audiogram (right ear denoted by O, left ear denoted by X), speech-recognition threshold 60 dBHL right ear, 60 dBHL left ear, 2004. (b) Audiogram, speech-recognition threshold 25 dBHL right ear, 15 dBHL left ear, 2008. Courtesy Daisy.

on fire and the warmth of the Holy Spirit inside of me." A conference speaker delivered a "word of knowledge" that God wanted to heal someone with hearing loss. Daisy did not hear the announcement (even though she was wearing hearing aids), but her friend nudged her and led her to the front of the church. After receiving prayer, Daisy was able to hear and repeat words spoken behind her without hearing aids. She later remarked that "what disabled me for 30 years, God healed in 30 seconds!! I haven't worn my hearing aids since." Daisy made an appointment with her audiologist to have her hearing retested. The audiologist reportedly exclaimed: "I can't believe this. This has never happened before. I've done these tests for a long time and I've never had this happen! I just can't believe this—you have normal hearing. You don't need hearing aids! So, tell me again, what happened?" Six months later, Daisy took her daughter to a prayer summit at the same church, and she, too, reported having a similar healing experience, discontinued using her hearing aids, and tested normal in both ears at her next audiology examination. As of 2011, Daisy attests that she and her daughter both have normal hearing.[57]

Unlike Patty, Bethany, and Daisy, most individuals who report healing at GA conferences do not seem to possess before-and-after medical records to shed light on their conditions. This is partly for the reason given by Dr. Crandall—that few doctors are interested in documenting miracles. Some individuals have mailed me copies of their medical records, but the records convey so little information that no definite conclusions can be drawn from them, even when paired with informant narratives. In a number of cases, individuals received prayer alongside conventional and alternative medical treatments, making it difficult to determine the relative influence of each healing modality. Other individuals attest to possessing medical records, but for one reason or another they have not produced them. In following up with leads from GA as well as other ministries, a typical pattern ensued: several weeks or months after a healing conference, the participant averred that healing was experienced at the time of the conference and had been maintained since then, that before-and-after medical records confirming the healing exist, and that the individual would be willing—even eager—to share these records with me. But after repeated phone, e-mail, and postal mail follow-up, no records were produced. Sometimes follow-up was greeted with apologies that a host of inexplicable life crises had intervened—but still no records, until I eventually lost touch with the contact.

There have been variations on this pattern—facilitated by the fact that ANGA cultivates a global community of perpetual conference seekers who can often be met and remet by chance at far-flung destinations. One example is Stan, who received prayer for healing at a Todd Bentley–James Maloney conference in Seattle, Washington in 2004. The conference DVD shows Stan responding to a word of knowledge for the disappearance of surgically inserted metal from his leg bone, after which he claimed to experience relief from associated pain. I met Stan in 2008 on an ANGA-affiliated Gary Oates Ministries trip to Brazil. Stan continued to attest to his healing, but the only medical information he could provide was that he had never returned to his doctor, because his leg no longer troubled him. He had, however, decided to start a new church in gratitude for his healing experience. While in Brazil I also remet Mimi, whose story of healing from asthma in 2004 at a Mahesh Chavda–Bill Johnson conference in Charlotte, North Carolina is related in chapter 6. Mimi reported still being healed, and I have subsequently seen her at several other conferences where the report remains consistent as of 2011. Mimi had, however, seen no need to return to her medical doctor for her breathing; she had only discarded her prescribed medications—and started running track, indeed, winning a college track scholarship.[58]

Stan's and Mimi's stories confirm the point suggested by the *Finger of God* film that ANGA culture defines "documentation" primarily in experiential terms. The epistemic weakness of overreliance on this experiential approach comes across through a healing testimony widely disseminated throughout ANGA-influenced networks in the 2000s—that of the Brazilian Davi Silva. Silva attested to having been healed from Down's syndrome at the age of six through his mother's prayers. Silva claimed, moreover, that medical documentation once existed but had not been preserved. In Silva's account, soon after his healing was recognized by elementary school officials, a team of Brazilian medical doctors asked to examine him because his recovery struck them as remarkable; Silva agreed on the condition that he be allowed to share his testimony. As a result of the testimony and the doctors' findings, they reportedly all decided to convert to pentecostal Christianity. Silva insisted that chromosomal tests were conducted when he was born and again after his healing. The first set of tests showed an extra chromosome—indicative of Down's syndrome—but the second set of tests did not reveal the extra chromosome. Silva's inability to produce medical documentation gave no pause to pentecostals who met him—because he was, in their words, a "walking miracle." During field research, I observed the frequently commented-on "evidence" that Silva was born with Down's: his palms are visibly creased straight across the middle, his face looks slightly rounded, and the position of his ears is relatively low on his head. Silva was to all other appearances a normal father of two who is a talented musician and a dynamic conference speaker. Silva's dramatic healing testimony made his other supernatural claims—for instance, that he regularly "visits heaven" to learn from angels the songs he writes—seem plausible to other pentecostals.[59]

The problem with Silva's narrative is that it is not factual. In 2010, eleven years after his testimony began to circulate in ANGA-related networks, Silva published a retraction, confessing that his healing story as well as other claims of supernatural experiences contain elements that he had fabricated: "I have included lies in almost all of these stories. Some of them are complete lies." Silva at first promised to publish a clarification of which elements were and were not factual but a month later declined to do so, resigning from his position at the ANGA-affiliated Casa de Davi, or House of David. (Nevertheless, ten months later Silva released a new solo musical album and announced his return to public ministry—with the backing of a Brazilian pastor, but not of Casa de Davi.) Unlike Kuhlman, who required medical documentation before endorsing healing testimonies, such has not been the customary practice in pentecostal ministries in the first decade of the twenty-first century. As part of the public retraction, Silva's associates defended themselves by stating that they never covered up his lies, they just never investigated his claims.[60]

Testimonies such as Silva's circulate by word of mouth and in print, often without any fact-checking efforts having been made. This is not to suggest that all such stories are false or even that many falsifications take place. Indeed, it is relevant here to note a tendency named by psychologists the *availability heuristic*. People tend to infer the probability of an imagined scenario on the basis of how vividly they can recall examples of such scenarios. Nevertheless, such judgments are often unfounded. Because most people can readily think of examples of high-profile ministry leaders committing fraud, it is assumed to be a frequent occurrence. There is, however, no evidential basis on which to conclude that Silva's dishonesty is the norm rather than the exception. Yet the tendency to accept at face value such dramatic claims as his without documentation opens the door for easy deception—while placing implicit pressure on others in the same interpretive community potentially to exaggerate their own experiences in order to appear comparably "spiritual."[61]

The disconcerting results of this pentecostal tendency to esteem most highly those who make the most supernatural-sounding claims can be illustrated by one further example of falsification. Frank is a fifty-something-year-old salesman who first traveled to Brazil in 2007. He told teammates that an injury, sustained in the 1980s, had permanently damaged his left eye. He had avowedly sought prayer from many itinerant healing evangelists without apparent benefit and had prayed for himself for healing every day for the last several years. On the fourth night of evangelistic meetings in Brazil, Frank heard one of his teammates testify to having just witnessed the restoration of a Brazilian woman's eyesight during the evening's meeting. Frank asked this team member to pray for his eyesight, too, even though it was by then one o'clock in the morning. Within a few minutes Frank was apparently reading, using his left eye—according to him and his wife who was also present—for the first time in nearly twenty-five years. I met Frank when he traveled on another international ministry trip, as he was telling everyone about his previous healing. He testified that his eye had remained healed, and that his vision was still gradually improving. Frank also claimed that, in the months since his healing, "manna" (the breadlike substance described in the Bible as materializing as food for the Israelites after their exodus from Egypt) had occasionally appeared in his open Bible, and "glory dust" (a goldlike substance that reportedly appears on people and objects and is interpreted by pentecostals as a supernatural phenomenon) had begun to appear all over his body—especially while he was engaged in evangelism. Similar claims are featured in the film *Finger of God*, which in all likelihood Frank and his teammates had all viewed. Observing Frank, I saw what looked like gold-colored glitter on his face and neck, as well as the tiny crackers that he produced and identified as manna. I also noticed that team leaders asked Frank, and only a select few additional team members, to preach for an evening church service, and that other team members looked up to Frank (who in any case has a dynamic personality) as an exemplar.[62]

I asked Frank for copies of medical records documenting his improved vision, and he mailed an optometrist's report on office stationery. The report states that in "02," Frank's visual acuity in his left eye (abbreviated "os") without correction measured "20/200." As of "07," his left eye acuity was "NOW 20/40." No further information is recorded. I followed up with Frank's optometrist, who confirmed that Frank was a patient and that he had been examined and that a report had been written on the date in question. The optometrist faxed me the office copy of the report—with two crucial pieces of information circled with the same note added and underlined next to each: "NOT OUR WRITING." The circled phrases are "02" and "NOW 20/40" (figure 3.11). When these details are omitted from the report, the meaning is entirely different from the version Frank sent me. As of 2007—three months after his alleged healing prayer experience—the visual acuity of Frank's left eye measured 20/200 without correction.

Perhaps Frank's vision was even worse before he received prayer in 2007, but he presented no evidence that this was the case. I contacted Frank to ask for an explanation of the discrepancy, and he responded that an office staff person, rather than the optometrist himself, had added the clarifying details. Perhaps, but the fax cover letter states explicitly that "the note indeed is from our office but has been altered." Frank did not respond to my subsequent, repeated efforts to contact him, making it hard not to conclude that he had intentionally falsified evidence of his healing testimony for reasons that remain obscure. If Frank falsified one aspect of his story, it may reasonably be surmised that he falsified others—such as the supposed "manna" flakes and "glory dust." Even if Frank was motivated by self-promotion, the altered optometrist's report is perplexing, because I had informed him that I was interested in publishing only de-identified medical records that would not reveal his identity to the public. Possibly Frank, not trained as a scholar, did not understand the magnitude of his deception—much as some prominent Christian leaders appear not to understand that plagiarism is a serious problem—and

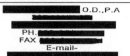

A

PH.
FAX
E-mail-

FAX COVER SHEET

To: CANDY Gunther Brown , PH.D.

Number of pages including this one _3_

Comment: RE: ▭ — The Note indeed is From our office but has been altered . What I have circled is not my writing.

Thank-you,

B

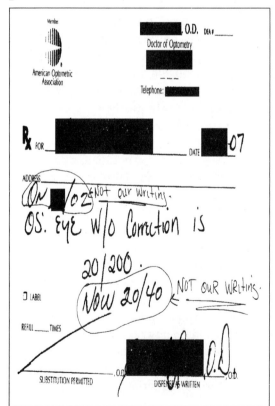

Figure 3.11a–b. Optometry records for Frank. (a) Fax from optometrist's office noting alteration of office record, 2010. (b) Annotated optometrist's note on prescription paper, 2007. Courtesy Frank's optometrist.

he was trying to "help" document pentecostal healing. Frank may also have felt embarrassed that the visual improvement he "really" experienced could not be medically corroborated.[63]

It is important that ANGA leaders and members *do* care a great deal about documenting healing experiences, but their understanding of documentation reflects a characteristically postmodern assumption that physical sensations and spiritual perceptions offer windows onto truth. Medical evidence might be a plus in this worldview, but it is generally viewed as inessential, even by GA and IM team members who by profession belong to medical and scientific communities. Dan, a retired radiologist whom I met in Brazil in 2007, prayed for a young man, who appeared to have a white cataract, complaining of vision problems in his right eye. Dan prayed for the man several times over a three-day period, over the course of which time the cataract appeared to shrink. When Dan could no longer see a white spot in the man's eye on the third day, and the man claimed improved eyesight, Dan declared the man healed, even though Dan lacked ophthalmic testing equipment.[64]

Global Awakening team members do typically attempt to assess people's physical condition before and after prayer—because they expect their prayers to make a tangible difference that can be tested right away. In contrast to the pentecostal Word of Faith model of claiming healing by faith while ignoring physical evidence to the contrary, GA team members encourage those receiving prayer to "test it out" and "try to do something you couldn't do before." George, the biomedical research scientist whose healing story opens chapter 4, administers informal before-and-after tests to those who request prayer for vision. When a ten-year-old boy approached George for healing of his eyesight in Brazil, George held up his hand and asked the boy if he could count how many fingers were raised. At first, the boy said he could not see anything. After a few minutes of prayer, he reported being able to see shadows. More prayer and, in George's words, "when I removed my hands again, he started seeing lights. I kept doing this—praying for healing and then asking to see if there was some improvement, and he kept getting improvement. After a while, he could count how many lights there were in the stadium—there were 5. Then I kept praying, and after a while longer, he could count how many fingers I was holding up, even from 5–10 feet away." Similarly, when a woman who had been diagnosed by her doctor with a degenerative eye disease requested prayer, George asked her what she could not see. She pointed to a bouquet of flowers six feet away and said that she could see that there were flowers, but that she could not see the petals. After a short prayer, she could see a few more details on the flowers. After another prayer, she could see the petals. George continued to pray until the woman could count how many fingers he was holding up from twenty feet away. In a parallel manner, George, following Clark and GA on a trip to visit IM in Mozambique, asked Sergio, who was presented by family members as having been deaf and mute since birth, to repeat words and sounds as George intoned them from behind Sergio's back. Sergio croaked responses, eliciting applause from the gathering crowd.[65]

Like George, other GA team members typically use the "count fingers" method to assess vision or make noises behind a person's head to evaluate hearing. Particular evidential value is placed on experiences that can be sensed by participants and witnessed by others, especially if there is a trophy that appears to provide evidence that a problem once existed but does no longer. These conditions seemed to be met at a 2007 conference in Rio de Janeiro, Brazil, when nine-year-old Pedro showed that his right leg was roughly $2\frac{1}{2}$ inches shorter than his left leg. Within a few minutes of prayer, Pedro felt his leg grow out, those around could no longer detect a difference in length, and Pedro left carrying his shoe lift in his hands. Often GA conference participants report feeling physical sensations such as heat or "electricity" during prayer or feeling pain move around before it disappears, or claim to see a vision—for instance of an angel performing surgery. Such experiences—attributed to supernatural agents such as the Holy Spirit or angels—constitute a significant form of evidence within GA's cosmology. For instance, a Brazilian woman who claimed to experience healing of pain in her right kneecap fell over during prayer and saw a vision of a "big storm spinning over her and then a bolt of lightning came out of the storm and touched her head. Then she saw an angel doing something in her side." Such visionary experiences, at least as much as medical evidence, constitute a form of proof persuasive within ANGA's culture.[66]

Global Awakening does not bring diagnostic equipment or medical personnel to conferences, nor is there any systematic effort to track whether people continue to claim healings the next day, let alone the next year. Yet GA regularly publishes what leaders call "trip statistics" of the numbers and types of healings experienced during each international ministry trip. The term *statistics* is a misnomer that reflects the group's aspiration toward scientific legitimacy. More accurately, team leaders take an unsystematic tally of how many people seem to experience healing or deliverance or convert to Christianity each night. Typically, the trip coordinator or a designee asks everyone on the bus after a meeting to raise one finger for each person in each of several categories. For instance, the official combined trip statistics for meetings in Rio de Janeiro and Imperatriz in 2007 reported: a total attendance of 27,560; 2,241 "physical healings"; 2,044 "sovereign healings" (that is, healings reported by waving one's hands overhead during en masse prayers and delivery of words of knowledge rather than during proximal intercessory prayer); 416 "emotional, inner healings and deliverances"; 212 "salvations/ rededications/called to ministry"; and 6,760 "blasted," or powerfully touched by the Holy Spirit. Separate numbers were recorded for categories of healing referred to in the New Testament or that seemed particularly miraculous: 17 "blind or legally blind seeing better than 80 percent"; 42 "deaf or mostly deaf ears now open and hearing"; 22 "tumors or cysts disappearing before our eyes"; 4 of "those who could not walk now walking."[67]

Trip statistics are inherently unreliable for multiple reasons—including inconsistent criteria for determining "healing" and implicit pressure to inflate the number and severity of conditions healed—because everyone can see how many fingers each team member raises. Desire to count a "biblical" healing (validating the group's legitimacy) may encourage reporting improvement of a less severe condition, such as difficulty walking without a cane, as an instance of the lame walking. Each team member has his or her own standards for what counts as a healing. Determining whether a condition is 80 percent better (the minimum level of improvement considered "healing" according to the guidelines established by Clark, in emulation of the Argentinian revivalist Omar Cabrera) versus 75 percent better is subjective. One team member admitted to saying a group prayer for four people when he ran out of time one evening and did not have an opportunity to test for improvement. "When doing stats," he reported, "I asked the Holy Spirit how many from that group had been healed for the report, and He said '2,' so I did [report that two were healed]." Even when team members do seek to evaluate results of their prayers more empirically, testing conditions such as hearing loss in a noisy room with no equipment is imprecise at best.[68]

Such "statistics" would scarcely be considered reliable by anyone trained scientifically. However, the primary audience is not scientists but other potential GA team members who want to travel where they, too, will be able to experience the miraculous. Mark, an expatriate American member of ANGA's Brazilian affiliate Casa de Davi, commented in an interview that the Brazilians have higher "integrity" in claiming healings and reported his belief that the Brazilians generally ignored GA's statistical claims. Nevertheless, during a stadium meeting in Londrina, Paraná, Brazil, Mark publicly testified that he had just experienced healing of a long-standing knee problem. He did not disbelieve that healings occur during GA meetings; he only resisted making claims that in his view exceeded the evidence. Understandably, Mark was, in his words, "extremely embarrassed" and "ashamed" when he later realized that he had himself been taken in by Davi Silva's unfounded claims even though he conceived of himself as tending "to be the 'scientific' sort."[69]

Another potential, and sometimes actual, risk of emphasizing statistics is the dehumanization of those receiving prayer for healing. The historian Amanda Porterfield has suggested that "recourse to scientific validation turns discussion of spiritual healing toward quantification of impersonal forces at work in disease and recovery and away from the emotional response to human suffering." One GA team member reduced the people he prayed for to their conditions, writing on the "testimony form" distributed by GA to all team members that he had "had 1 knee, 1 set of feet and one stomach pain healed." He wrote at greater length about praying for "Mr. Blind. . . . He was a short, roly-poly guy with an absolutely delightful spirit about him—a joy to be with. Kind of like a really cute little puppy." In this testimonial, the person seeking prayer, whose name was not recorded, is condescendingly compared to an animal. More often, testimonials speak respectfully of the individuals receiving prayer, but the risk of objectification seems inherent (though it can be resisted) in the quest for "documentation," however defined—whether by prayer groups, medical professionals, committees investigating spiritual healing claims, or even academic researchers, such as the present author.[70]

Conclusion

Medical and religious practitioners have long debated the value of medical records in documenting claims of religious healing. Regardless of how medical documentation is constructed, it cannot prove—though in certain cases it may disprove—that prayer heals anyone. Medical records are often sketchy and ambiguous in meaning. Doctors jot down notes quickly and skip details that may seem significant to patients. Even if patients believe their recovery occurred through prayer, sociological research indicates that few will say so to their doctors, because such patients expect a skeptical response. Doctors' opinions express subjective, though informed, evaluations. Even apparently objective laboratory reports and radiographic films require human interpretation; thus, patients often seek a second opinion. What even the most complete medical records can show is that a medical expert previously diagnosed a patient with a disease or disability; no medical interventions—or none that were expected to be curative—were administered by that provider; an expert can no longer detect clinical evidence of the diagnosed problem; such a recovery is statistically rare, given the diagnosis, prognosis, and any treatment; and there is no obvious medical explanation for how the healing occurred, given the current state of medical knowledge.[71]

What cannot be proven, within the paradigm of medical science, is that prayer had anything to do with improvements in signs and symptoms or even that the problem has been permanently "cured," because many conditions, such as cancers, unpredictably recur even after an interval of years. The medical category of *spontaneous remission* signifies an unexpected improvement that may or may not turn out to be permanent; the label does not constitute an explanation of cause or mechanism, and indeed may discourage investigation of anomalous recoveries. On rare occasions, doctors may be quoted as saying a recovery is "miraculous," but they are either simply stating that they cannot account for a recovery or, if they are genuinely invoking supernatural agency, they are no longer speaking in their capacity as medical professionals.

Medical records, when available, are nevertheless valuable as one among several methods of examining healing claims. The potential of the medical lens for revealing certain things about health and disease has generated enduring, though ambivalent, interest among pentecostals and those investigating their claims in modern and postmodern cultures. Comparison of medical records from before and after prayer can offer a scientifically informed perspective on whether someone claiming healing showed improved health. Failure to consider medical documentation has sometimes resulted in the dissemination of patently false claims. Scattered records collected from pentecostals between the 1960s and 2011 suggest that certain individuals claiming healing did exhibit medically unexpected recoveries. Yet the relative scarcity of medical documentation and inherent gaps in the information that medical records can convey also indicate the importance of finding supplementary windows onto healing claims. Accordingly, the following chapters proceed empirically to perceptions of healing experiences, measurements of health changes, and longitudinal assessments of individual and social outcomes.

CHAPTER 4

How Do Sufferers Perceive Healing Prayer?

✦

George first traveled with Global Awakening on an international ministry trip to Cuba in 2004. His primary motivation for going was frankly a quest for his own physical healing—of a brain tumor for which no medical treatment was viable and for which the prognosis was grim. In the six months since the diagnosis, George had been aggressively seeking intercessory prayer for healing at a series of North American pentecostal conferences located in every region of the United States and Canada. Almost every time ministry teams prayed for him, George perceived a powerful touch from the Holy Spirit—he fell over, cried, laughed, sensed heat, and vibrated as if he had grabbed an electrical wire. Every three months he returned to his medical doctor for another MRI, hoping for medical confirmation of his healing—but he was repeatedly disappointed. Instead of giving up, George went to more conferences to seek more prayer. As intercessors prayed for his healing, they also prayed for an impartation of spiritual gifts in order that George might minister healing to others. That sounded good to George, but he was preoccupied with his own need for healing.[1]

Still, when Randy Clark encouraged the fifteen hundred attendees at GA's 2003 Voice of the Apostles conference to consider joining the prayer team that would minister in Cuba, something resonated with George, and he decided to go. In Cuba, George prayed for a man who could see only 2 feet in front of him without glasses and 4 feet with glasses; after fifteen minutes of prayer, he appeared able to see 20 feet without glasses—and in gratitude accepted an invitation to become a

Christian. Among several others who attested to experiencing healing through George's prayers in Cuba was a woman whose doctors had sent her home to die of ovarian cancer following unsuccessful radiation therapy. She had a large, palpable tumor on her ovary, was emaciated from being unable to eat, and was too weak to walk. During prayer, she sensed heat, fell over, regained strength to walk—and could no longer find the tumor.[2]

When George returned home, he began to pray for other people's healing at every opportunity. On a visit to his mother, he met one of her friends—who revealed that he had found a tumor on his stomach and had noticed, with some alarm, that it was growing larger. After 10 minutes of prayer, the tumor seemed smaller, and after a few more minutes of prayer, it could scarcely be palpated. When George checked back with this man a month later, he reported that the tumor had completely disappeared. Meanwhile, George's mother—who had witnessed the effects of her son's prayers—marveled, "It's all about Jesus," and decided on the spot to renounce decades of involvement in "New Age" spirituality and return to the Christian faith. George continued to frequent pentecostal conferences—and to travel with GA and other ministry groups to several destinations in Latin America and Africa—at first seeking prayer for his own healing, but increasingly praying for other people. George also came to devote many of his evenings and weekends to praying for people who sought him out, some of whom had themselves traveled long distances in search of prayer for healing.[3]

Meanwhile, George regularly returned to his doctor for MRIs. Because George was by profession a biomedical researcher, he understood his prognosis. The expected course for his low-grade glioma was gradual but virtually certain growth over the span of months to years, generally leading to death within several years regardless of treatment. The first few scans confirmed the initial diagnosis. But after two years of failing to detect any growth—rather, an apparent diminishment in the size of the lesion—George's doctors became increasingly puzzled, although they never used the word "miracle." Eight years later, George remained symptom free, and his most recent MRI report omitted the term "tumor." George accounts for his good health as resulting from the cumulative effects of many prayers for healing. Although not dramatically healed at any one of the many pentecostal conferences he attended, George believes that each prayer contributed to his healing.[4]

Why Conduct Empirical Research?

Over the course of this study, I have met many individuals such as George who attest that they have been healed through prayer. Assessing empirical outcomes of prayer remains a challenging project. The previous two chapters revealed limitations both of randomized, controlled trials of distant intercessory prayer and of the collection of medical documentation in support of healing claims when either approach is used as the primary method for assessing the empirical effects of prayer practices. George's anecdote highlights these limitations. Although he did solicit prayer from distant intercessors, George considered the proximal prayers he received at pentecostal conferences to have been more obviously influential. He often sensed something physically, such as heat or electricity, while receiving proximal prayer, but he could not point to any definite effect from the distant prayers. George's medical records also require interpretation. Although he has a series of MRIs collected over a seven-year period, the absence of a predicted disease progression does not by itself explain why his case did not follow the usual course.

It is important to be clear about the scope of what any one type of data or method can and cannot demonstrate. Previous survey researchers have sometimes attempted to use their data to answer questions—such as whether prayer "really" results in healing—that this type of data is not suited to answer. Not finding compelling medical evidence of miraculous healing in the data, some scientists have construed healing claims as reducible to psychosomatic improvements or cases of misdiagnosis. The British Medical Association survey that opened chapter 3 provides an apt example. An investigative committee predisposed to disbelieve religious healing claims concluded that the surveyed doctors had failed to provide evidence of healing. What such findings reveal is the limitation of the selected research method as applied to the question asked rather than providing conclusive evidence about the efficacy of prayer.

This project approaches the problem of interpreting religious healing practices by employing several distinct yet complementary methodological perspectives, and keeping in play multiple working hypotheses. As the scientific theorist John R. Platt advised in 1964, "Beware of the man of one method or one instrument, either experimental or theoretical. He tends to become method-oriented rather than problem-oriented. The method-oriented man is shackled: the problem-oriented man is at least reaching freely toward what is most important." In a related vein, the well-respected geologist T. C. Chamberlin, writing in 1897, advocated the scientific method of "multiple working hypotheses" as an antidote to the "habit of precipitate explanation" followed by an "unconscious pressing of the theory to make it fit the facts, and a pressing of the facts to make them fit the theory." As a result of this unfortunate propensity, even though science proceeds most efficiently through competition between two or more hypotheses, in practice most scientific research is driven by a single ruling hypothesis. Chamberlin explains that "we are so prone to attribute a phenomenon to a single cause, that, when we find an agency present, we are liable to rest satisfied therewith, and fail to recognize that it is but one factor, and perchance a minor factor, in the accomplishment of the total result." Albert Einstein similarly modified the oft-cited principle of "Occam's Razor"—that the simplest explanation tends to be the most accurate—by urging that "the supreme goal of all theory is to make the irreducible basic elements as simple and as few as possible without having to surrender the adequate representation of a single datum of experience." In an effort to represent the data adequately, this project has avoided relying exclusively on any one reductionist explanation of healing prayer practices, instead viewing these practices through multiple lenses. Patterns emerge as the resultant series of images are layered into one composite picture.[5]

This chapter and the next two build on each other to model a way of studying healing practices by integrating quantitative and qualitative empirical research methods developed in the social and natural sciences, informed by theological analysis of how participants practice prayer in their social contexts. The goal of this inquiry is to provide insight into how certain pentecostals construct the meanings and outcomes of healing prayer, and to understand better the processes through which healing practices exert individual and social effects. This chapter uses written surveys to assess pentecostal *perceptions* of illness and healing—such as George's perception that he was progressively healed through prayer at pentecostal conferences. Recognizing gaps in the questions answerable with survey data, chapter 5 employs a prospective clinical study to *measure* the effects of proximal intercessory prayer on two specific health outcomes: hearing and vision. Chapter 6 uses ethnographic and textual methods to trace the longitudinal implications of healing experiences for informants' long-term beliefs and actions. Integrating the findings yielded by these diverse research approaches allows investigation of *intersections* between perceptions and measurable effects and development of a theory to interpret the social implications. This project does *not* isolate the mechanisms by which any empirical effects may occur. Neither does this research answer the philosophical-theological question of whether any effects prove or disprove the actual existence or activity of "God" or any other suprahuman force. Instead, these chapters seek to assess and, where possible, quantify perceived and measurable effects of pentecostal healing practices on individual health outcomes and subsequent self-concepts and social behaviors.

Scope of Empirical Research

The empirical research presented in the second half of this book offers a series of distinct, yet complementary perspectives on a type of in-person, direct-contact, proximal intercessory prayer that frequently occurs at GA and IM healing conferences in North America, Brazil, and Mozambique. Prayer for healing takes place in a great many contexts, not just pentecostal conferences, but such conferences do consistently feature healing prayer, and people who need healing seek out such conferences for this reason. The decision to single out GA and IM events in particular—out of numerous similar pentecostal conferences—stemmed in part from the relatively high level of influence these groups exert in certain sectors of global pentecostalism, but also, more pragmatically, from the willingness demonstrated by group leaders to allow and facilitate empirical studies by outside researchers.

This last point about accessibility is not a trivial one. Several other high-profile pentecostal groups, including the offices of the International Association of Healing Rooms in Spokane, Washington, Santa Maria, California, and Valparaiso, Indiana; Bethel Church in Redding, California; Fresh Fire Ministries in Abbotsford, British Columbia; and the Assemblies of God Ignited Church in Lakeland, Florida have all rebuffed research efforts presented in a similar manner. A possible explanation for the greater receptivity of the selected groups is that GA was already in the habit of attempting to collect "trip statistics" that purportedly quantify healings at each conference, and the organization had made limited efforts to track down medical records confirming healing claims. Although GA was not particularly effective at statistical reporting or collection of third-party verifications, it is crucial that seeking such corroboration was a value for Randy Clark, GA's director. Clark, who is interested in the history of healing movements and attuned to perception of legitimacy by the medical community, was aware of empirical investigations of Wimber conducted by the social anthropologist David Lewis and of the Toronto Blessing conducted by the sociologist Margaret Poloma. Clark doubtless hoped that independent investigation would add legitimacy to his ministry. Iris Ministries leaders were not especially interested in investigations, but neither did they oppose them. Shielded from criticism by their remote location, IM leaders seemed to care relatively little about outsiders' perceptions. This organization's decision to allow systematic investigation may have stemmed in part from direct encouragement by Clark—as a pentecostal network leader—to accept outside scrutiny. After my research group measured changes in several subjects' auditory and visual acuity before and after proximal intercessory prayer, Heidi Baker commented that "God didn't seem to mind" researchers taking measurements, adding that she "hadn't been sure" that God would permit it—a concern that harks back to the prayer-gauge controversy of the nineteenth century.

Inherent in conducting ethnographic research is the possibility that the researchers will affect the practices of the communities under study, thereby biasing the results. Global Awakening probably did step up its efforts to look for before-and-after medical records in support of healing claims, although notably it still did not produce many illuminating records—especially compared with the extensive portfolios collected by the healing evangelist Kathryn Kuhlman in the 1970s. Overall GA practices did not noticeably change between initial contact in 2003 and the end of the study in 2011. Iris Ministries, with whom we had much more limited contact, continued with business as usual when researchers were present. Apart from the specific meetings during which IM leaders allowed us to take clinical measurements, the group seemed to have been relatively unaffected by investigations; it was notable that IM leaders were unwilling to add unplanned healing practices at certain meetings in the United States where I wanted to test the effects. To complement observations and conversations with group members, I collected and analyzed formal survey responses, using a combination of quantitative and qualitative methods.[6]

Such anecdotes as George's do not constitute scientific proof of cure, let alone provide evidence of divine causation. But research has brought to my attention many such cases in which an observable—at least to the person claiming healing—change in physical condition, often accompanied by a profound alteration of demeanor, took place during or shortly after prayer. And for some informants I have been able to track the effects of these changes for as long as eight years. From the perspective of many such individuals, they experienced healing, and this experience prompted a reorientation of worldview and a transformed sense of life purpose. I have also met informants who are still seeking healing, who have to all appearances given up, or who have died of their health problems during the course of this research. As the religious studies theorist Victor Turner puts it so well, "Obviously, there is much that can be counted, measured, and submitted to statistical analysis. But all human act is impregnated with meaning, and meaning is hard to measure, though it can often be grasped, even if only fleetingly and ambiguously." What many informants grasped was a sense of apparent divine love and purpose for their lives perceived in their successful—and sometimes even in their unsuccessful—pursuit of healing. But given that scholars, the present author included, do like to count, measure, and where possible submit data to statistical analysis, an effort has been made to do this as well.[7]

Description of Survey Research Methods

I developed a written "Healing Survey" to ask GA and IM conference participants about past healing experiences, current need for healing, use of medical and spiritual approaches besides prayer, and whether they perceived healing during the current conference. The preconference and postconference questionnaires consist of a total of twenty-seven questions (see appendix). I distributed the survey (in English and Portuguese, the national language of Brazil and Mozambique) at seven GA conferences in Toronto, Ontario; Harrisburg, Pennsylvania; St. Louis, Missouri; Rio de Janeiro, Rio de Janeiro, Brazil; Imperatriz, Maranhão, Brazil; Londrina, Paraná, Brazil (with the ANGA affiliates Gary Oates Ministries and Casa de Davi); and Pemba, Cabo Delgado, Mozambique (in partnership with IM). All surveys were completed anonymously, but North American subjects were given the option of filling out a contact card if they wished to participate in a follow-up telephone interview. I completed 68 semistructured telephone interviews with North American conference participants. During field research, I also conducted dozens of informal interviews with Brazilians, Mozambicans, and North American conference attendees and international ministry trip participants. This survey used a convenience sample, and caution should be exercised in generalizing findings to all pentecostals (table 4.1). It is also quite possible that respondents would have answered differently had the questions been worded in other ways—or had some respondents not been concerned about providing answers that would maximize their chances of experiencing healing or meeting presumed researcher expectations. Yet the survey responses do offer insight into how certain participants in ANGA networks socially construct their experiences of healing prayer.[8]

Table 4.1.   Number of Returned Surveys by Subject Group and Region.

	Preconference	Postconference
North Americans	**328**	**251**
Ontario	62	57
Pennsylvania	126	112
Missouri	56	42
International Ministry Trips	**84**	**40**
Brazil	62	31
Mozambique	22	9
Brazilians	**593**	**259**
Rio de Janeiro	114	48
Imperatriz	173	63
Londrina	306	148
Mozambicans	124	86
Total including Mozambicans	1045	596
Total excluding Mozambicans	**921**	**510**

Choices and Challenges in Coding Health Problems and Healing Claims

My research group translated Portuguese survey answers into English and entered all surveys into a database, and I coded responses for quantitative analysis. I categorized types of illness and healing as physical, mental/emotional, and spiritual because pentecostals (as well as many other people attracted to a variety of holistic healing philosophies) typically distinguish among body, mind, and spirit while also viewing all three as interconnected. Following pentecostal usage, I coded as "mental/emotional" conditions such as depression and fear. I classed substance addictions and prostitution as spiritual problems (respondents spoke of being "freed from the spirit of prostitution" or the "spirit of nicotine"), but eating disorders as physical and mental/emotional (overeating is often attributed to "emotional wounds," but linked with physical complaints such as back pain). I recognize the complexity of such conditions (for many of which cultural and sociopolitical forces are deeply implicated) and that my categories are artificial and my placement choices debatable. I do not mean to imply that conditions coded as mental/emotional or spiritual are less serious than those coded as physical or to suggest that certain illnesses are "merely" psychosomatic. I also created subcategories, for instance classifying types of physical problems as back pain, stomach problems, or cancer.[9]

I attempted to code conditions as more or less severe, but it soon became apparent that placing too much stock in such categorizations is deeply problematic. From the perspective of the researcher, a condition such as a headache may appear to be a minor problem because generally not life threatening; however, from the perspective of a person in chronic, debilitating pain, a headache can be very serious. One Brazilian rated "myopia and astigmatism" as a level 10 problem (on a Likert scale of severity from 0 to 10); it is possible that this individual did not have corrective lenses and therefore rated the condition as more debilitating than would have a North American with the same visual acuity who had corrective lenses. Similarly, a reported past healing that "I lived for the world now I live for Jesus" may seem relatively inconsequential to the researcher but is of the utmost importance to the person reporting such an experience. I was concerned about respecting the integrity of respondents' experiences. At the same time, it seemed important to evaluate when responses to particular survey questions signaled a misunderstanding of the survey questions or of medical diagnoses. For instance, several respondents indicating that a doctor had given them a "terminal" prognosis were, it appears, reporting on non-life-threatening conditions such as dental cavities or hypothyroidism.

For comparison purposes, I roughly categorized conditions as "non-life-threatening," "serious," and "life-threatening." Even conditions coded as non-life-threatening might be extremely bothersome and life altering, such as reports of "strong pains," chronic migraines, severe visual impairments, and the poignant claim that "my back hurts. It has been years that I don't know what it is to live without this pain and my shoulder hurts too." This last respondent rated the severity of pain as a 10, but reported a doctor's diagnosis: "He said that there was nothing wrong with me." In failing to classify this condition as serious, I do not mean to invalidate the suffering experienced but only to denote that it does not appear likely to shorten life span. I classed as "serious" conditions affecting the internal organs, diagnosed as requiring surgical intervention, and/or of at least one year's duration, especially where the potential seems to exist that the condition may reduce life expectancy. I coded as serious: "I suffered of bronchitis and asthma for over 23 years," a "weak heart," and ovarian cysts that doctors advised removing. "Life-threatening" conditions include cancer and HIV. In attempting this categorization, I reiterate the concern that such classifications be used only to make rough comparisons, not to dismiss any reported symptoms as unimportant.

Indeed, the depth of suffering described by survey after survey—even those reporting "non-life-threatening" conditions—leads me to question the common tendency of researchers summarily to dismiss healing claims as either trivial or preposterous. For example, the well-respected historian of evangelicalism George Marsden has little to say about divine healing practices in his survey textbook, *Religion and American Culture,* apart from noting that pentecostal televangelists "typically provided healings for innumerable small ailments among the viewing audiences, were upbeat, and promised health, wealth, and success to their supporters." If small claims are typically discounted as trivial, large claims are as often rejected as incredible. Grant Wacker, an eminent historian of Pentecostalism, is one of the very best scholars in this field. Yet even Wacker writes dismissively that healing evangelists "routinely claimed healings that seemed not so much miraculous as simply preposterous. Decayed teeth were filled, halos photographed, screaming demons tape-recorded, and bloody cancers coughed up and put on display." Some of our respondents made comparably striking claims—for instance, recovering from being run over by a car at age eleven after being declared "legally dead." Whether such claims seem "preposterous" may depend on the prior assumptions of the interpreter. Regardless of whether scholars are convinced of their "miraculous" character, it seems to me problematic to dismiss rather than analyzing what respondents present as deeply meaningful experiences of suffering and liberation.[10]

Quantifying the number of healings reported is complicated for theological reasons. Some pentecostals, particularly those influenced by the global Word of Faith movement (popularized by the Oklahoma-based Kenneth Hagin since the 1960s), think they must claim healing "by faith" after receiving prayer, whether or not they experience an improvement in symptoms (or else risk "losing" their healing because of unbelief). Others, including the GA and IM leadership, insist that healing testimonies should be based on physically sensing a reduction in symptoms (generally the standard is 80 percent improvement or better) and/or being able to do what one could not do before the healing. The survey asked respondents how they knew they were healed. I coded responses as being "by faith" alone, perception of a spiritual experience at the time of prayer (including physical sensations of heat or "electricity" or seeing a "vision"), and/or sensate (that is, discernable by the senses) improvement in symptoms. When counting the number of respondents who experienced healing, I ran two sets of analyses—including everyone who said they were healed (less restrictive, or "claim," criterion), and only counting those who specified a sensate improvement in symptoms (more restrictive, or "improvement," criterion). The less restrictive group might be said to have claimed "healing," whereas the more restrictive group also experienced at least partial, albeit possibly temporary "cure." In order to account for the pentecostal perspective that there are degrees of healing (and cure), I distinguished those who reported that their symptoms had improved "completely" from those who indicated improvements of "almost completely," "more than half," "about half," "less than half" or "not at all," and I also looked at changes in symptom severity rated on a 0-to-10 Likert scale.[11]

What the Healing Surveys Reveal

Quantitative and qualitative analysis provides information about the types of conference participants who are more likely to report needing, expecting, and experiencing healing, as well as shedding light on the nature of these experiences and the social processes through which healing prayer is constructed.

Demographics

The demographic profile of survey respondents is consistent with previous research characterizing the Toronto Blessing as largely a middle-class, Caucasian, relatively young movement in which women are predominant. North American respondents reported a median education level of a college degree and a median annual income between $40,000 and $59,000. Considering North Americans and Brazilians together, most respondents identified as Caucasian (table 4.2). Most international ministry trip (IMT) participants came from the United States (table 4.3). The median age was forty to forty-nine years. More women (62 percent) than men completed surveys.[12]

Table 4.2.   Ethnicity/Race of Global Awakening Conference Participants.

	Brazilians	North Americans
White (branco/a)	98	268
Black (negro/a, preto/a)	28	9
Brown (pardo/a, moreno/a, mulato/a)	43	
Asian	3	30
Native American/Indian	2	3
Latino/a		12
Other	3	

Table 4.3.   Nationalities of International Ministry Trip Team Members.

	Rio/Imperatriz, Brazil	Londrina, Brazil	Pemba, Mozambique
United States	66	55	30
South Africa			9
United Kingdom		4	
Norway	1		1
Germany			1
Singapore			1

Although GA aims to attract non-Christians to its conferences (and views healing as an evangelistic tool), the group did not seem to succeed in this goal at the surveyed conferences. The survey asked respondents whether they were Protestant, Catholic, or "other"; to list any denominations or orders with which they "feel connected"; and to circle whether they identified with Christians who are Charismatic, Pentecostal, evangelical, and/or liberal. Most respondents identified as Pentecostals (295) or Charismatics (151), with smaller numbers of evangelicals (144) and liberals (101). Most also circled or listed multiple Christian subgroups with which they identified. Probably many would have agreed with the individual who expressed affinity with "all that believe that Jesus is the only Lord." Protestants (697) were much better represented than Catholics (43). Several individuals specified having left Catholic or Jewish groups to affiliate with Protestant churches. As one respondent from Londrina, Paraná, Brazil phrased the still widely held Protestant sentiment that many Catholics are not "real" Christians, "I was Catholic—now I come to this church; I want to serve God." Both GA and IM claim to draw more non-Christians when hosting outdoor evangelistic outreaches; this could not be confirmed, and it would be very difficult to conduct survey research at outdoor events.

Using the statistical procedure of multiple regression analysis to test several factors simultaneously, I found that demographic variance (including race, nationality, education, income, age, gender, and pentecostal identity) failed to predict healing needs, expectations, or experiences.[13] The only exception is that older North Americans were more likely to need healing and to experience a sensate improvement in symptoms.[14]

These findings do not support deprivation or utilitarian models of healing. The now-classic deprivation thesis holds that people with lower education and income levels, and nonwhites, are more likely to seek and claim to experience pentecostal healing (reflecting the presumably greater credulousness of these populations). In examining healing claims at Vineyard conferences, the social anthropologist David Lewis largely adhered to the deprivation model, adding a utilitarian component. Finding that fewer young people needed healing, but a higher proportion of young people experienced healing, Lewis reached the theological conclusion that "when God does choose to heal, it is often because he still has purposes to fulfill on this earth in the lives of those whose bodies are restored in some way." The present findings do not indicate that less-educated, poorer, nonwhite, or younger people are statistically more likely to report healing.[15]

Past Healings

The survey asked Brazilian and IMT respondents, "Have you ever received divine or spiritual healing of an illness, pain, or disability?" and "If 'yes,' please describe your most significant healing experience." Consistent with large-scale surveys of pentecostals, a majority of respondents—59 percent of Brazilians and 84 percent of IMT members— reported previous experiences of "divine healing." Most past healings (80 percent) were of physical rather than mental, emotional, or spiritual problems. Multivariate regression analysis does not indicate that past healings are predictive of need, expectation, or experience of healing. The only and surprising exception is that IMT members who reported a past healing were less likely to report experiencing a sensate improvement in symptoms at the current conference. Yet IMT members and Brazilians alike interpreted past healings as significant life events that even years later contributed to ongoing meaning making and identity formation.[16]

Narrative descriptions suggest that numerous respondents attributed multiple past recoveries to divine intervention. Although asked to describe their "most significant healing experience," a number of individuals listed several divine healings. An IMT woman in her forties listed healing of "hearing—UTI—knees—back pain," and another IMT woman in her fifties specified "polio, arthritis, endometriosis, etc." A Londrina woman in her thirties enumerated "healing from asthma, scoliosis, astigmatism, renal problems." An Imperatriz, Maranhão, Brazil woman in her fifties recalled more generally that "I received many cures, like my spinal column, headache and others." An Imperatriz man in his seventies made a still broader declaration that he had received divine healing for all of his past ailments: "I received many cures. Spinal column, deafness, prostate, and every time I have an illness Jesus Christ has healed me." Given decades of prior experience, whenever this man needed healing, prayer seemed an obvious recourse.

Past healing experiences seem to have made a deep impression on respondents who remember them as evidence of God's superintendence throughout the course of their lives. A woman in Imperatriz recalled that "17 years ago I was healed from a disease the doctor did not know what it was. About a year ago God healed my kidneys." A Londrina woman remembered that "I was healed from asthma a few years ago. I fell under the anointing and when I got up I was healed." A woman attending a GA conference in Missouri attested that she had been "healed of MS, Depressive Disorder, & Anxiety Disorder ALL AT ONCE 10 years ago. I have the MRI films of before and after with the reports." Another Imperatriz woman attested, "I was cured of gastritis 8 years ago. I was cured from sinusitis and a problem with my spinal column on the same day 10 years ago and I continue liberated up to now by the Grace of God." For this respondent, both the moment of experiencing healing and the subsequent decade's freedom from the condition attested to divine concern.

Memories of healings appear to be so vivid that individuals recalled seemingly minor details such as when and where they were healed or who was praying. A Londrina man specified that "I was healed from a lesion on my right shoulder in 2007 during a prayer time in a Sunday night service." A woman in Rio recalled that "yes, many years ago in a ministry in Apacentar de Nova Iguacy, I was healed from depression." Similarly, an IMT woman in her late teens recalled that "I was radically and miraculously healed of asthma 10 min. after Bobby Conner [a well-known "prophetic" leader] prayed for me at [an ANGA conference] my 8th grade yr." This woman attested to having become interested in traveling with GA because of this past healing experience.

A number of individuals looked back on past healings as validating their decisions to convert to pentecostal Christianity. An IMT member in Mozambique recalled that "after being saved God delivered me from a 25yrs alcohol addiction." Similarly, a woman joining an IMT in Mozambique detailed that "I smoked from the age of 11. I became a Christian when I was 23. I had tried for years to quit—I even smoked through pregnancies. I could not quit. About 2 weeks after I got saved they had an altar call for people to be delivered of a habit. I did not think to go up—but my sister nudged me. So I went. The pastor prayed for me—laid hands on me and commanded a spirit of nicotine to come out. I was not familiar with these terms but I left the church that night not having any desire to smoke. I even carried cigarettes with me for a month just in case. It has now been 25 years—and I have never had the desire, not even once." In this narrative, salvation was the necessary but insufficient precondition for healing; deliverance from a demonic "spirit of nicotine"—although an unfamiliar concept for this new Christian—avowedly freed her from physical dependence on nicotine. Similarly, a Londrina woman associated healing with the religious rite of passage that symbolized her full affiliation with Christianity: "I was healed from back pains on the day of the baptism." For such individuals, healings were not isolated events but memorable landmarks of spiritual progress.

Researchers facing the daunting task of sifting through countless similar-sounding claims may be tempted to dismiss healings of apparently "minor" conditions, such as back pain, as relatively insignificant. Yet even such minor healings may seem quite significant from the perspective of the person needing and experiencing healing. A woman who traveled with GA on an IMT to Brazil recalled that "the Lord healed me of back pain 7–8 yrs ago." Likewise, a British man who joined an IMT to Brazil in 2007 remembers that "I had muscle spasms in my upper back with pain about 35 yrs ago and was prayed over and received total healing in the mid 70s." For each of these respondents, healing from back pain was an unforgettable experience, not a trivial one. Indeed, people reporting healings do not always differentiate so clearly among major and minor conditions as researchers are likely to do. Thus, an IMT woman in Brazil recalled being healed "many different times—most significant—diverticulitis 13 days in bed without improving—went to healing service, had hands laid on me and was well the next day (went back to doctor for colonoscopy and told us no longer had diverticulitis after inflammation experience and healing)." This respondent continued, without emphasizing a difference in severity, that "also on the way to this trip had severely painful ingrown toenail—received prayer by team members and is completely healed in one day." From the perspective of this IMT member, both instances similarly indicated divine superintendence.

Past experiences of complete or even partial healing encouraged respondents to seek further prayer. One Londrina respondent cataloged healings received when "I came here for the first time: Eye—dislocation of the retina. Back—paralyzed right leg. Psoriasis (half way). Thyroid (half way). Obesity." This person had returned to receive more prayer for the thyroid and psoriasis (a skin disease). A woman attending a GA conference in Pennsylvania attested to having received partial healing from multiple sclerosis, but she was seeking more prayer, because "I still can't function as I desire." Another Pennsylvania attendee reported that she had "rec'd some healing" from chronic immune deficiency syndrome, but she was back for more prayer, because "it isn't complete." Respondents reporting complete healing of non-life-threatening conditions also returned for more prayer if subsequently afflicted with life-threatening diseases. For instance, an Imperatriz woman formerly healed of chronic migraines was currently seeking healing from Hodgkin's lymphoma.

Overall, responses indicate that past healings are both commonplace and memorable experiences in the lives of pentecostals surveyed. From the vantage of the individual recalling such a healing, even a relatively minor recovery may be imbued with deeply significant and enduring meanings.

Current Needs for Healing

The preconference survey asked all subjects, "Do you need healing for any illness, pain, or disability?" A total of 659 people, 72 percent of all those returning questionnaires, answered that they did. Brazilians were no more likely than North Americans to report needing healing. Most respondents (94 percent of North Americans and 83 percent of Brazilians) in need of healing reported physical problems, rather than mental or emotional or spiritual ones. The need most frequently expressed—accounting for 37 percent of those reporting a problem—was for healing of "pain" in some part of the body, such as the back, shoulder, or neck (17 percent); head (7 percent); knees (5 percent); feet (3 percent); hips (2 percent); or arms (2 percent). These findings are consistent with national U.S. surveys reporting the prevalence of pain.[17]

Respondents cited diverse physical problems of varying levels of severity, with significant differences between Brazilians and North Americans. The most common problems related to vision (8 percent), the cardiovascular system (6 percent), the stomach (5 percent), the respiratory system (5 percent), the reproductive system (4 percent), the skin (3 percent), the throat (3 percent), allergies (3 percent), hearing (2 percent), diabetes (2 percent), cysts or tumors (2 percent), the thyroid (2 percent), the kidneys (2 percent), the teeth (2 percent), infections or inflammation (2 percent), or hernias (1 percent). Only 1 percent noted cancer diagnoses. The median level of self-reported symptom severity on a 0-to-10 Likert scale was 5 for both Brazilians and North Americans, but Brazilians reported higher mean Likert scores overall.[18] Both Brazilians and North Americans reported considerably more non-life-threatening than life-threatening conditions. However, North Americans were more likely to report both non-life-threatening and life-threatening problems.[19] This may indicate that Brazilians on average had more serious health problems, but those North Americans with the most serious conditions made special efforts (and had the financial means) to travel to conferences in search of healing.

Scholars of North American pentecostalism have noted a late-twentieth-century shift in emphasis from physical to "inner" or "emotional" healing as medical care has improved and the field of psychotherapy has burgeoned.[20] Brazilians were surprisingly more likely than North Americans to report a primary need for mental, emotional, or spiritual healing.[21] One woman in Londrina noted that "Jesus healed me from depression through a study about inner healing and spiritual warfare." Another Londrina woman wrote in English, "I [sic] inner healing session after the abortion" and then went on to describe the circumstances in Portuguese. Nineteen Brazilians (3 percent of all needs reported), but no North Americans, sought healing from depression. Of the 2 percent of respondents who wanted healing from addictions, 9 of 11 were Brazilian. Brazilians were also more likely to report a need for healing of marriages and relationships with family and friends (1 percent). One Imperatriz woman described "pain in my heart (but it is sentimental) for not having someone next to me (my husband). Because I have been betrayed, I sometimes feel that my heart aches but I already forgave the one who betrayed me." Such accounts are consistent with research on Brazil showing that alcoholism, domestic strife, and abandonment of families by men are major social problems.[22]

The number of needs reported and the poignant detail in which they were described suggest that need for healing contributed to the appeal of the surveyed conferences. This is consistent with the religion scholar Andrew Chesnut's conclusion that health crises are the primary reason that Brazilians affiliate with pentecostalism. In contrast, scholars of North American pentecostalism have found that most adherents are first attracted to the pentecostal worldview rather than initially coming with a specific need for healing. The current findings do not contradict such results. Yet only one respondent stated that he had *not* come to the surveyed conference seeking healing: a local man attending a GA conference in Ontario noted that he had "several needs of healing but did not come specifically for healing." Other individuals who acknowledged that their health problems were not life threatening nevertheless affirmed a strong desire for divine healing. For example, an IMT woman stated that her chronic breast cysts were "so far all non-cancerous, but I would love to be healed." Even if not the primary or only draw, many North Americans as well as Brazilians attended surveyed conferences seeking healing.[23]

To summarize, current need for healing was a major source of concern for many pentecostal respondents. It is striking just how much human suffering the collected surveys reflect. Some conditions were of short duration and relatively minor severity—such as headaches that had started earlier in the day—but other problems had caused difficulties for decades or threatened death. Even if not life threatening, both chronic and acute health problems appeared to be the source of great pain, inconvenience, and embarrassment.

Healings Reported at Surveyed Conferences

The postconference survey asked all subjects, "Did you receive healing (complete or partial) for any pain, illness, or disability at this conference?" Fifty-two percent of those who answered this question responded in the affirmative. Brazilians and North Americans were equally likely to report healing. Those who answered "no" to this question, or who implied a negative answer by not returning the postconference survey, should not be overlooked. For these individuals—the majority of conference attendees—the suffering described on the preconference surveys presumably continued or intensified as expectation may have turned to disappointment, confusion, anger, or despair.[24]

Most respondents claiming healing reported improvement of a physical problem. Previous studies have suggested that those claiming healing at pentecostal conferences typically report partial healing of relatively minor conditions, mostly of a mental, emotional or spiritual nature, rather than being cured of major physical problems. In his study of Catholic Charismatic healing, the anthropologist Thomas Csordas argued that "spiritual healing . . . serves as a kind of 'consolation prize'" for those who receive no other type of healing. "If the all-benevolent Lord does not see fit to grant a physical healing, for example, He will 'at least' grant a spiritual healing. Thus, spiritual healing performs a crucial role as a hedge against the failure of healing prayer."[25] The present study did not find that respondents who wanted healing of a physical problem were likely to experience healing of a mental, emotional, or spiritual problem instead. Only three respondents who wanted physical healing instead reported mental/emotional or spiritual but not physical healing. Three other respondents wanted mental/emotional or spiritual healing but reported physical healing instead. For instance, a Londrina man wanted healing for "ringing in my ears/fear of not believing in God." He listed his expectation of receiving healing as 5 on a 0-to-10 scale. Perhaps this individual had in mind a fear of not being healed—which worried him that he might not have enough faith to be healed. After the conference, he reported being "almost completely" healed of "ringing in the ears, hypertension, stomach"; he did not mention being relieved of his fear, although the physical healing experience may have implicitly alleviated his fears. Some reports of mental/emotional healing may have reflected a desire to be able to report some condition as healed, as in the case of a woman from Londrina who wrote: "I do not know if I can call it a healing, but before I was very timid and by the grace of the Lord I was healed." North Americans

(84 percent) were more likely than Brazilians (80 percent) to report healing of physical as opposed to mental, emotional, or spiritual problems (just as North Americans were more likely to report needing physical healing).[26] For both groups a majority of healings reported were of a physical nature.[27]

The problems reported as healed tended to include the same problems people came to the surveyed conferences wanting to have healed. Scholars have suggested that pentecostals generally redefine their health problems as more minor retrospectively in order to be able to claim some degree of healing. On the basis of her study of 160 participants in Baltimore, Maryland Charismatic and New Age healing groups, the sociologist Deborah Glik has argued that "the majority of respondents claimed some degree of healing, associated mainly with symptom alleviation rather than cure." According to Glik, "redefined health problems were often less serious, less medical, more chronic, and more 'emergent' than those initially defined, and respondents who redefined problems were significantly more likely to claim a healing experience." Glik noted a "pattern of discrepancy" between "problems initially presented" and "those for which healing was claimed."[28] In contrast, the current study found that most respondents claiming healing (69 percent) reported being healed of at least one of the conditions they had listed as needs at the beginning of the conference. Most respondents (78 percent) claimed healing of just one problem, but 22 percent reported healing of more than one condition, and 6 percent reported healing of three or more problems. Table 4.4 gives the following breakdown of respondents reporting being healed of:

Table 4.4.   Comparison of Preconference Needs and Postconference Healing Claims.

	Same +	Same –	Same +/–	Total Same	Diff. –	Diff. +	Total Diff.
Brazilian	21	7	3	90	23	16	39
North American	11	6	0	76	21	15	36
Total	32	13	3	**166**	44	31	**75**

- all the same needs listed on the preconference survey plus other problems (same +)
- a subset of needs listed on the preconference survey (same −)
- a subset of needs listed on the preconference survey plus other problems (same +/−)
- at least one problem listed on the preconference survey (total same)
- problems instead of those listed on the preconference survey (diff. −)
- problems even though no needs were listed on the preconference survey (diff. +)
- problems other than any listed on the preconference survey (total diff.)

An important factor in explaining the relatively numerous instances of people claiming healing of a different condition than that indicated on the preconference survey is the common pentecostal practice of delivering "words of knowledge." Leaders as well as lay conference participants frequently announced problems that they believed God especially wanted to heal at that time. Typically, those reporting healing after responding to a word of knowledge explained: "I didn't think about getting prayer for this." Although scholars are correct in observing that many words of knowledge delivered in pentecostal conferences are relatively nonspecific, it is also worth noting that many of the preconference descriptions people gave of the conditions they needed healed are also quite general, such as back pain or a headache. There was a fairly close match in the kinds of conditions indicated in words of knowledge and the sorts of problems that people wanted healed when they arrived at the conferences.[29]

The types of conditions reported as healed on the postconference survey were roughly comparable to the types of conditions people listed as needs on the preconference survey. Table 4.5 shows the total numbers of people reporting specific needs for healing on the preconference survey with the numbers indicating whether or not they were healed of specific conditions on the postconference survey. Only

Table 4.5. Comparison of Types of Conditions Reported as Needs and as Healed.

	Need	Healed	Not Sure/ Not Healed
Pain	243	153	51
Back/shoulder/neck	121	72	20
Vision	51	6	19
Headaches	46	29	9
Cardiovascular system	42	11	14
Stomach	36	10	9
Knees	34	26	8
Respiratory system	32	13	8
Reproductive system	26	6	7
Legs	26	12	7
Skin	23	2	7
Feet	22	14	8
Throat	21	2	3
Depression	19	5	5
Allergies	18	0	3
Hearing	16	7	6
Infection/inflammation	16	2	3
Hips	16	11	1
Diabetes	15	2	6
Cysts/tumors	15	5	1
Thyroid	13	2	3
Arms	13	5	2
Kidneys	12	3	5
Teeth	11	3	4
Mental/emotional/inner healing	11	9	4
Addiction	11	2	2
Obesity/eating disorder	8	1	1
Hands	7	5	2
Hernia	7	1	2
Jaw	6	2	3
Insomnia	6	1	2
Cancer	6	2	4

about half as many people returned postconference surveys as returned preconference surveys, and it may be assumed that most of those not returning a postconference survey did not experience healing.

Researchers have commented, sometimes disdainfully, on the relatively minor character of many of the healings reported at pentecostal conferences. Claims of diminished pain or increased mobility are all but impossible to measure or submit to outside verification. Such claims are among the easiest to explain as resulting through natural mind-body interactions. Accurately identifying the mechanism of healing generally makes little practical difference for the person who sensed pain before and now feels better. (Indeed, in order for mind-body interactions to *work*, it may be necessary for the person to perceive a divine process.) But more scientifically oriented interpreters are understandably likely to hypothesize that other similar-sounding claims probably reflect a similarly naïve misinterpretation of data that can better be accounted for within more mundane explanatory frameworks.[30]

The severity of conditions healed approximately matched the severity of conditions people wanted healed. It is true that a larger proportion of the people surveyed reported healing from pain than from cancer, but it is also the case that a larger proportion came to the conferences complaining of pain than of cancer. A series of statistical tests shows that, on the whole, respondents were no more likely to report being healed of a condition with less severe symptoms, of shorter duration, or that was of a less life-threatening nature than the needs listed on the preconference surveys.[31] It is important to note that certain types of condition are more conducive than others to self-evaluation of whether healing has occurred in the short time frame of a single religious service or even a multiday conference. For instance, it was easier for individuals to tell whether their back pain or headache felt better than to know whether diabetes, thyroid deficiency, or cancer had been cured. Thus, an IMT man wanting his thyroid healed answered that he was "not sure" whether he was healed, because "I would have to go to my doctor for tests." Similarly, a Missouri man indicated that he could not answer how much his condition had improved because he had "never had symptoms of heart valve problem." Likewise, a respondent from Rio seeking "spiritual health and whole mental health" was "not sure" whether healing had resulted because it was "still premature." Postconference healing reports are constrained by what individuals could sense shortly after prayer, before they had opportunity to return to their doctors or to see how they fared over time.

Respondents generally reported sensate improvements, but not total "cures." The survey asked individuals not only whether they were healed, but also to indicate how much healing they had experienced ("not at all," "less than half," "about half," "more than half," "almost completely," "completely"), and to quantify the severity of their symptoms before and after prayer on a 0-to-10 Likert scale. For those reporting healing, the median degree of healing claimed was "almost completely," or 3 on a Likert scale. Our findings did not confirm a claim made by other researchers that conference attendees tend to experience higher degrees of healing for mental/emotional than physical problems. Rather, there was a trend toward respondents with more serious or life-threatening conditions reporting a more complete degree of healing than respondents with non-life-threatening conditions.[32]

All in all, the data show that the typical respondent claiming healing— perhaps in response to a word of knowledge—experienced an "almost complete" reduction in pain related to the same physical problem noted on the preconference survey as in need of healing.

Evidence of Healing

The postconference survey asked, "How do you know that your condition has been healed?" Most respondents (87 percent) specified a sensate improvement in physical symptoms. Scholars have noted that pentecostals construct a holistic concept of healing that may not require a biomedical standard of "cure."[33] For the surveyed pentecostals, whether I used less or more restrictive criteria for counting "healing," there were significant correlations with higher degrees of improvement in physical problems. In other words, respondents may have understood healing holistically, but this holistic view included an ideal of sensate improvement in physical symptoms.[34]

Brazilians were more likely than North Americans to claim healing without sensate improvement, based on "faith" and/or a spiritual experience at the time of prayer, or by faith alone.[35] One respondent from Londrina claimed healing from heart and hearing problems "by faith, and the 'fire' I felt during the prayer." This individual's heart condition may not have caused any symptoms that could be gauged during a religious service. More striking is that the individual also claimed healing of a hearing problem without noting improved ability to hear. Similarly, a North American man attested to healing of asthma, noting that he had trouble breathing only during an asthma attack. Because he was not having difficulty at the time of prayer, he reported healing based on faith alone: "I just know, trusting God. I got prayed for and just believe I was healed." This kind of Word of Faith approach of claiming healing by faith regardless of symptoms is relatively rare among pentecostals surveyed because ANGA leaders strongly discourage it.

The pentecostal leaders studied construct healing primarily as sensate improvement in symptoms. Randy Clark regularly urges conference attendees and IMT members to report healing only if the person receiving prayer feels an 80 percent or greater reduction in symptoms or becomes able to do something he or she could not do before prayer. Clark's reason for the 80 percent standard, borrowed from the Argentinian pentecostal healing evangelist Omar Cabrera, is that if people think they must wait for 100 percent improvement they will worry so much about some possible last remnant of symptoms that they will never claim healing. In many instances, Brazilian as well as North American survey respondents noted the disappearance of symptoms after prayer. A woman from Rio de Janeiro described her healing as "a simple experience—my sister prayed and the symptoms that I was feeling disappeared." Such lay conference participants, like ANGA leaders, define healing as disappearance, or at least decrease of symptoms.[36]

Some respondents who reported no physical improvement or a minimal reduction in symptoms circled "not sure" when asked whether they had been healed. (They were counted as "not healed" for purposes of analysis.) Such individuals seemingly wanted to avoid making a "negative confession"—a phrase commonly employed in Word of Faith circles in which it is believed that spoken words shape reality in positive or negative ways—by admitting that they had not been healed, but they also wanted to avoid claiming healing that had obviously not oc-curred. A participant in GA's Pennsylvania conference acknowledged that her arthritic knee pain was "not at all" improved, but she circled "not sure" because "the Lord spoke to me & said you have to walk your healing out. . . . because I believe what my God says—I can't see it—it hasn't changed—I believe it will." Another woman in Pennsylvania who circled "not sure" noted that "my hip pain did not leave but Heidi [Baker] had a word [of knowledge] for hips and Randy [Clark] had it for ligaments under the left knee & down the leg—I believe they are mine even though I can't prove it now. I'll know as time goes on." Some Bra-zilians reasoned similarly, such as one Londrina man with pain in the right shoulder who circled "not sure," elaborating that "I was healed, but I need to move daily on the name of Jesus." Before the conference, he rated the severity of his problem as a "10." He left blank the postcon-ference question asking the current severity—perhaps to avoid making a negative confession.

To sum up, most but not all respondents—and more North Ameri-cans than Brazilians—claimed healing on the basis of sensate physical changes. Those who wanted to avoid making a negative confession tended to report that they were "not sure" rather than definitively an-swering whether they were or were not healed.

Expectation of Healing

If concerns about avoiding making a negative confession may have tempted some respondents to overreport their level of experienced healing, the same concerns may also have resulted in a tendency to underreport need for healing. Some respondents exhibited a strong concern about avoiding answering survey questions in ways that might suggest lack of faith (presumably reducing their chances of being healed), whereas others readily admitted that their faith was limited. One Missouri man answered the preconference question "Do you need healing for any illness, pain, or disability?" by circling "yes," but also inserting "the complete manifestation of" before the printed word "healing," and appending: "by Faith in what Jesus did I'm healed." This man rated the severity of his asthma symptoms as 8 out of 10 for how bothersome they had been in the past week. He reported healing on the postconference survey. Judging from his preconference responses, one might have expected this man to claim healing "by faith," but instead he cited the physical evidence of "better breathing" and quantified that his Likert symptom level had gone down to a 3, and that he felt "more than half" better. By contrast, a Missouri woman acknowledged on her March 2006 preconference survey that "I've had pain in my left hip since Sept. 2004." She rated her expectation of healing at the conference as 7 out of 10 (coded as "not sure"). Yet she reported at the end of the conference that "the pain is gone. It all seemed to be so simple and unexpected." The first of these respondents went to great lengths to affirm "faith" on his preconference survey, whereas the second acknowledged doubts. Yet both experienced healing evidenced by improvement in symptoms.

Popular conceptions of "faith healing" typically portray faith (or the power of suggestion) as the crucial ingredient in spiritual healing. Jesus reputedly told certain supplicants that their faith had made them well but chastised others for lack of faith. In the current survey, reported expectation of healing did not statistically predict healing experiences.[37]

Survey responses do suggest differences in how North American and Brazilian respondents constructed faith. North Americans who said on the preconference survey that they expected healing were less likely to admit of plans to visit a doctor in the future if not healed, and there was a trend toward their being more likely to report an improvement in symptoms on the postconference survey.[38] Brazilians were, overall, more likely than North Americans to rate their faith levels as high.[39] In fact, 73 percent of Brazilians rated their expectancy of receiving healing at the given conference as 10 out of 10, compared with just 7 percent of IMT participants attending these same conferences.[40] Brazilians were, however, no more likely than North Americans to report experiencing healing.

Survey questions about expectation cannot get inside the heads of respondents to identify whether or how strongly they "really" expected healing. Brazilian respondents may not have had any higher actual faith levels than the North Americans surveyed, but Brazilians may have been acting from a cultural context (influenced by globally disseminated Word of Faith teachings and the locally prominent

Universal Church of the Kingdom of God) that predisposed them to feel a stronger need to "prove" their faith by how they responded to the survey. This points to a larger limitation of the entire survey project—that analysis must be based on how respondents chose to present themselves to the researchers, which may not clearly reflect self-concept or behavior.

Analysis of the available evidence suggests that, for both Brazilians and North Americans, faith and expectancy may be less significant in predicting healing than either pentecostal or biomedical theories have supposed.

Explanations of Illness and Healing

Survey questions probed how respondents understood the causes of illness and healing. As the sociologists Meredith McGuire and Debra Kantor note, "A bodily experience has no inherent meaning; meaning must be applied, drawing upon a range of culturally available explanations." The preconference questionnaire asked subjects "How do you explain the cause of the condition you described?" Respondents drew on a mix of biomedical and spiritual explanations, but how individuals answered the question did not predict expectation or experience of healing.[41]

Most respondents (91 percent) recognized the role of natural causal agents. Many also posited the involvement of spiritual factors. For instance, an IMT woman in Brazil attributed her irritable bowel syndrome to a combination of "not eating right, not exercising enough, stress and inability to let go of past sins." A Brazilian man seeking healing for his knee acknowledged his doctor's diagnosis of "inflammation," but added that the root cause was his sin of "criticism." Other respondents similarly interpreted medical diagnoses within a larger worldview in which the spiritual and physical realms are interconnected. For a problem diagnosed by doctors as "stress," a respondent from Rio de Janeiro elaborated "spiritual warfare, stress and witchcraft," blaming past involvement in a number of African-Brazilian religious traditions: Umbanda, Candomblé, spiritualism, Catholic folk healing, and psychic surgery. It is not, however, the case that Brazilians invariably attributed physical or even mental disorders to evil spirits. For example, a Londrina respondent sought healing from the medically defined problem of "psychosis." Conversely, some North Americans identified spiritual causes of medically diagnosed conditions, as when a Missouri respondent attributed asthma to an "Evil Spirit (curse)." Such individuals accepted the accuracy of medical diagnoses, but framed them within comprehensive spiritual explanatory models.

The common tendency to associate sickness with sin validated religious choices if healing followed repentance but occasioned frustration when individuals remained sick even after renouncing their sins. A man from Rio recalled that "at age 15 I had epileptic seizures. When I returned to Christ, I was healed." A Londrina respondent similarly reported that "my back was healed. I had backslidden for many years. My posture was correlated." By contrast, a woman from Rio with a hearing problem voiced perplexity that "I am at a good place in the Spirit" but had not been healed.

A few respondents who had not yet experienced complete healing attributed their afflictions to "God's will," a common teaching in historic Catholic and Protestant churches, but one that ANGA theology explicitly rejects (instead arguing that Satan is the source of sickness and God is the source of healing). A respondent from Londrina who reported having previously been healed of several other problems, including a dislocated retina, a paralyzed leg, and obesity, but not thyroid deficiency or psoriasis, concluded, "May the will of God be sovereign." A Missouri woman expressed uncertainty about God's will to complete her healing; she had already been "healed supernaturally from Lupus. Not sure about healing for inner ear [drum, a residual effect of lupus], because it keeps me humble & remembering how far I have come." One Londrina woman explained the death of her husband a year before by redefining the experience not as failure, but as the "ultimate" healing: "My husband and I prayed much for his healing, but unfortunately he came to die on 6.28.07. It really shook me and I separated myself from God. But Praise God that today I understand that though he was not healed physically, his soul was healed and he is with God. Today I can pray again, speak of the gift of healing, and I am asking for God to guide me." Respondents who remained ill or who experienced the loss of loved ones searched for explanations that would allow them to minimize what psychologists call *cognitive dissonance*, or uncomfortably conflicting ideas, in order to retain their belief in God, divine love, and God's general will for healing.[42]

When respondents did experience healing, they often identified the cause as divine love. One respondent from Rio recalled that "I had back pains and one day through prayer and love I felt a heat on my back and I noticed that I was healed." A Pennsylvania woman similarly attributed her healing from an eating disorder to "God's Power—love." A Londrina woman explained that "I suffered of bronchitis and asthma for over 23 years. I was healed as I received the love of God, for the illness has its roots in the emotional level. I believed that God had favorite children. I was born in a Christian home and everyone was healed except for me. With this revelation, the bronchitis and asthma never came back." In this woman's evaluation, a revelation of divine love for her personally had healed her emotional, and consequently her physical, afflictions. Other respondents characterized their healing as resulting from "God's great love," "the love of Christ for me," that "God met me and knows me," "God touched me," "Jesus lives and heals," or cited "faith in God," the "supernatural," or a "miracle."

In response to the postconference survey question "How do you explain your healing?" not a single respondent gave a naturalistic explanation. Most respondents both cited natural causes for their illnesses and spiritual causes for their healings. A majority directly credited God with healing, although Brazilians were more likely than North Americans to single out the importance of their own faith without also mentioning divine activity.[43] One Pennsylvania man, far from crediting his own faith for healing from back and ankle pain, affirmed that it "had to be divine Holy Spirit. I didn't do anything except receive." Whether respondents credited their own faith, divine intervention, or a combination did not predict expectation or experience of healing.

In sum, respondents understood sicknesses as resulting from both natural and spiritual factors but credited healing subsequent to prayer to divine activity and human faith. Respondents commonly interpreted healing as an expression of divine love. Differences in explanations of illness and healing did not predict expectations or experiences of healing.

Attitudes Toward and Usage of Prayer

Although the overall percentages of people reporting healing at the conferences surveyed are relatively small, such a finding would not surprise many pentecostals. Often, pentecostals receive prayer on multiple occasions for a given problem before claiming complete healing, believing that the healing process usually occurs over time (sometimes as brief a span as ten minutes, sometimes as long as ten years) and that even if the healing itself is instantaneously recognized, in many cases much groundwork has already been laid. This model of "persevering" prayer contrasts with another influential pentecostal model, the Word of Faith view that prayer should be offered only once for any one problem before claiming healing by faith, lest repeated prayer denote lack of faith and thus block healing.

The pentecostals surveyed took the position that failure to continue praying for one's needs until physical symptoms were "completely" resolved diminished the likelihood of ever experiencing complete healing. If a typical GA participant is not healed of a problem at a single conference, more prayer will be sought at other conferences and church services. Hence, it is unsurprising that cross-sectional studies by previous researchers—for instance William Nolen's visit to a single Kathryn Kuhlman service in 1973—have yielded rather unimpressive empirical findings. Longitudinal studies are also needed to follow the course of individuals over months and sometimes years in their pursuit of healing through prayer for more serious maladies. In such a project, it is important to be wary of the *post hoc, ergo propter hoc* fallacy commonly committed by pentecostals in their self-interpretations. Most people recover from most health problems regardless of treatment, and treatments often work for reasons—such as the placebo effect and other psychosomatic mechanisms—other than users think. Stories like George's, which opened this chapter, are nevertheless extraordinarily revealing. Surveyed at any single conference, George would have been unable to report any degree of healing, although after attending many conferences he reported as a cumulative effect a major, medically unexpected recovery.[44]

Pentecostal theology envisions more serious conditions as generally requiring prayer of greater frequency or duration than that requisite for minor problems. The claim of a woman from Londrina is noteworthy in this regard: "I fought with a reading problem from 2002 to 2004 and I was healed at a prayer marathon after being prayed for 49 times." Such "marathons" reflect the practice of "soaking prayer" popularized by the Catholic ANGA-affiliated Francis MacNutt. For MacNutt, prayer is comparable to radiation therapy in its cumulative effects, because there are presumably levels of "more" and "less" anointing, difficulty, and healing. Pentecostals commonly acknowledge that healing is not always immediate and that it may not be clear why healing occurs when it does. A woman from Imperatriz recalled, "I received the cure of migraine headaches I had from the time I was a child until I was 15. I suffered from the ailment constantly. One morning in the worship service at my congregation I received the cure." Often pentecostals report some measure of "improvement" rather than complete healing after a given prayer, believing that such improvements are often progressive and lead eventually to total healing. Francis MacNutt has estimated that in the many conferences he has conducted, on average one quarter of attendees are healed completely at the time, one quarter report no benefit, and one half experience a measure of improvement. This fits with the present finding that the typical respondent claiming healing improved "almost completely." From the perspective of a pentecostal needing healing, any improvement can be interpreted as a sign of God's love and as an encouragement to pursue further prayer.[45]

Most of those reporting a need for healing at the beginning of a surveyed conference (76 percent) had already received prayer for their conditions, and most planned to continue praying for the same condition if not healed at the current conference (92 percent). Of those who received prayer before, 35 percent had experienced some lasting improvement, 19 percent had initially improved but the symptoms had returned, and 46 percent had experienced no improvement. North Americans were more likely to report a sensate improvement in symptoms at the current conference if they had received prayer for the condition previously and planned to continue praying if not healed during the surveyed conference.[46] There were no significant correlations between past or future prayer and healing for Brazilians, perhaps because prayer was a more universal strategy.

Although respondents reported praying for their own healing, many emphasized the importance of receiving intercessory prayer from others. An Imperatriz man noted that currently "I don't have any illness but sometimes when I get a pain I order it to leave my body and soon I am cured." Several Brazilian respondents specified the names of visiting American healing evangelists, such as Randy Clark and the ANGA-affiliated Gary Oates, whose prayers had apparently led to past healings. Others emphasized the very ordinariness of the people praying and the circumstances under which healing was experienced. A woman from Londrina "had lots of migraines, we went to the hospital regularly when my nose bled. In a simple church I was healed; this was decidedly what happened." Similarly, an IMT woman in Brazil reported healing of a vitreous detachment that could not be fixed and that kept her from "seeing well out of the right eye." She had received "numerous prayers" on various occasions, but one day "a lady laid her hands on the eye, prayed quickly and it was healed. I felt nothing." A woman from Imperatriz did not even know right away that she was healed "in 2006 when a beloved American brother prayed for me. I was healed, however, I only realized when I got home." Although most respondents emphasized the value of proximal, in-person intercession, a few noted that they were healed while praying along with televangelists. An Imperatriz man recalled that "once I had a very sore throat. I prayed with the pastor on television and when the prayer was finished the pain had totally passed." Certain Protestant respondents acknowledged that they were healed through the prayers of Catholics— while simultaneously revealing an anti-Catholic bias. A woman from Imperatriz noted that "I had a balance disorder from an ear infection. I was very dizzy and could not stand on my feet for too long. I would fall from side to side. One day a Catholic sister prayed for me. I had a lot of faith and independent of her religion I was cured." From this woman's perspective, healing did not validate the beliefs of the person praying but instead reflected God's compassionate response to the faith of the person seeking intercession.

In total, responses suggest that surveyed pentecostals tend to view prayer as a strategy that should be, and often is, employed repeatedly for the same condition, because prayer appears to be cumulative in its effects. Proximal intercessory prayer is valued as particularly efficacious.

Attitudes Toward and Usage of Medicine

Respondents did not generally express antimedical views. Most Brazilians (83 percent) as well as most North Americans (81 percent) who needed healing had already visited a doctor for their complaint, although North Americans exhibited a trend toward having made more medical visits for the same problem.[47] North Americans who had not been to a doctor were more likely to experience an improvement in symptoms at the surveyed conference. It was interesting that North Americans who planned to visit a doctor if not first healed through prayer were less likely to expect healing but more likely to experience healing during the surveyed event.[48] This may suggest that North Americans perceived (even unconsciously) some tension between faith and medicine and that prayer was most effective for conditions that were bothersome but not sufficiently serious to require immediate medical attention. No significant correlations could be found in the Brazilian data.

Brazilian respondents tended to credit God with all healing, whether or not physicians were involved. An individual from Imperatriz attested to a previous divine healing of a "renal problem, serious operation, I trusted the Lord and was healed." It is impossible for a researcher to evaluate whether this individual's faith had anything to do with surviving the operation. But from the perspective of the person reporting the healing, the nonexistent evidential value of the example is entirely beside the point. This individual's purpose in attesting to divine healing was to express gratitude to God, not to provide proof to skeptics. Brazilians did not in every instance credit God with unexpected medical healing. A man from Rio marveled that, following an accident that had forced the surgical removal of several vertebrae, "the doctors said that I would be a paraplegic and today I walk and drive." This man did not classify his better-than-expected recovery as "divine healing." He answered "no" to the question about whether he had ever experienced divine healing and indicated an intention to continue seeking prayer for greater mobility of his neck.

Brazilian respondents were more likely than North Americans to articulate the idea that prayer is superior to medical treatment. A woman from Imperatriz refused to accept her doctor's negative prognosis as determinative. She recalled that "when the doctor told me I had an incurable disease I did not accept it and I went to the doctor of all doctors Jesus Christ. He heard my prayer and I was completely healed." Other Brazilians noted that they sought prayer before going to the doctor. A Londrina woman remembered that "three years ago I was overwhelmed with severe menstrual cramps. One day during my menstrual cycle, I had severe cramps and I was ready to go to the doctor, and I decided to stay with a sister and she prayed and I never again felt cramps." Because this woman felt herself healed through prayer, she did not go the doctor.

Brazilians who had been to a doctor often sought prayer instead of following through on taking prescribed medications or undergoing advised surgical procedures. One Brazilian respondent after another said of their doctors, "he prescribed medicine but I did not get it"; he said I should "take the prescribed medication for the rest of my life, but I do not take it"; or "he prescribed medication for me to take and I did not take it." Even when the prescribed medications were simple antibiotics to treat an infection, Brazilians did not always fill prescriptions (whereas North Americans—who generally either have health insurance or easy access to inexpensive generic drugs—did consistently note using prescribed pharmaceuticals). Brazilians failed to carry through with recommended operations, for instance reporting that "it has been more than a year that I have had this lump [hernia] the size of a ping pong ball. . . . [The doctor] scheduled the surgery one year ago but I still have not had the surgery." Likewise, in a case of severe myopia, "there is no cure without surgery and it would cost 8 thousand reais [approximately $4,500] and it might be more." Financial constraints, rather than principled objections, seem to have been a major reason Brazilians did not take their doctors' advice. Brazilians sought prayer for healing in part because they had no viable medical options.

Brazilians did express religious objections to the use of unconventional medical alternatives. The preconference survey asked, "Other than prayer, had you ever tried alternative medical or spiritual remedies for healing of this condition?" One individual from Imperatriz admitted to having previously resorted to Umbanda, Kardecist spiritism, spiritualism, African-Brazilian prayer leaders, and Catholic folk healers "when I wasn't an evangelical Christian." As for future plans, the respondent indicated "prayer" alone. Several other Brazilians who described plans to use alternative medical or spiritual remedies specified that what they meant was "only Jesus," "more intimacy with God," or that "God is my medicine." In contrast, some North American respondents expressed greater acceptance of alternative medicine. A North American who had used chiropractic, massage, naturopathy, acupuncture, herbs, and homeopathy to cope with multiple sclerosis specified that "all my healing has come from alternative medicine" and indicated an intention to continue using alternatives alongside prayer and conventional medicine. A Southern Baptist IMT woman, just a month before traveling with GA to Brazil, had visited an herbalist for "detox" to treat her psoriasis; if she was not healed during the present conference, this individual noted an intention to continue using prayer and alternative therapies, but not conventional medicine. There were no statistically significant correlations between use of alternative medicine and needs, expectations, or experiences of healing.[49]

All told, Brazilian and North American respondents used medical treatments alongside prayer. Brazilians tended to rely more heavily on prayer, in part because they could not afford expensive medical interventions.

Conclusion

The survey responses presented and analyzed in this chapter illumine how certain suffering individuals constructed prayer for healing in the context of GA and IM healing conferences. Many of the Brazilians and North Americans surveyed attended pentecostal conferences with a personal need for healing in mind, despite having previously sought help through prayer and conventional or alternative medicine. Respondents remembered past divine healing experiences and attested to sensate improvements in physical symptoms at the surveyed events. These findings lead to the question of how pentecostal perceptions of the effects of healing prayer compare with measurable outcomes.

CHAPTER 5

Can Health Outcomes of Prayer
Be Measured?

✦

Preaching from a makeshift bamboo platform in a typical mud-hut village in northern Mozambique, near the southeast coast of Africa, Heidi Baker issued a *promessa*, or promise: "Bring me your deaf, and Jesus will heal them, in confirmation of the truth of the gospel." The moon was almost full on this clear, tropical winter night. In the comfortable 80-degree weather, most of the thousand-person, predominantly Muslim village had come out. They were attracted by the showing of the *Jesus Film*, in the local Makua language, on a portable projector and screen with the help of generator-powered stage lights and a booming sound system. "Bring me your deaf!" Mama Aida, as Baker had come to be known, repeated in ringing tones in both Portuguese and Makua. A young adult man, Jordan, was soon brought by his father and a quickly gathering crowd of villagers, all of whom chimed that Jordan had been deaf and mute since birth. Before Baker prayed for him, on this particular evening she had given permission for a western research group to test his hearing, using a portable audiometry machine that administered tones of increasing intensities through headphones. The audiometer produced tones all the way up to 100 decibels hearing level (dBHL) in each ear—louder than a motorcycle—but there was still no response by the subject. Using gestures, Jordan replied negatively to his father's query as to whether he had heard anything.[1]

Baker put her arms around Jordan and prayed for less than a minute, commanding his ears to be opened in Jesus's name. She then asked Jordan to repeat after her as she spoke from behind his line of sight: "Jezush," "Hallelujah," and clapped her hands and snapped her fingers at increasing distances. Jordan imitated the words in a hoarse, raspy voice, and clapped and snapped after Baker, to the apparent amazement of the crowd, who insisted that he had never before heard or spoken at all. My research group reinstalled the headphones and tried to explain to the subject how to press the audiometer's response button as soon as he heard a tone. Jordan pressed the response button when some of the tones reached 60 dBHL (0 dBHL being perfect hearing)—not terrible, given that the ambient noise from the commotion of the crowd and the still-playing sound system remained around 80 decibels sound pressure level (dBSPL). But unless the subject was constantly reminded to press the button when he heard a tone, he apparently forgot the instructions in the excitement of new sensory input and an interested crowd of villagers, missionaries, and researchers all focusing their attention on him. Jordan seemed to press the button consistently whenever we reminded him that he should press the button when he heard a sound, but otherwise he did not press the button. He responded more reliably when instead asked to imitate the tone when he heard it, or when asked after each tone (or nontone, silences that tested for false-positive responses) whether he had heard anything.[2]

Explaining how to take a hearing test in the context of an illiterate culture to someone apparently unaccustomed to the communication of complex ideas seemed to present more of a challenge than the researchers had anticipated. Alternatively, Jordan's hearing had not improved, but he only appeared to respond to tones because he coincidentally pressed the button or made sounds when tones were being administered. In either case, the audiometer repeatedly aborted its automated protocol due to inconsistent responses. After switching to the manual mode and getting a few false positives mixed in with some consistent responses, we finally gave up after forty-five minutes of trying to measure the subject's hearing, and excluded the results from the analysis. Nevertheless, it seemed obvious to everyone present that Jordan was repeating sounds in his environment, whereas a few minutes before he had appeared oblivious even to very loud noise. At the platform, Baker gave an altar call for "salvation from sin," and a number of people in the crowd responded. The following morning, two Muslim men sought out the small village church, wanting to convert to Christianity because they had heard about the apparent miracle. Did Baker's prayers result in a cure of deafness, and was it "miraculous"? How can scholars account for this apparent success of healing prayer—despite the failure of western technology to measure it?

Context and Study Design

Mozambique is a country that has suffered a long history of political instability and natural disasters, including droughts and famine. The nation won independence from Portugal in 1975, but colonial domination soon gave way to civil war between a Marxist government (the Frelimo party) and a resistance movement (the Renamo party). Guerrilla warfare destroyed roads, schools, and hospitals. More than a million land mines maimed (and caused potentially lethal infections in) civilian villagers. Until the signing of a national peace agreement in 1992, Mozambique ranked as the world's economically poorest country. The economic situation had improved somewhat by the early twenty-first century, but there was still only one doctor for every forty thousand people. Without widespread immunization or treatment for rampant diseases such as malaria, half the nation's children were dying before they reached age five. The AIDS epidemic had orphaned an estimated two hundred thousand children. In religious terms, the nation is mixed in composition; a 2007 census found 28 percent Catholics, 28 percent Protestants, 18 percent Muslims, and 26 percent in other categories; the Muslim population is concentrated in the northern provinces.[3]

Heidi and Rolland Baker arrived in Mozambique in 1995, having secured government permission to take charge of a dilapidated orphanage in the capital city of Maputo, in southern Mozambique. When officials from the Department of Education became aware that the Bakers were using the orphanage to proselytize, they issued an eviction notice. Over the next five years, the Bakers and their struggling organization, Iris Ministries, founded other small, nongovernmental children's centers in several cities. After flooding devastated much of the country in 2000, IM's relationship with government officials improved dramatically. The Bakers' location in Mozambique, combined with their connections to a global pentecostal community that had financial resources made them more effective than large aid organizations such as the United Nations World Food Program (with whom IM cooperated) in getting emergency relief to refugees in certain remote areas. Iris Ministries was one among many international aid organizations that responded to the crisis, but IM's contributions made national and local government leaders—not to mention starving, diseased refugees—more receptive to its initiatives, even if economic aid came with a religious agenda. As IM's position in Mozambique stabilized, the group expanded its outreach activities into the northern, largely Muslim provinces.[4]

Northern Mozambican villages generally consist of a collection of between a few dozen and several thousand mud huts without electricity or running water (figure 5.1). Village culture is nonliterate; clocks, calendars, and modern technology are unknown, and few people have even a general idea of their own ages. During a typical village outreach, several Mozambican and western IM team members drive several hours from the ministry base in the small seaside city of Pemba, Cabo Delgado, in northern Mozambique, over primitive roads that see little vehicular traffic—or they fly a small airplane to cover longer distances. Occasionally, IM staff are joined by short-term western volunteers, such as the GA team that was visiting during our research. The combined team sets up portable audiovisual projection equipment, with which IM attracts a crowd of between several hundred and several thousand people by singing to keyboard accompaniment and showing a local-language film (very much a novelty in these areas). An IM leader stands up to preach that Jesus came to forgive sins and heal diseases— often prefacing the message by inviting the "deaf" and "blind" to the platform to receive prayer for healing (figure 5.2).

Iris Ministries leaders are not the only persons to perform proximal intercessory prayer, or PIP—in-person, hands-on, intercessory prayer to God for healing. Other Mozambican and western IM—and in this case, GA—affiliates also pray for healing. This happens during evening outreaches and daytime "medical clinics," in which IM staff

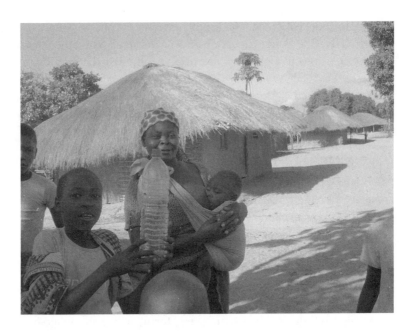

Figure 5.1. Impiri, Cabo Delgado, Mozambique is a typical mud-hut village. An empty plastic water bottle obtained from a Global Awakening visitor seems photo worthy to one young villager, 2009. Photograph in author's collection.

members set up a tent from which a medical doctor and several nurses, with the help of Mozambicans and other westerners, distribute basic pharmaceuticals and administer PIP. Attendance at medical clinics is much lower than at evening meetings (several dozen people, most of whom are seen in private), and emotional stimulants such as loud music and public healing displays are minimal (figure 5.3).

Mozambican and western IM team members all use a similar procedure in praying for healing. They usually spend between one to fifteen minutes (more rarely an hour or more) administering PIP. They place their hands on the recipient's head or shoulders and sometimes embrace the person in a hug, keeping their eyes open to observe results. In soft tones, they petition God to heal, invite the Holy Spirit's anointing, and command healing and the departure of any evil spirits in Jesus's name. Those praying then ask recipients whether they were

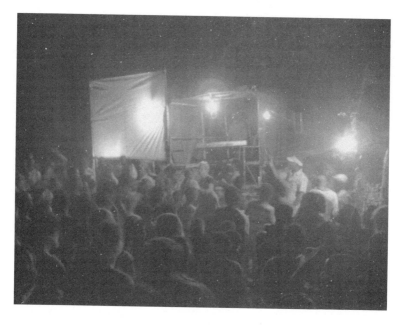

Figure 5.2. Attracting a crowd in Chiuré village, Cabo Delgado, Mozambique, 2009. Photograph in author's collection.

healed. If recipients respond negatively or that the healing is partial, intercessors continue PIP. If the response is affirmative, intercessors conduct informal tests, such as asking recipients to repeat words or sounds (for instance hand claps) intoned from behind the head or to count fingers from roughly one foot away. If recipients are unable or only partially able to perform tasks, intercessors continue PIP for as long as circumstances permit—generally no longer than fifteen minutes.

In designing a clinical study—to assess what, if anything, changes measurably when people pray for and report healing in such a context—I wanted to isolate conditions that were less susceptible to psychosomatic improvements than the condition, rheumatoid arthritis, selected by Dale Matthews in his study of direct-contact, proximal prayer (introduced in chapter 2). I wanted to focus on conditions for which we could measure psychophysical thresholds (the lowest sensory levels that subjects can reliably detect), rather than relying exclusively on

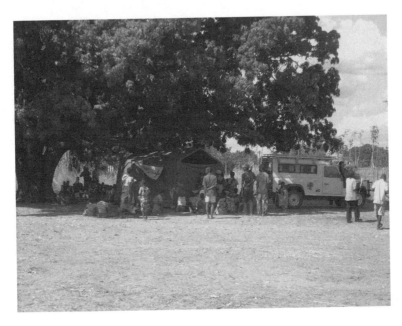

Figure 5.3. Iris Ministries sets up a medical tent to offer basic pharmaceuticals alongside prayer, Namuno village, Cabo Delgado, Mozambique, 2009. Photograph in author's collection.

self-reports of symptom severity. But I was also interested in conditions for which self-reporting played some role (as opposed to a condition such as asymptomatic hepatitis C, which can be assessed only by blood tests), because I wanted to compare perceptions of healing with measurable effects of PIP. It also seemed advantageous to be able to compare the magnitude of any effects with similar research on the effects of hypnosis and intentional suggestion, since it has been proposed in the scholarly literature that any effects of in-person prayer may be attributable to unintentional hypnosis or suggestion. Testing hearing and vision fit these criteria. Compared with a condition such as rheumatoid arthritis, auditory and visual impairments are relatively less sensitive to, although not unaffected by, psychosomatic factors. Indeed, researchers have investigated effects of suggestion and hypnosis on vision and hearing and claimed significant results. The effects of suggestion seem to be correlated with the intensity and duration of the healing encounter. It is noteworthy that in the Matthews study, subjects each received six hours of in-person prayer, whereas in the present study interventions were considerably briefer—in many instances less than one minute total.[5]

Hearing and vision are regularly singled out for prayer at IM and GA conferences. Indeed, in pentecostal circles, the IM codirector Heidi Baker is widely perceived as a "specialist" in prayer for hearing and vision. Baker herself claims that she has the strongest "anointing" for healing of the deaf during village outreaches in the predominantly Muslim province of Cabo Delgado, Mozambique. Baker asserted during an interview in the summer of 2009 that every deaf Mozambican she had prayed for in Cabo Delgado in the past two years had exhibited at least some improvement in hearing. By contrast, Baker reports having spent a year praying for every blind person she could find (more than twenty) without seeing any of them healed, until she prayed for three blind women on each of three consecutive days. All the women happened to be named Mama Aida (Baker's own Mozambican name), and all of them reportedly experienced healing. (Baker interprets the coincidence as God's way of showing her that she was spiritually "blind" and that the similarly blind western church needed "to see what God is doing among the poorest people on earth." As a result of this experience, Baker began accepting invitations to speak in churches outside Africa.) Baker claims that now many, but not all, blind Mozambicans receive their sight following prayer; her organization provides housing, food, and other care for those not yet healed. Healing of the blind and deaf are also often reported at GA conferences in Brazilian cities. Indeed, when GA reports trip statistics of healing (through methods that bear no resemblance to actual statistical analysis), they make separate tallies for the number of "deaf or mostly deaf" and "blind or legally blind"—within which categories a wide range of levels of impairment are included. The category of "legally blind" makes no literal sense as it was used, for instance, in the context of a convention in Recife, Pernambuco, Brazil in 2006, but rather indicates a generalized recognition of some visual impairment that is less than total blindness.[6]

It is important to understand precisely what pentecostals are claiming when they assert that someone has been "healed" of blindness, deafness, or, for that matter, any other condition. The term *healing* is used to denote improvement, not necessarily a change from total absence to total fullness of function. Thus, a false dichotomy is created by asking the common question of whether someone with auditory or visual impairments is or is not "healed" after prayer. In our study, most improvements measured occurred somewhere along a continuum; most subjects were not totally blind or deaf before prayer, nor had their vision or hearing reached a clinical standard of perfection by the end of prayer; nevertheless, measurable improvements could be noted in several instances.

Groups such as IM and GA emphasize prayer for hearing and vision for several overlapping reasons, all of which relate to how impressive it sounds to claim to cure the blind and deaf. These are, indeed, serious conditions that are relatively common in the two-thirds world. The World Health Organization estimates that 80 percent of the 278 million people who now have significant hearing impairments and 90 percent of the 285 million people with significant visual impairments live in the developing world. Very few of these people can obtain hearing aids, corrective lenses, surgery, or any other medical assistance. From the perspective of those seeking compelling healing testimonies, praying for improvements in hearing and vision offers the advantage that bystanders can immediately tell whether those receiving prayer—people generally known by lifelong community members actually to have the problems claimed—are newly able to hear or see stimuli in their surroundings. It is more difficult for skeptical observers summarily to dismiss improvements in these conditions, compared with a complaint such as back pain, as falsely perceived in the emotional excitement of the moment or as the product of merely "functional" improvements through "psychosomatic" processes of suggestion. Perhaps most important of all, in the worldview shared by GA and IM, Bible passages specifically refer to healing of the blind and deaf as evidence of the coming of the kingdom of God. For this last reason in particular, there is likely a tendency to exaggerate the levels of visual and hearing impairments before prayer and to exaggerate the levels of improvement after prayer in order to validate the IM and GA ministries. Thus, in evaluating such claims, outside verification of self-reported "statistics" of how many deaf and blind are healed is imperative. Our study, though limited in its implications by field conditions, is a first step toward empirical investigation.[7]

We began with the null hypothesis that PIP would have no significant effect on subject outcomes. At research sites in Impiri, Namuno, and Chiúre villages and Pemba city, Cabo Delgado, Mozambique; Barretos and São Paulo (São Paulo), and Uberlandia, Minas Gerais, Brazil; Seattle, Washington and Chicago, Illinois, we assessed auditory and visual acuity before and after PIP, using a handheld audiometer (with sound meter) and vision charts (16′ and 20″ "Tumbling E"), (figures 5.4 and 5.5).[8]

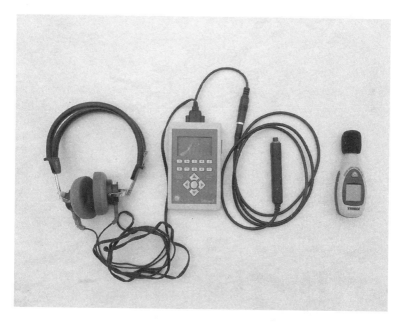

Figure 5.4. Audiometer and sound meter used for measuring hearing thresholds and ambient noise. Photograph in author's collection.

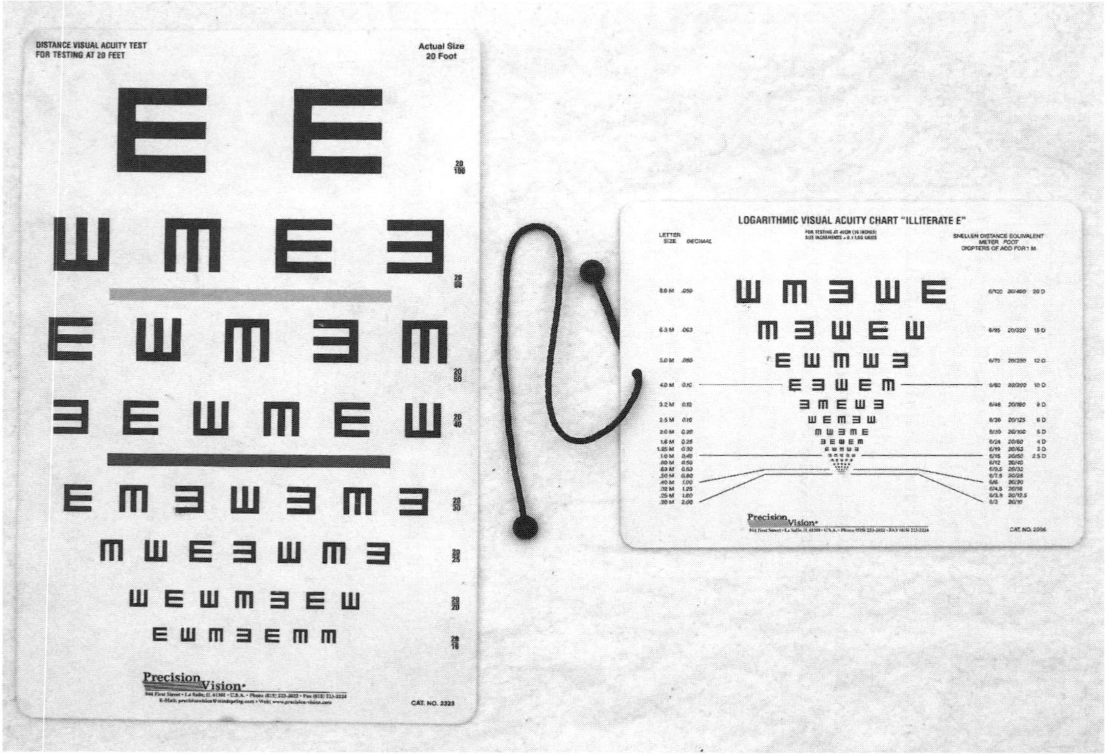

Figure 5.5. Tumbling E vision charts for use at 16′ and 20′ to measure vision thresholds of illiterate subjects. Photograph in author's collection.

In Mozambique, every consecutive subject was included in the study who received prayer for vision or hearing loss and assented to diagnostic tests (all subjects assented). Measurements were taken immediately before and after PIP. The results of this research have been published in the peer-reviewed *Southern Medical Journal,* but the findings are reported more fully here and interpreted within the framework of a broader research program. We prospectively evaluated a consecutive series of 24 Mozambican subjects (19 males, 5 females) reporting auditory (14 subjects) and/or visual (11 subjects) impairments who received PIP; one subject reported both hearing and vision impairment. No subject ordinarily wore hearing aids or corrective lenses.[9]

Hearing and Vision Measurement Methods

In measuring hearing thresholds, we followed the standard Carhart-Jerger protocol. That is, wearing over-the-ear headphones, subjects were administered a 3 kHz tone (a series of three beeps) well above the subject's threshold. The hearing threshold, or lowest intensity sound that subjects could reliably detect, was determined by administering a moderately loud tone and, if this did not elicit a response, progressively increasing the intensity to verify ability to respond to instructions; then the intensity was reduced to well below threshold. The intensity was increased systematically by 5 dBHL until a response was made, then the threshold was verified by lowering the intensity by 10 dBHL at a time and increasing it by 5 dBHL until a response was made. The maximum intensity that could be generated by the audiometer was 100 dBHL. Subjects whose pre-PIP hearing thresholds exceeded 100 dBHL were assigned a conservative 105 dBHL threshold for subsequent analysis. Participants responded by button press or verbal confirmation when they heard a sound. Some participants needed prompting to indicate whether or not they heard a sound, apparently due to difficulty following directions with the unfamiliar equipment—few if any of the villagers had ever seen a similar device. In these cases, prompts were periodically given intentionally when no sound was presented in order to detect false-positive responses (that is, reporting hearing a tone when none was administered). To avoid overestimating sensitivity, we excluded three subjects from further analysis due to false-positive responses; in the case of at least one of the excluded subjects—Jordan in the opening anecdote—there is more to the story than what this summary dismissal conveys, given that Jordan was newly able to imitate sounds in his surroundings.[10]

Cultural context and field conditions required modifications in protocol. After using the audiometer response button with the first subject, Jordan, and noting that other subjects also seemed perplexed by the response button, we switched to primarily using verbal responses (such as imitating the "beep" sound), recognizing that the unfamiliar equipment was confusing to the subject pool. Due to time constraints (that is, IM leaders were unwilling to allow major interruptions in the flow of their meetings), hearing thresholds were measured for all subjects only at 3 kHz (part of the frequency range of human speech) in each ear separately instead of across the whole frequency spectrum; we took additional measurements as time allowed. Also because of time constraints, some subjects reporting problems only in one ear were tested only (pre- and post-PIP) in that ear. A total of eighteen ears in eleven individuals with hearing impairments were analyzed. Measurements could not be conducted in an acoustically isolated room due to the remote field locations. The high ambient noise (AN) from the nearby crowd of people also presented a considerable challenge to measurement accuracy. Ambient noise was measured with a sound meter in dBSPL in order to investigate whether its fluctuations presented a potential confound in the before- versus after-PIP measurements. Ambient noise was measured separately during pre- and post-PIP testing, with minimum and maximum AN recorded during each subject session.[11]

We measured visual acuity using 16″ (6 subjects) and/or 20′ charts (5 subjects). We used the 20′ chart for elderly subjects who had no major difficulties with the 16″ chart but who reported distance-vision problems. Subjects were tested using both eyes together, or with each eye separately, as time allowed. The minimum measurable acuity was 20/400 on the 16″ chart and 20/100 on the 20′ chart. A premeasured string was used to hold charts at the appropriate distance. As researchers pointed to each letter, subjects pointed or verbally indicated which direction it faced; researchers did not confirm whether responses were correct, making it less likely that subjects memorized the chart. Due to field-imposed time constraints, those subjects who self-reported improvements were given priority for retesting after PIP; we lacked time to retest two of eleven subjects, so we reported them as unimproved.

Quantitative Results: Mozambique

We found a highly significant improvement in hearing across the eighteen ears of eleven subjects (figure 5.6).[12] Two subjects showed hearing thresholds reduced by over 50 dBHL. Ambient noise was very high during testing (50–100 dBSPL), but AN (85 dBSPL), calculated for each subject individually as the average of the minimum and maximum noise during measurement, was unchanged between pre- and post-PIP tests, indicating that AN was not likely to be a confound.[13] The average 3 kHz threshold after PIP was 49.4 dBHL, which was slightly high, perhaps due to high AN.[14]

Significant visual improvements (both difference and ratio of before versus after) were seen across the tested population (figure 5.7a).[15] Three of eleven subjects improved from 20/400 or worse to 20/80 or better, and one subject improved from unable to count fingers at 1′ (20/8000) to 20/125 (figure 5.7b). All but one vision subject was tested in broad daylight; the remaining subject was tested after dark, with illumination provided by stage lights and a flashlight; the lighting level did not appear improved between the pre- and posttest (conducted less than one minute later), making it unlikely that variable lighting was a confound.

Both auditory (p < 0.003) and visual (p < 0.02) improvements were statistically significant across the tested populations. Generally, the greater the hearing or vision impairment pre-PIP, the greater the post-PIP improvement.

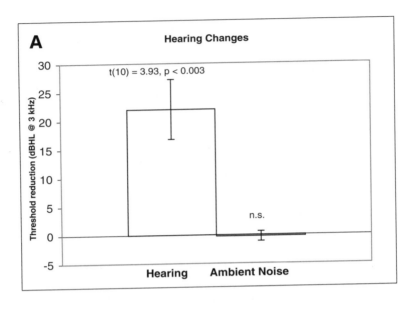

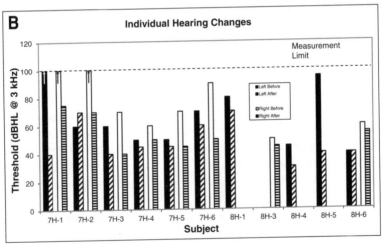

Figure 5.6a–b. Mozambique hearing measurements. (a) Hearing thresholds at 3 kHz were significantly improved across the population. Improvements cannot be accounted for by reductions in ambient noise. (b) Hearing threshold changes ranged from 10 dBHL increase to over 60 dBHL improvement.

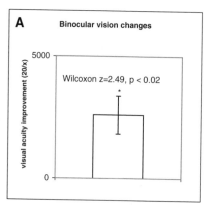
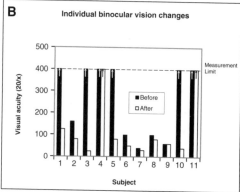

Figure 5.7a–b. Mozambique vision measurements. (a) Binocular visual acuity increased significantly across the population. (b) Individual improvements ranged from no change to an improvement from >20/400 to 20/25.

Quantitative Results: Brazil

Although we found statistically significant changes in both hearing and vision after PIP administered in Mozambique, we still did not know whether these results would generalize to other individual intercessors, regions, and cultural groups. One particular IM leader, Heidi Baker, was involved in administering PIP in 13 out of 25 interventions. To investigate replicability, we performed a follow-up study at GA meetings in urban Brazil, using the same measurement methods for hearing and vision employed in rural Mozambique.[16]

Healing services in Brazil are typically conducted in urban churches or outdoor sports arenas. Many attendees are poor (GA provides bus service from *favelas,* or urban squatter areas) and have little access to reliable medical care, but electricity, mobile phones, and sanitation services are generally available, and a basic level of education is common. Brazil's economy has grown since the country gained independence from Portugal in 1822 and formed a republican government in 1889, supported by abundant natural resources, well-established transportation networks, and rapid urbanization. Although still classified as a developing country, Brazil has the eighth largest economy in the world as judged by gross domestic product. A substantial rich-poor gap means, however, that many of the benefits of economic growth have not reached the nation's poor majority. Pentecostalism thrives among the impoverished. Although nearly three-quarters of the population (74 percent) identify as Catholic, Protestant churches, two thirds of which are Pentecostal, had attracted 15 percent of the population by the 2000 census; approximately 2 percent of Brazilians acknowledge practicing African-Brazilian religions or spiritism. Local pentecostal leaders are conscious of their rivalry with traditional healers who promote religions such as Umbanda and Candomblé or devotions to Catholic saints. Although a competitive religious climate heightens the social significance of public healing displays, GA has contributed to a shift in emphasis in pentecostal churches from leaders toward laity in the role of praying for healing.[17]

Global Awakening teams model democratized prayer practices. A typical GA international ministry trip team consists of a handful of leaders accompanied by dozens of lay western pentecostals. In our study, Randy Clark administered PIP to only one of the forty-one subjects analyzed. All and only those individuals tested both before and after PIP were included in the analysis. Of those, two subjects were excluded due to failures in measuring AN during testing. A total of eighteen auditory subjects were analyzed, with both ears for each subject included individually as separate measurements (figure 5.8).

At 3kHz, the results showed a significant population reduction in hearing thresholds.[18] This finding must be treated with caution, however, because AN also showed a reduction, from an average of 60.4 dBSPL before PIP to 52.2 dBSPL after PIP. This AN reduction was also significant.[19] Thus, it is unclear whether the reduced hearing thresholds were the result of reduced AN or improved hearing. To investigate this further, the threshold reduction was correlated with AN in the subset of ears showing reduced hearing thresholds (n = 16). Although the correlation was positive, it was not significant.[20] Therefore it remains unclear how much of the threshold reduction can be attributed to reduced AN and how much can be attributed to other factors.

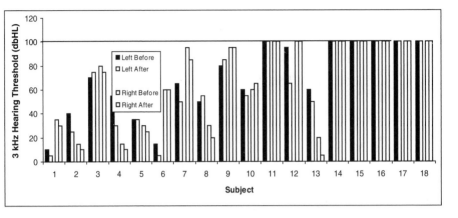

Figure 5.8. Brazil hearing measurements. Results from replication study in urban Brazil, showing the degree of hearing-threshold improvement at 3kHz.

We found more clearly significant effects for visual acuity. A total of 23 pre- and post-PIP visual measurement pairs were taken (6 left, 6 right, 11 both eyes). The ratio of before versus after acuity was calculated for each measurement pair (figure 5.9).

The null hypothesis of no improvement in visual acuity after PIP (acuity ratio = 1) was tested, and the acuity improvement ratio[21] was significantly greater than 1.[22] These results are consistent with a significant population improvement in visual acuity after PIP. Overall, the results from the follow-up study in Brazil replicate the findings of significant improvement in visual acuity as reported in Mozambique.

Quantitative Results: United States

At first glance, it may appear preferable to conduct studies of hearing and vision in a country such as the United States, where most people with impairments have received regular testing, the records for which could be readily procured, and where it would be easy to perform post-PIP tests under controlled conditions, for instance, in an acoustically isolated room. Both IM's Heidi Baker and GA's Randy Clark regularly

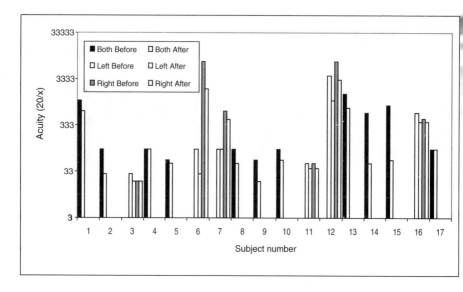

Figure 5.9. Brazil vision measurements. Results from replication study in urban Brazil, showing acuity before and after PIP on log scale. Note subjects 14 and 15, who improved from 20/600 or worse to 20/60 or better.

speak at pentecostal healing conferences throughout North America. Both claim, however, that they witness many more dramatic improvements in places such as Mozambique and Brazil than they do in more developed countries, arguing that "anointing" and "faith" tend to be lower where medical therapies are more widely available (but also insisting that healings *should* be equally available in the western world). One factor in the higher rate of claims made outside North America is that there is a larger pool of people for whom to pray. Many more people have untreated auditory and visual impairments in developing countries. In industrialized areas, not only do fewer people have impairments to begin with but most of those who do already wear hearing aids or corrective lenses or have had surgery or other interventions to improve their conditions. North Americans typically pursue prayer for their hearing or vision at most as a "second thought," not because healing is desperately needed, but because dispensing with medical aids would be more convenient or would provide a "testimony." (See though, in chapter 3, the cases of Joy, a U.S. woman who did present medical records indicating improved vision after prayer, and Daisy, a U.S. woman whose hearing test results were better subsequent to prayer.)[23]

We administered six pretests to five American and one Norwegian GA team members in Mozambique, all of whom wore hearing aids or corrective lenses. Only three of those tested actually sought prayer for healing during the conference, none of them from Baker. Moreover, it was unclear that any of those who did seek prayer for ear or eye conditions would have done so had pre- and posttesting not been offered. An unexpected obstacle was that one subject did not want to remove her contact lenses, since she had not brought extra cleaning solution— necessary, in case the prayer did not work; another subject realized after testing that he had forgotten to remove one of his hearing aids for the test.

We administered several dozen pre-PIP hearing and vision tests at a pentecostal conference in Chicago, Illinois sponsored by the Toronto-offshoot HUB (His United Body) Ministries, where Heidi Baker was the scheduled speaker. Baker, as is typical of her North American appearances, did not actually pray for healing for conference attendees. In Baker's words, her "ministry is different in the U.S."—focused on motivating privileged westerners to live sacrificial lives of love. None of the pretested subjects returned for posttests or testified in the meeting to healing of visual or auditory problems. It also is unclear how many of them sought or received prayer for these conditions—or would have, had the very fact of on-site testing not suggested the idea. Only one Chicago subject was blind, and none was deaf. Baker nevertheless asserted that four deaf children had been healed during a similar conference in Boston, Massachusetts the previous week, although I did not succeed in contacting anyone in Boston who could confirm the report. Baker's claim was frustrating from a research standpoint because I had actually made plans to conduct similar tests in Boston during the specified event, but Baker's personal assistant had denied me permission on the grounds that Baker does not normally pray for healing when in the United States. Baker's host in Chicago, Nancy

Magiera, extended permission despite the earlier refusal, and once personally contacted, Baker agreed—and, indeed, told me, "you should have been in Boston last week."

We also measured vision and hearing at a GA conference in Seattle, Washington; only two of seventeen pre- and posttested subjects exhibited measurable improvements. It is again unclear how many of them sought prayer specifically for healing of these conditions during the conference, or how many would have, had not the availability of "free testing" encouraged them to do so. Thus, the presence of the researchers and the introduction of testing procedures seemed to present more of a confound in U.S. settings than in Mozambican and Brazilian contexts. In the latter, prayer for severe auditory and visual impairments is regularly performed in crowded settings, and the presence of a few more people, even with novel mechanical devices, exerts relatively little effect on the behavior of intercessors or prayer recipients. I would like to see further testing in developed countries, but there are important advantages to more natural prayer settings even though the field conditions are difficult.

Comparison of Results to Suggestion and Hypnosis

Studies of PIP, by their nature, expose subjects to suggestions that their conditions will improve. Could the changes we measured be attributable to suggestion or hypnosis? One previous study showed that a few minutes of suggestion led to statistically significant visual acuity improvement, but the effect was so small that a subject would not be able to read one line smaller on the standard Snellen visual acuity chart. Several studies of hypnotic suggestion showed an average 2 or 2.5 times increase in visual acuity, with the largest reported improvement from 20/200 to 20/20, despite no measurable changes in ocular refraction. Other studies reported no improvement in vision or auditory thresholds after hypnotic suggestion. A 2004 review article summarizes the results of suggestion and hypnosis studies as failing to demonstrate significant improvements in vision or hearing. The average visual acuity improvement measured in Mozambique was over tenfold, significantly higher than in suggestion or hypnosis studies (figure 5.10)[24]

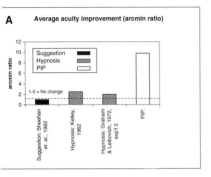
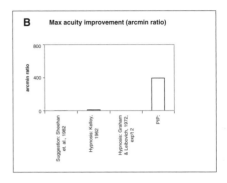

Figure 5.10a–b. Comparison with suggestion and hypnosis. (a) Studies of hypnotic suggestion and suggestion without hypnosis have found small but statistically significant improvements in visual acuity. The magnitude of effects across the population was significantly larger in PIP than in suggestion and hypnosis. (b) The maximum improvement in visual acuity for PIP was larger than the maximum improvement reported for suggestion and hypnosis.

Qualitative Analysis of Hearing Data

For several clinical subjects, we were able to supplement quantitative measurements with qualitative analyses based on interviews and observations. Three hearing subjects presented with particularly notable characteristics. Martine is an elderly Mozambican woman brought to IM for both hearing and vision impairments during an evening outreach in Namuno village. Before PIP, she made no response at 100 dBHL in either ear at 3 kHz. After PIP, Martine responded at 75 dBHL in the right ear, 40 dBHL in the left ear. Martine reported that she could not read the 20/400 line of the 16″ vision chart with both eyes together; she did not exhibit any improvement in visual acuity after Baker administered PIP. We had a rare opportunity to retest Martine the following morning—it is extremely difficult to conduct follow-up, given that villagers quickly disperse after meetings, leaving no "address," let alone possessing phones—when Martine came to IM's medical tent to receive additional PIP for her eyes. It was notable that Martine's hearing threshold remained unchanged in the left ear compared with the previous evening's post-PIP level, but the right ear seemed further improved—with a new threshold of 30 dBHL. Interestingly, pentecostals claim that healing is often progressive, and that improvements may begin or intensify hours or days following PIP. Despite having received PIP the previous evening, Martine still reported being unable to read the 20/400 line of the vision chart. After ten minutes of additional PIP by IM-affiliated Mozambicans and westerners (Baker was not present), Martine accurately read the 20/80 line of the vision chart.[25]

Martine's case is illuminating for several reasons. First, it helps to answer the question of whether those who exhibit improvements immediately after prayer ever "remain healed" the next day, once emotional stimulants have died down. This subject's hearing threshold not only remained improved, but actually improved further overnight—although only in one ear, the one that still "needed" further improvement. This is, of course, only one case and does not answer the question of whether "healings" are always enduring, nor does it answer whether this particular improvement was permanent. It would have been desirable to retest Martine's hearing a week or a month or more later, but the field conditions made this unfeasible. I hope that future studies will be able to include such longitudinal follow-up. Second, it is noteworthy that Martine's hearing, but not her vision, improved immediately following Baker's PIP; this is consistent with Baker's own claim that she has more anointing for the healing of hearing than eyesight. It is also interesting that Martine's vision did improve following additional PIP by other IM affiliates, suggesting that the effects of PIP may not be limited to a narrow group of intercessors and consistent with the pentecostal claim that ordinary practitioners can effect healing. This case also suggests that some people who do not improve following PIP may yet improve if additional PIP is subsequently administered, whether because of cumulative effects of additional prayer or differences among intercessors, or because the subject is better prepared for (or "has more faith" in) the intervention. The pentecostals studied often advise those still needing healing after prayer not to give up on account of prematurely drawing the conclusion that healing must not be "God's will." Similarly, the unhealed are often encouraged that they need not refrain from seeking further PIP because it seemingly exhibits lack of faith (a position common in the Word of Faith movement).[26]

One of the most intriguing cases we came across is Gabriel, a thirty-seven-year-old Brazilian man tested in the city of Uberlandia, Minas Gerais, Brazil. Gabriel had at the time worked for GA for five years as a translator and Brazilian national coordinator and had attended many healing conferences. On the day we were conducting hearing tests, GA's director, Randy Clark, was teaching a group of Brazilians how to pray for healing, using his translator, Gabriel, as an example. As Gabriel recounts his experience, Clark had said:

> "for example if [Gabriel] here had a problem with his ear and I'll pray for him," and he put his hand on my left ear, . . . I said, "you know Randy if you are going to demonstrate that, I have a problem with the right ear so if you could pray for that." He said, "Oh sure, this is good. So you actually have a problem. Let's see how it goes." So he starts to pray for me, teaching the church how to do it, praying for me. And then I started to feel heat. And it started to feel like a little ant started to crawl up and down the inner ear, deep down inside. And I still feel it tingling right now. I think it is an on-going process. . . . He said "more Lord," and I felt it jump to four [ants]. "More Lord" again and it jumped to about ten. He said, "more Lord" and it was about twenty . . . and it was like a whole ant nest was here crawling. And then it became a tingling. It just became a tingling. And then it was very hot, very hot, very hot. And then it suddenly became very cold as if someone had come with like a mint or something very fresh in the mouth and then blew. Very cold. And I also felt a cold hand on my shoulder. And I looked back and no one was there; it was just Randy touching my ear. So exactly the moment that I felt this cold hand on my shoulder, Randy said, "yes Lord, thank you for your angels. They are here with us helping in this healing." . . . And then at the end of the prayer I felt like when you clean your ear. It was very itchy, very itchy. And you know when you clean it with a q-tip and it hurts, you pressure [sic] too hard, that is the feeling I had. Okay, so people start to talk to me and I could hear better so it started to hurt a little bit and I was covering it, you know, for a while. . . . and I can still feel it is a little tender, there is still movement in there. So I think it is not over yet.

This account is unusually detailed in describing how the PIP experience felt: heat, cold, a sensation like that of the touch of a cold hand (interpreted as an "angel" at Clark's verbal suggestion), sounds so loud that it hurt, and most interesting of all, the tingling and itching of a growing ant colony. This interview was conducted four hours after PIP was administered. In a similarity to the progressive nature of Martine's case, Gabriel expressed the belief that effects of PIP were residual and that the healing was an "on-going process" that was "not over yet." This was a rare instance when it was possible to follow up by e-mail one month later and to conduct an interview two years later at GA's 2011 Voice of the Apostles conference in Pennsylvania: Gabriel reported that his hearing had remained improved and that he could still "tell the difference." Before-and-after hearing tests at 500 Hz, 3 kHz, and 6 kHz revealed reduced hearing thresholds in both Gabriel's right and left ears—with the single exception that the right-ear 3 kHz threshold remained unchanged. This is important, because in a more time-pressured situation the protocol was to test only at 3 kHz in the ear in which a problem was claimed—in this case the right ear, which would have led us to conclude that there had been no change in hearing thresholds despite the subject's perceived improvement. This case suggests the value in future research of testing multiple frequencies in both ears whenever at all possible given the field conditions.[27]

Maria is a thirty-one-year-old Brazilian woman in Uberlandia whose hearing was tested before and after PIP on one day—and re-tested the following day, with slightly lower thresholds the second day, consistent with the idea of "progressive healings." This example stands out because the numerical changes measured in pre- and posttests were subtle, especially in the right ear. Taken by themselves, they might reasonably be dismissed as not indicating any real change given that AN also diminished. Yet Maria claimed that after PIP she could hear her son's voice for the first time. She reported that she had been sleeping normally the day after receiving PIP when, in the words of a translator, "she woke up with a sound and then she got very, very worried with this different sound. And she was so happy because she could listen. She got scared to hear this sound. And she calmed down after that and she cried. And the sound she heard was this boy and she was so, so emotional because she was listening to the son and for the first time she could hear her son. And she cried and wept." In this instance, interview data provides an important complement to quantitative measurements in evaluating the effects of PIP on hearing, suggesting that even minor changes in measured thresholds can have a significant experiential impact.[28]

Qualitative Analysis of Vision Data

Several vision subjects provided additional details in interviews that complement the quantitative measurements. Maryam is an elderly Mozambican woman brought to IM during an evening outreach in Impiri village who reported that her vision had been "very bad" "for a long time." Maryam did not have an opportunity to observe other apparent healings, because she was the first person who came forward for prayer in that vicinity. After Maryam could not identify any characters on the 16″ vision chart, Baker asked her to count the number of fingers she held up from approximately 1′ away (20/8000); Maryam said she could not see the fingers. Baker hugged Maryam and briefly (spending less than one minute) administered PIP. Baker again held up fingers, and Maryam counted them accurately. She was then able to read as far down as the 20/125 line of the vision chart with each eye singly. Because this incident took place at night, under relatively weak artificial lighting, there is no way of knowing how well she could have seen in daylight. Maryam's right eye, which was observably discolored white, remained discolored after PIP; Baker herself commented on this anomaly (Baker claims that sometimes she observes a change in eye coloration—from white to gray to brown—after prayer, but no such claims were made during the time when we were present), simply stating that she did not know how the woman could see out of that eye. Maryam reported that she felt very happy—and she looked happy—because, in her words, before she could only see a little, but now she could see much.

We measured a similarly large change in visual thresholds during an outreach event conducted in broad daylight at which there was no "emotional" music or preaching and Baker was not herself present.

Michael is a young adult Mozambican man who came to a morning medical clinic in Chiuré village set up by IM from the back of a truck parked alongside an unpaved road. Michael came seeking prayer for his vision; he waited in line while another man received PIP for neck pain (and reported healing), but Michael did not observe any other subjects having their vision tested. Before PIP, Michael could not read the 20/400 line of the 16″ chart with both eyes together. After PIP of approximately five minutes duration by western IM affiliates, Michael read the 20/125 line with both eyes; after several additional minutes of PIP, he read the 20/40 line. Michael then announced that he wanted to be baptized immediately, since Baker and other IM leaders were then at a nearby river baptizing new converts. Before he had a chance to go, Baker returned to the vicinity and, hearing Michael talk about being healed, used his recent experience as a point of departure to preach to a gathering crowd of Mozambicans who had not been at the river; several in the crowd promptly converted to Christianity and asked to be baptized without delay.

Consistent with the predictions of *Hernstein's matching law*—that those seeking a benefit explore multiple sources in proportion to expectation of reward—Makuas, like many other Africans, typically employ an experimental approach to healing, visiting *curandeiros, feiticeiros,* Muslim spiritualists, and Christian healers. In times of health crisis, Mozambicans often have nowhere to turn besides traditional healers who may employ a combination of herbal medicine, divination, and spiritism. Following an experience in which Mozambicans perceive the Christian God to be a particularly effective healer, subjects appear more likely to affiliate with Christianity (though perhaps not exclusively).[29]

Other material considerations also contribute to conversions. In seeking converts, Baker frequently calls traditional healers "thieves," because they charge for their services, and emphasizes that IM does not charge for performing healing rituals. Apparently unaware of any medicinal value of herbal remedies, Baker demonizes traditional healers as profiteering from "witchcraft." From the perspective of Mozambican villagers, Baker herself may appear to be a powerful prophet healer, differing from those she sets up as rivals (many of whom are also women who envision themselves as spiritual "mothers" to their "children") only in the degree of material and spiritual resources she seems able to mobilize. In addition to offering free prayer for healing, bush outreaches include free meals for the community, and are often accompanied by distribution of food and clothing and occasionally by the digging of a water well. (IM brought food and clothes to Impiri, and Baker promised to dig a well there.) At the conclusion of two of the three bush outreaches observed, local churches presented to IM a thank offering of noncash goods including fruit and live poultry (articles of high value to these villagers); in both instances, Baker responded by presenting to the village a cash offering of considerably greater value. Thus, reciprocity was maintained while IM portrayed God as bestowing more gifts than were demanded in return. Although some Mozambicans welcome Baker's healing rituals and financial largesse, for others—including traditional healers and Muslim village leaders—she and Iris Ministries constitute threats to livelihood and political-religious power.[30]

Despite stereotypes of pentecostals blaming those not healed for lack of faith or holiness, I witnessed no such behavior by IM or GA members (although contact with Mozambicans was too limited to evaluate local interpretations). Sonia is an elderly, blind, Mozambican woman who did not exhibit healing. Baker recognized Sonia when she was brought to her at a Pemba conference. Baker had apparently prayed for her many times before. Nevertheless, Baker spent an unusually long time on stage hugging, crying, and praying for Sonia in spite of her seeming resistance to healing—and the public nature of this repeated failure.

In Brazil, there were likewise several particularly interesting cases. A few Brazilian subjects whose visual thresholds measurably improved after PIP described physical sensations at the time of prayer as well as reporting a perception of being able to see more clearly. Ana is a sixty-seven-year-old Brazilian woman tested in São Paulo who read the 20/100 line with her left eye during the pretest and the 20/30 line with her left eye during the posttest. Ana reported feeling heat in her eyes while people prayed for her and said that pressure in her ears (which she felt relieved) had affected her vision. When she opened her eyes after PIP, Ana reported that the people close to her looked totally different, and she could see clearly as she never had before.

Other subjects similarly reported sensations of heat, either localized to their eyes, as with Ana, or more generally throughout their bodies. Julia is a forty-eight-year-old Brazilian woman tested in Barretos, São Paulo, Brazil, who, with both eyes together, read the 20/60 line during the pretest and the 20/20 line during the posttest. Julia reported that during prayer she felt intense heat in her body. Before PIP, she could not see the details on faces or read the Bible without glasses, but after PIP she could do both. Similarly, Yasmin is a sixty-eight-year-old Brazilian woman tested in Barretos who with her left eye read the 20/100 line during the pretest and the 20/50 line in a posttest administered the following day; after receiving additional PIP, she was retested that same day and read the 20/30 line. With her right eye, Yasmin counted fingers at 1' (20/8000) during the pretest and at 4' (20/2000) during the posttest. She reported that during prayer she started to feel a lot of heat in her body. Yasmin's vision remained improved the day after receiving PIP and further improved after additional PIP. Although measurements for both eyes improved post-PIP, Yasmin still could not see well with her right eye at the time of retesting. It is uncertain whether further PIP would have resulted in additional improvements.

Some subjects reported no physical sensations such as heat during PIP, yet they perceived that they were able to see better afterwards. Vitória is a thirty-eight-year-old Brazilian woman whose vision was tested, both eyes together, in Uberlandia. During the pretest, she could count fingers from 9' (20/2667) away. During the posttest, she could read the 20/60 line on the eye chart. Vitória reported that as soon as she opened her eyes after receiving PIP, she found that she could read the name badge of the person who had been praying for her, that everything became clear, and that the pain she had been experiencing from straining to see was gone. The GA team member who prayed for her reported that when Vitória had come for prayer her eyes were squinted together; Vitória had told him that she was experiencing pain from forcing her facial muscles to strain to see, and that something was wrong with her corneas. Other subjects offered fewer details about the nature of their problems or their experiences during prayer, but simply reported being able to see better following PIP. Beatriz is a sixty-one-year-old Brazilian woman whose vision was tested, both eyes together, in Uberlandia. During the pretest Beatriz could count fingers at 13′ (20/2000). During the posttest, she could read the 20/50 line of the vision chart. Beatriz reported that she could see much more clearly.

Directions for Future Research

My research group conducted a small, preliminary study that suggests the potential for developing a new line of inquiry into the clinical effects of proximal prayer. When we published the quantitative results of the Mozambique research—"Study of the Therapeutic Effects of Proximal Intercessory Prayer (STEPP)"—in a peer-reviewed medical journal, the article generated widespread interest and some sharp criticism. Although the tone of certain critiques implied a more than scholarly personal stake in the issues, respondents did raise a number of important considerations that are relevant to designing the next phase of trials.[31]

First, critics raised questions about controls in the STEPP research. This concern breaks down into two questions, namely, "Was there a control group?" and "Did the investigators control for possible confounds in the results?" There was no control group that received a sham prayer intervention. For the study design, we followed recommendations of a 1998 report—*Scientific Research on Spirituality and Health*—published by the National Institute for Healthcare Research (NIHR, not related to the National Institutes of Health [NIH]). According to the NIHR report:

> The first step is to conduct small, or pilot, studies to establish the feasibility and safety of the proposed intervention. Next, one might proceed to small, uncontrolled trials to establish efficacy as well as the size of the effects of such interventions. Then, individual-site (i.e., at a single hospital or clinic), controlled studies could be conducted, followed by large multi-site randomized, double-blind trials to examine the effectiveness of these interventions in the appropriate clinical settings.

Panel members agreed that studies conducted in this area should always utilize the "null-hypothesis." In other words, studies should hypothesize that there is no effect for religion or spirituality on health and then try to disprove it by showing a significant difference or effect associated with a specific religious or spiritual factor or intervention.

The STEPP article describes an early phase in the line of investigations called for by the NIHR report. In particular, the report identified a "critical research need" for studies conducted in their natural "religious and spiritual settings," as opposed to hospitals or clinics, in order to preserve ecological validity. We conducted our study in natural settings where intercessory prayer is commonly practiced and where practitioners assert the greatest effects. We followed the report recommendation of beginning with small, pilot studies using what the NIHR called a *one group pretest-posttest design* to establish the feasibility, safety, and efficacy of interventions before proceeding to larger-scale, controlled trials. As the NIHR report notes, "although this design provides little protection against the various threats to internal and external validity, it may be an important first step in determining treatment efficacy." We followed the further guideline that all such preliminary studies should use the null hypothesis.[32]

Instead of employing a separate control group, we used a widely accepted study design known as a *within-subjects design*. This design has the advantages of being less costly in terms of required number of subjects and affording greater statistical power for some tests, but the disadvantage of affording less control over potentially confounding variables, such as placebo effects. We chose a within-subjects design as more appropriate for a small preliminary study of effects that, to our knowledge, have never been rigorously shown previously. The goal of the preliminary study was not to isolate a particular mechanism as responsible for the effects but rather to test whether such effects can be found at all. A within-subjects design is the most efficient way to test this question. There is a long tradition of using within-subjects designs for a variety of psychophysical studies including testing vision and hearing, even with relatively small numbers of subjects.

The results of these studies have been (and continue to be) published in well-respected journals, including the flagship *Science* magazine. Now that preliminary research has suggested the existence of an effect, it would be appropriate to use a *between-subjects design*, one that does utilize a separate control group, in developing more refined protocols.[33]

The NIHR report suggests that a next step in studying an intervention's effects on nonurgent medical conditions (such as hearing and vision loss, for which briefly delaying experimental interventions is not ethically problematic) might be use of a *randomized control-group pretest-posttest design*. In such a study, subjects would be randomly assigned to receive immediate treatment or no treatment, in this case PIP, until after pre- and posttests had been administered. Subjects in the *wait-list control group* would, after a short delay and study posttest, also receive PIP, after which their hearing or vision would be retested. Researchers could instead administer sham prayers or a different, touch-based, spiritually inflected intervention, such as Therapeutic Touch, to subjects in the control group. This approach may not, however, be optimal because the concept of sham prayer is inherently vague. Also, there are ethical, informed-consent problems with assigning subjects to receive a different type of spiritual intervention than they have requested, especially because many pentecostals have religious objections to practices such as Therapeutic Touch. The wait-list control-group design also seems preferable because it permits researchers to conduct sequential experiments using the same sample. Subjects in the wait-list group are their own controls for the second set of tests, doubling the effective sample size and also increasing statistical power due to the removal of the between-groups variance.[34]

Complete double-blinding is not feasible in a study of proximal prayer, because it would lack both construct validity and ecological validity. Although the STEPP protocol did not include blinding, in support of experimenter reliability, several audition subjects showed no measurable improvement despite self-reported improvement. It would be desirable to implement a measure of blinding in any follow-up research. First, the researchers conducting hearing or vision tests could remain in a mobile clinic (sound insulated and light regulated, thereby providing the additional advantage of a more controlled testing environment) adjacent to the site where PIP is administered, and be blinded to whether subjects are in the experimental or control group and whether (or how many times) they have received PIP. Second, the pentecostals administering PIP could be blinded to whether subjects are in the experimental or control group and whether (or how many times) they have received hearing or vision tests. Third, the subjects seeking prayer could be blinded to whether they are in the experimental or control group; subjects in both groups would receive PIP and hearing or vision tests, although the sequencing would necessarily be different. A different group of researchers from those conducting tests could assign subjects randomly to study groups and escort them between PIP and testing sites. Although some level of blinding should be implemented at the next stage, researchers can learn from distant prayer studies that there are drawbacks to attempting to apply every standard established in experimental drug research rather than developing methods that are tailored to the particular nature of the phenomena under consideration.

A further question about controls is whether the STEPP research controlled for possible confounds in the results. We did control for potential confounds, such as differences in ambient noise during before and after testing. We also compared our results with results from previous studies of intentional suggestion and hypnosis to examine the relative strength of such effects. In future studies, the researchers might use themselves as controls by testing their own hearing in conditions of low and high AN. Effects of AN might also be mitigated by using ear buds instead of supra-aural headphones and by conducting all hearing tests in a sound-insulated mobile clinic.

A second type of concern expressed by reviewers of the STEPP article is that subjects may have been "plants" preselected by the group under study. This would have been difficult to accomplish, since subjects were recruited by loudspeaker announcements made to the population at large, inviting anyone with hearing or vision impairments to come or be brought forward to participate in the study. Every consecutive individual who approached the study site to participate and assented to the protocol was included. Critics also implied that the STEPP study included only those who self-reported improved vision and/or hearing, thereby biasing the results. This was a prospective study. Every subject who assented and received intervention was posttested and reported. Interventions did not continue indefinitely until subjects reported improvement. Most interventions lasted between one and fifteen minutes.

Reviewers further suggested that the investigators relied on self-reports of improved hearing or vision. This is not the case. The study was conducted in order to avoid the common tendencies of basing healing claims on self-reports or crude tests of counting raised fingers or responding to hand claps. Instead, the study evaluated subjects using standard medical hearing and vision testing equipment and procedures. We measured no improvement for several audition subjects even though they self-reported improvement. Several other vision subjects neither self-reported improvement nor showed measurable improvement. Because there was not time to retest two subjects, we reported them as unimproved. We excluded three subjects from analysis because of unreliable data, that is, false-positive responses during audiometric testing. Even so, and even with a small sample size, we found large enough effects in individual subjects and consistent enough effects across the study populations for the results to reach the level of statistical significance for both hearing and vision. Note that a small sample size does not mean that the results are ungeneralizable. It is more difficult to achieve statistical significance with fewer subjects, yet even with this more challenging condition, we still measured effects that are highly significant for hearing and significant for vision. This suggests that the underlying phenomena have larger effect sizes.[35]

The STEPP article, which focused on clinical effects of PIP, did not attempt to explain mechanisms by which functional improvements occurred. It is possible that suggestive elements of the study contributed to improved function. Subjects may have been motivated (perhaps unconsciously) to try to produce worse performance on pretests and/or improved performance on posttests. It is unclear, though, that even motivated subjects would have been able to improve their visual acuity or reduce their hearing thresholds by the magnitudes measured simply by trying harder. If this scale of improvement were achievable, even temporarily, visual and hearing impairments would not be such serious health problems. Moreover, it seems unlikely that such a motivational dynamic significantly affected the results for three reasons. First, Mozambican traditional healers often charge more money when a healing is successful; given this social expectation of healing exchanges, subjects might be predisposed to minimize rather than maximize reported improvement. Second, although participants may have expected healing, they lived mostly in religiously mixed, largely Muslim, communities; a number of participants may not have been Christians, and would not necessarily be predisposed to believe in pentecostal healing. Long-term research on the global expansion of pentecostalism suggests that many of those who self-report healing subsequent to pentecostal prayer were not Christians at the time but later affiliated with pentecostal groups because of perceived healing experiences. Thus, participating in a Christian healing ritual may have been viewed experimentally—much as a Christian might try Buddhist meditation—and may have entailed more social costs than social benefits. Third, producing a hold-back effect in a hearing test would be challenging, because subjects reliably would have to feign a narrow hearing threshold over the repeated passes of the standard Carhart-Jerger method. This would be difficult (though not impossible per se), especially for the generally uneducated Mozambican subjects.[36]

Practice effects may have contributed to some observed improvement, but these would also be present in hypnosis studies to similar degrees and therefore may not fully account for the larger effects observed here. Furthermore, the amount of practice was minimal at best. Subjects with measurable hearing thresholds experienced the test tones of a given frequency only a few times in each ear, in keeping with the Carhart-Jerger method. In some cases, the threshold-verification pass of the Carhart-Jerger protocol revealed a lower pre-PIP threshold than the initial pass, apparently due to practice effects, and so the protocol continued until the measured pre-PIP psychophysical hearing threshold was stable. In this way, any existing practice effects were already largely accounted for in the pre-PIP test. Subjects with no measurable hearing threshold pre-PIP were deemed deaf in the corresponding ear(s) if they both self-identified as deaf and exhibited no tone response or visible startle response even to tones of 100 dBHL, in which case it is unclear how such an experience might constitute practice. Likewise, visually impaired subjects were allowed minimal experience with the eye chart during the pre-PIP test. They were asked to read as far down the eye chart as they were able to a single time, and care was taken not to reveal the smaller lines below their pre-PIP acuity threshold prior to the post-PIP test. It seems reasonable that subjects whose pre- and post-PIP visual thresholds differed by only one or two lines on the eye chart may have been exhibiting practice effects. It seems much less likely that subjects who went from being unable to read a single line (in which case it is unclear that this experience constituted practice) to reading far down the chart were exhibiting practice effects.[37]

Certain critics of the STEPP article implied that Mozambicans and/or Brazilians are inherently more susceptible than North Americans to effects of suggestion and/or religious excitement. This proposition dangerously borders on racism and neocolonial cultural arrogance. It should not be assumed that Mozambicans or Brazilians are simply more suggestive than North Americans. It should also be noted that some of the subjects measured did not receive PIP during a large evening religious meeting but during daytime medical clinics in which the emotional influences of music, crowds, and related stimuli were greatly reduced. More directly to the point, the protocol did not rely on subjects to tell the researchers whether they thought they could see or hear better after prayer; we measured exactly how well they performed on pre- and post-PIP hearing or vision tests.

In future research, it would be advantageous to supplement measurement of psychophysical hearing and vision thresholds with objective tests of ear and eye function and physical examinations of ear and eye health. This might allow us to diagnose the etiology of auditory or visual impairments and/or assess whether structural changes occurred. For hearing, an otoacoustic emissions (OAE) screener could be used to test cochlear and middle-ear function independent of subject responses; this objective test reduces potential confounds, such as placebo effects, but cannot replace audiometric testing, because it does not provide an accurate assessment of hearing thresholds. An otoscope could be used to examine outer- and inner-ear health, for instance, by looking for otitis media and otitis externa. For vision, an autorefractor and retinoscope could be used to measure refractions independent of subject responses; this objective measure reduces potential confounds, such as placebo effects, but does not replace information provided by vision charts. Eye health could be evaluated using a retinoscope, for example, to detect corneal irregularities and degree of cataract formation, and an ophthalmoscope, for instance, to detect diabetic retinopathy, glaucoma, and macular degeneration. Such tests may be useful in ruling out one or more potential mechanisms for demonstrated effects in order to narrow the range of possible mechanisms to account for the phenomena.[38]

Follow-up with subjects in developing countries, for the purpose of assessing long-term effects, can be extremely difficult. At a medical clinic the next day, we managed to retest one Mozambican subject who initially received PIP at an evening meeting; her measured improvements remained, and we measured additional improvement following further PIP in this setting. We retested several Brazilian subjects the following day, and improvements remained and/or further improvements could be measured. We also followed up with one Brazilian subject one month later and again two years later; he self-reported that his hearing was still improved, although we did not have an opportunity to retest his hearing. In future studies, subjects might be offered a small incentive to return to the research site for retesting the following day. All subjects recruited in the United States and non-U.S. subjects who have regular access to telephones, e-mail, and/or postal mail could be asked for their contact information so that researchers can contact them one month and six months later to inquire whether they have perceived any changes in their conditions. These subjects could also be asked to sign medical-records release forms, allowing researchers to request records from their health-care providers related to hearing/vision from before and after studied PIP interventions.

In sum, future studies might be designed to employ additional controls, test whether impairments with certain etiologies are more susceptible to improvement through PIP, probe the mechanisms by which PIP produces effects, and assess whether improvements are long term.

Conclusion

The research program that commenced with the STEPP article has not solved every problem in studying the empirical effects of prayer, but it does suggest a potentially fruitful research direction. The initial study has three main findings. First, Mozambican and Brazilian subjects did exhibit improved audition and/or visual acuity subsequent to PIP interventions. Second, the magnitude of measured effects exceeds that reported in previous studies of suggestion and hypnosis. Third, although it would be unwise to overgeneralize from these preliminary findings for a small number of PIP practitioners and subjects collected in far from ideal field conditions, future study seems warranted. Further research might discover principles about when, how, and, why PIP works that could eventually lead to clinical applications for use in contexts where access to conventional treatment is limited. The implications are potentially vast, given World Health Organization estimates of the hundreds of millions of people living in the developing world who currently suffer from auditory and visual impairments without receiving any treatment.

Although there would be substantial obstacles to seeking eventually to apply what is learned from further research, poor global health is an enormous problem, and little help is being offered by conventional medicine to many of those who are suffering. The proposal of studying PIP does not imply that pentecostal prayer is effective for the reasons that religious participants think it is. Whether PIP has measurable effects is an empirical question, and we did an empirical study to begin to answer this question. Complex mind-body interactions are in play, as are many methodological challenges to doing this kind of study. Such practices and states of mind as touching, human emotion, and positive thinking all affect mind-body connections in ways that science is only beginning to understand. Much more research is needed to determine the mechanisms by which any effects (positive or negative)—whether from PIP, other kinds of emotional touch, or spiritual healing practices in other religious traditions—take place. The fact that we do not yet understand the mechanisms underlying the effects does not invalidate the findings per se, but does indicate the need for additional research.[39]

Regardless of the mechanisms, and regardless of the personal philosophical and/or religious beliefs of researchers, efforts can be made to investigate a wide range of therapeutic interventions that may in some way promise relief—without any bridging of the "nonoverlapping magisteria" of medical research and religious healing. This research program questions the logical rationale behind taboos of otherwise valid empirical questions and investigates prayer practices using the same empirical methods of hypothesis testing and statistics used in any other branch of science. In so doing, the project draws no unwarranted conclusions about the underlying mechanisms of PIP effectiveness but only reports that there is an empirically observable effect that deserves follow-up on empirical and ethical grounds.

These empirical results do not imply theological conclusions, for instance, that doctors should pray with their patients or refer them to pentecostal meetings. Dr. John Peteet makes a similar important point in his editorial on the STEPP article: "Critics nevertheless remind us that separating helpful spiritual practices from their traditions has both practical and ethical risks." Yet, Peteet continues, "Whatever their views about the efficacy of healing prayer and about whether it belongs in the armamentarium of medicine, clinicians and believers share core commitments to healing whenever it is possible, and to meaningful acceptance when it is not." If empirical research continues to indicate that PIP may be therapeutically beneficial, there are ethical and nonpartisan public-policy reasons to encourage related research. It is a primary privilege and responsibility of medical science to pursue a better understanding of therapeutic interventions that may—even indirectly, by teaching principles—advance global health, especially in contexts where conventional medical treatments are inadequate or unavailable.[40]

The results of this prospective trial suggest that *something* is going on in pentecostal PIP and that researchers have an opportunity to learn more about what exactly that is and whether and/or how applications might eventually be developed that can be of practical clinical benefit. As with every other category of data pertaining to the effects of prayer practices, there are limits to the information that clinical measurements can provide. One important question that remains is whether the people who exhibit cross-sectional measurement changes are affected in any lasting way. This question leads to the approach of longitudinal follow-up.

CHAPTER 6

Do Healing Experiences Produce Lasting Effects?

.✦.

The head-on collision occurred just five minutes after eighteen-year-old Randy Clark had been challenged by his drug buddy Geofry: "Clark, come on—admit it! You know that if we were in a wreck right now and you died, you'd go to hell!" Another friend, Joe—who also got drunk and stoned daily—chimed in: "Yeah—that's right!" Clark, who was being ribbed for "getting religion," had just rededicated his life as a Christian and insisted, "No, Joe—I wouldn't go to hell. But how about you?" Just then an oncoming car knocked the teenagers' vehicle off the road. It flipped end over end three times, hit a telephone phone, and landed upside down in a ditch. Joe died instantly. Clark, pulled out from where he was pinned inside the vehicle, remained in a delirious, semiconscious state for four days. Several of his ribs were broken, his facial bones crushed, his digestive track was paralyzed, and his spinal discs had been compressed, causing nerve damage. Despite prescribed narcotics, the pain was excruciating. The doctors warned that too much movement could result in permanent paralysis and that, at best, Clark could expect to remain hospitalized for between seven and eleven weeks.[1]

Clark was already familiar with the idea that God heals. When he was five years old, his grandmother suffered from a painful, swollen goiter. One day, she "heard the voice of the Lord" tell her to go to her bedroom and pray. As she did so, "It felt as if a hot hand went down my throat." The goiter instantly vanished, never to return. Interviewed in 2008, Clark recalled this incident as the first defining moment in his life. Clark also remembers being fascinated by watching Oral Roberts's healing services on TV. These memories stayed with Clark while he was growing up, yet he turned to drugs and sex, responding to an altar call for salvation at age sixteen, but returning to his former habits until the day of the car accident. As soon as Clark regained alertness, he requested a Bible—which he could only read through mirrors, because his injuries required him to lie flat in bed. He prayed, "Lord, You spared my life! I should be dead now, but You spared me. I give my life back to You. I'll do anything You want me to do, but please don't call me to preach!" Clark prayed for his healing, as did relatives and church members. Within a few days, doctors expressed surprise at the rapidity of his recovery. Plans to transfer Clark to a better hospital were canceled, because his digestive tract regained movement; the doctor who came to set his broken jaw left without doing anything, exclaiming "it's already set"; all the pain left his spine overnight. Although he had been warned not to move lest he become paralyzed, Clark—by now certain that God was healing him—got out of bed and began to walk. Alarmed, nurses ordered him back to bed, but he rejoined that since God had healed him, God would not allow him to become paralyzed. Clark left the hospital within three weeks.[2]

There is no way to "prove" Clark's claim that God healed him. People sometimes recover more rapidly than doctors expect for a variety of natural reasons. It is, however, possible to examine how Clark constructed his experience and to trace effects of this *perceived* divine healing on him and, indirectly, on people he influenced. Almost as commonplace as claims of healing through prayer is the skeptically posed question, Do those who testify to having been healed *stay* healed? Most people have heard reports of a physically challenged person dramatically rising from a wheelchair during an emotionally charged healing service, only to collapse back into the chair, exhausted, at most a few hours later—no better and perhaps worse off than before. There are inherent limits to the research methods employed in the previous two chapters—surveying people's perceptions and measuring objective changes immediately after a healing experience. This chapter employs complementary approaches, using ethnographic and textual methods to study longitudinally the effects of healing experiences on expressed attitudes and behaviors over the course of time. The previous chapters analyze statistically the effects of healing practices at particular conferences. This chapter instead focuses on case studies of individuals who have pursued healing for themselves and others through long-term participation in a broad spectrum of nondenominational pentecostal conferences, regular church services, and private devotional activities that mark the daily and weekly rhythms of the transnational healing networks brokered by such organizations as GA and IM. The job of the ethnographic researcher is facilitated by the global character of pentecostal networks. Many of the same individuals frequent events in scattered locales, making it relatively easy to follow up with clusters of individuals over months and years simply by attending major pentecostal events that constitute gathering points for members of this translocal community.

Interpreting pentecostal narratives is, however, by no means easy or simple. Many of the pentecostals studied are storytellers who love to testify about their experiences—often with an agenda of converting or exhorting the listener, bringing glory to God, and reaffirming the testifier's identity as a child of God who has an intimate relationship with the divine. Unwritten rules or conventions govern what should or should not be included in a healing narrative. Because the purpose of testimony is to instill faith, narrators—consciously or unconsciously— self-censor admissions of continuing symptoms or doubts, and external censors (ministers and Christian publishers) are unlikely to publicize accounts that report failures, include obvious inconsistencies, or otherwise fail to provide a compelling apologetic for divine healing. Any recollected account is necessarily a created story that is in a sense fictional, rather than an objective report of "just the facts." Testimonies, whether in oral or written form, are not stable, but may change over time or depending on audience or circumstances. This chapter does not take for granted the truthfulness nor allege the falsity of pentecostal narratives, but instead uses accounts of healing as provisional windows onto the meanings narrators construct and articulate and the social processes through which these meanings are transmitted and possibly contested and revised.[3]

For most of the following narratives, I have been able to draw on a combination of published or informally circulated testimonials and a series of observations and personal interviews conducted over the course of as many as eight years. Rather than isolated examples, the case studies selected reflect the ripple effects of healing experiences within fluid relational networks. Typically, one person's perceived healing experience shapes other people's quests for healing and their long-term beliefs and behaviors. This chapter accordingly begins with transformational experiences of the network leaders Randy Clark and Heidi Baker, from there tracing out lines of influence on other individuals who have in turn affected still others. The goal of this chapter is not simply to illumine the experiences of particular individuals or to situate them in their social networks, but more broadly to model the relational processes through which healing practices facilitate the spread of global pentecostalism.

Randy Clark: Lighting Fires

Shortly after his release from the hospital in 1970, Clark gave a testimony about his healing experience at a church youth service, purportedly initiating a six-week-long revival. Almost everyone in the local high school attended nightly services; two hundred fifty persons publicly "professed faith"; and eleven—including Clark—believed themselves "called" into ministry. Clark did become a Baptist pastor near his hometown in southern Illinois—although his rocky path included financial struggles and resistance from Christians who considered him disqualified by a divorce and remarriage. In 1983, while listening to a sermon about a woman who had been subject to bleeding healed by Jesus that typically "spiritualized" the Bible story (Mark 5:25) rather than emphasizing the healing per se, Clark had a strong impression that God was telling him to begin teaching that God still heals today. Since Clark knew little about healing beyond his own experience, he contacted the Vineyard's founder, John Wimber, whose California-based ministry was by this point attracting national and international attention. Clark attended a Wimber conference (at which the Korean megachurch pastor David Yonggi Cho also spoke), and Wimber sent a team to conduct a conference at Clark's Baptist church. Clark avowedly received an impartation of gifts of healing through the laying on of hands. Members of his church began to experience healings—despite the congregation's cessationist doctrine that God had stopped per-forming miracles of healing after Christianity was firmly established. This new pentecostal emphasis generated so much controversy that Clark soon resigned and planted a new, smaller church that joined the Vineyard movement.[4]

Clark moved from Illinois to St. Louis, Missouri, the healings petered out, and Clark entered what he later called the "desert years" of 1986 to 1993. Then Clark attended a conference in Tulsa, Oklahoma led by Rodney Howard-Browne, the South African missionary to the United States best known for bringing to pentecostalism a "laughing revival." Clark had been reluctant to attend the event, because it was hosted by Kenneth Hagin's Word of Faith movement, whose theology—that positive confessions of faith are the primary ingredient in attain-ing healing (and financial prosperity)—he disdained. Clark was also unimpressed by phenomena such as laughter. From his reading of the eighteenth-century revivalist Jonathan Edwards, the "real evidence of revival is not phenomenon or lack of phenomenon, it's the fruit." So he asked a friend who had been to Howard-Browne's meetings two weeks before what the fruit had been. The answer satisfied Clark: "I have seen more healings in the last two weeks than in the previous eight years combined." By this point, Clark felt so desperate for a "touch from God" that he had been fasting from food for two weeks, saying, "I'm not going to eat until You touch me!" Although everyone around him at the conference seemed affected, Clark did not feel anything until the final morning, when Howard-Browne prayed for him. Clark fell backwards and found that he could not get up for forty-five min-utes and that he himself had started laughing (one of just three times in his life, even during and after the Toronto Blessing, that Clark says he felt spiritually inebriated). Then Clark stood in line again and again for more prayer. When he returned to his St. Louis Vineyard congregation—which he had been leading on a "seeker-sensitive" model that gave no emphasis to spiritual gifts—people started falling, laugh-ing, and reporting healings, and the same thing happened when Clark attended the next Vineyard regional meeting. As reports of these un-usual phenomena spread through the Vineyard network, John Arnott, the pastor of a Vineyard church in Toronto, Ontario, invited Clark to speak at his church for a series of four services in January 1994. This marked the beginning of the Toronto Blessing.[5]

Seventeen years later, healing remains a major theme in Clark's revivalism—which he envisions as *Lighting Fires* (to quote the title of his autobiography)—everywhere he visits. On average, Clark has been away from his wife and four children preaching 180 days out of every year. Clark reflected in 2008 that "since '94, the biggest sacrifice and the most painful thing I know is that in my experience as a father I've lost half of my children's childhood." Yet, Clark does not regret the sacrifice because "healing has been a huge thing in my life.... I've always had a heart for ministry because I was almost killed at 18.... Healing has been this rock, has been the critical thing for me." Almost every time Clark preaches, he prays for an impartation of spiritual gifts, especially healing, to his audience. Clark's perceived healing experience twenty-two years before Toronto set off a chain of events with unpredictably wide ramifications. Yet the extensive reach of Clark's influence has admittedly come at the expense of being present for his own family, who may not always have felt loved in the process.[6]

Heidi Baker: Stopping for the One

One of the countless individuals influenced by Clark through the Toronto Blessing is Heidi Baker, who is today highly regarded by many Christians worldwide for her work among the poor in Mozambique, Africa. She is also well known as an itinerant evangelist who calls audiences in the western world to "spend time in the presence" of God and to "stop for the one" and show love. When Baker first visited Toronto in 1996, she was a self-described "burned-out" missionary who felt emotionally and physically exhausted. After eighteen years of missionary work in Asia, England, and Africa, she and her husband, Rolland, had planted four churches, and they were struggling to provide food for 320 orphaned children. Working eighteen-hour days, Heidi Baker had been on antibiotics six times in two months with infections and dysentery and had just been diagnosed with pneumonia and possible tuberculosis. During the first TACF service, Baker's fluid-filled lungs opened up and she could breathe effortlessly for the first time in weeks.[7]

Baker returned to Toronto in 1998 for further recharging. This time, Clark prayed for Baker, telling her, "God is asking, 'Do you want the nation of Mozambique?'" Clark prophesied that "the blind will see. The crippled will walk. The deaf will hear. The dead will be raised, and the poor will hear the good news." Baker avowedly felt the "heavenly fire of God falling on me. I was so hot I literally thought I was going to burn up and die. For seven days I was unable to move." She had to be carried even to the washroom, needed help to drink water, and was for most of that period unable to speak. Responding to critics of such phenomena, Baker insists that experiences of God's power are critical to experiencing long-term fruitfulness: "It is not frivolous to see people stuck to the floor—it is not frivolous to see people crying—it is not frivolous to see people shaking and quaking and feeling the power of God. I want you to know that unless God touches you, you will not go in his power and you will not see what he wants you to see." After Baker's intense experience in Toronto, she returned to Mozambique with new energy and passion—although some of the Bakers' greatest challenges still lay ahead. Fifteen years later, the Bakers had planted an estimated ten thousand churches and provided homes for ten thousand orphaned children—as apparently miraculous healings and multiplication of food fueled church growth in predominantly Muslim areas of one of the poorest countries in the world.[8]

As with Clark, healing was a major theme in Baker's life long before the Toronto Blessing. Before she was born, Heidi's at-the-time nominally Catholic and Episcopalian parents had been barren and, in desperation, prayed to God, "If you give us children, we'll give them to you." They adopted a son, who died. They unexpectedly conceived Heidi, but when she was four years old, she contracted encephalitis and was in a hospital intensive-care unit for a month. Her parents again prayed, "If you will spare our daughter, you can take her and you can use her and you can have her for your glory." Heidi did recover and grew up in a wealthy home in Laguna Beach, California, but she struggled with dyslexia and was placed in a class for special learners. When she was sixteen years old, in 1976, she was living on a Choctaw Indian reservation in Mississippi as an American field-service student when someone invited her to attend a Pentecostal revival service. Heidi responded to the Navajo preacher's altar call for salvation, the follow-ing day experienced "baptism in the Holy Spirit," and four months later was healed of dyslexia. After this last experience, Heidi shed the thick glasses that had magnified print without aiding comprehension, and became a straight-A student and award-winning speed reader. Shortly before her healing, Heidi had a visionary experience in which it seemed that God said, "I am calling you to be a minister and a mission-ary. You are to go to Africa, Asia, and England." She began by preach-ing on the streets and leading outreaches into poor communities in Southern California and Mexico.[9]

In 1980, Heidi married Rolland Baker, a third-generation Pentecos-tal missionary born and raised in China. Two weeks after their mar-riage, they left for Indonesia as missionaries. For several years, the Bakers took dance-drama teams around Indonesia and to the Philip-pines, Taiwan, and Hong Kong. After losing their visas because the Indonesian government did not like their proselytizing, the Bakers went to live among the poor in Hong Kong. The Bakers spent a total of twelve years in Asia, by the end of which time Heidi had become very sick and was diagnosed with myalgic encephalomyelitis (ME), or chronic fatigue syndrome, and later with multiple sclerosis (MS). The Bakers nevertheless believed God was telling them that it was time to go to En-gland, where they both pursued Ph.D.s in systematic theology at King's College London, while starting a church among street people.[10]

The Bakers' next stop was Mozambique, then known as the poorest country in the world. Meanwhile, Heidi received prayer for healing from MS—without apparent benefit—from every, in her words, "poster boy" itinerant evangelist on the conference circuit. For years, she was "not just a little sick, but super-sick. I was in a lot of pain all the time. I couldn't walk for long periods and often couldn't even lie still and read. . . . I would have to hold onto the pulpit in order to preach be-cause I was so weak. . . . Through that suffering a great compassion was birthed in me—a compassion for anyone who is hurting." During the last six months of her illness, Baker was paralyzed on one side and blind in one eye. She experienced healing one day as a group of Mo-zambican children gathered around to pray for her, pushing her face into the dirt in their enthusiasm. As of October 2011, Heidi Baker is an exceptionally fit fifty-two-year-old who dances, runs, lifts weights, and snorkels.[11]

Baker has, however, experienced other bouts of sickness along the way. Significantly, Baker has been hospitalized for methicillin-resistant Staphylococcus aureus (MRSA)—a life-threatening bacterial infection—a total of seven times. Each time the infection got worse and proved harder to treat, even with the strongest antibiotics available. The last time was in 2005, when she spent thirty-two days hospitalized in Malaysia and South Africa. The doctors gave her little hope of recovery—telling her they were "so sorry," but there was "nothing they could do" and that she should "just prepare to die." Baker recalls that one doctor said, "You can write your tombstone. You need to consider putting things in order." The only hope offered was that if she traveled to a specialized hospital in the United States, surgeons might be able to cut out the infection. While hospitalized in South Africa, Baker felt her faith encouraged by listening to the ANGA Revival Alliance affiliate Bill Johnson's sermons on healing on her iPod three times. All the while, she got sicker and sicker.[12]

Finally, with Rolland's help, Heidi pulled out her IV and checked herself out of the hospital. She told her doctors that she was going to see a "top specialist" in Toronto—by which she meant Jesus. Heidi had been invited to preach at TACF, but "no one thought I would [preach] because I was dying there." Baker believed God had given her a message from the book of Zechariah, and that if she preached it in Toronto she would be healed. Wracked with pain, she struggled up to the pulpit and preached

about becoming a resting place. That's our goal in ministry. Not how many churches you build or how many people you reach, but that we would become the resting place for Him. And . . . . if we're in the presence [of God] that God would cause us to see the temple rebuilt, and we are the temple, and if we're really rebuilt and the Holy Spirit totally fills us then there's no room for sickness to stand. . . . And I started speaking the Scripture: "I will be a wall of fire round about you declares the Lord and the glory within." And the fire hit me from my head to my toes . . . three times. And those open, oozing

sores—that 32 days of Vancomycin and Zyvoxid could not heal—
the Lord closed them up that day. I was totally, completely, instantly
healed.

Sensing that God was telling her that "now I want you to dance," she
stopped preaching and began worshiping and thanking God and dancing across the stage—while a videographer filmed her for the conference DVD. In this video, which I reviewed, Baker appears weak when
she begins to preach, but seems to exhibit increased energy as she
continues her two-hour-long sermon, which concluded after 11:30 p.m.[13]

At 5:00 a.m. the next morning, Baker avowedly put on the running
shoes that Rolland had bought for her while she was hospitalized—as
a symbol of faith. She ran for an hour "with no weakness, no exhaus-
tion, completely healed from MRSA. . . . The scars are there to this
day, but the wounds closed up as I was preaching." To satisfy her
mother, Baker followed up two days later at the emergency room of
the prestigious Hoag Hospital in Newport Beach, California, where
there are specialists in the treatment of MRSA. On seeing the South
African hospital's paperwork, the staff rushed to prepare Baker for
surgery, but she insisted that they "look at the 'infection' first." The
examining doctor said: "This is healing up well. You won't need an
operation. . . . You don't need to be in the hospital. The scars look bad,
but they'll go away. What are you doing here? What is this letter [from
the South African specialist]?" When Baker explained what had
happened in Toronto, the doctor reportedly commented, "This is a real
miracle!"[14]

Baker signed a medical-records release form allowing me to ask for
her complete file from Hoag Hospital (and reproduce the records
here). Figure 6.1a shows that Baker walked into the emergency room
on October 22, 2005—two days after she preached in Toronto. The
form notes that she had been hospitalized in Malaysia and South
Africa for MRSA and that she was taking the antibiotics Vancomycin
and Zyvoxid. The nurse who examined Baker eleven minutes after her
arrival observed small sores, rash, and boils, and noted that the patient denied that these were painful. Figure 6.1b indicates that this
nurse referred Baker to a doctor who examined her and found "healing

wounds," "no abscesses," "no pus," and "wounds closed." The doctor's clinical impression was that the patient's wounds had resulted from an "infection" he identified as "MRSA." He sent her "home," rather than admitting her to the hospital, noting that her condition was "improved." Figure 6.1c shows that Baker had a laboratory test done two days later, the result of which was "no staphylococcus aureus isolated." This medical file confirms some of the basic details of Baker's story— namely, that she did, in fact, follow up with the hospital she specified on the date she indicated, that the medical professionals who examined her were convinced that she had had MRSA but that she no longer required hospitalization, and that laboratory tests showed no evidence of remaining staphylococcus bacteria.

Baker looks back on her healing from MRSA as a milestone in her ministry. She learned the principle of "thankfulness and rejoicing. Often, when we are prayed for, we feel a little better, but maybe are aware that we are not *fully* healed. We always tend to look for instantaneous, complete healing, instead of rejoicing in the fact that God has touched us. In that hospital I learned to give thanks for every little bit of healing God gave as he gave it." The experience of having to persevere in praying for healing also gave Baker a "revelation about worship and warfare—how that, if we would worship, we would defeat the enemy; how that sickness was from hell, from the darkness; and how to take authority over sickness. We have to love the person but really hate the sickness, because sickness comes from the enemy; it doesn't come from God. . . . And when I began to worship and take authority with great faith for healing—not with my focus on the Devil, but on God—suddenly there was an increase of deaf being healed. There'd be four or five in a night healed of deafness. I saw an increase in Mozambican illnesses being healed." Baker reached the conclusion that "the battles we win against sickness here are won for others more than ourselves," and interpreted her own suffering and subsequent healing as a catalyst for others to experience healing.[15]

Rolland Baker has also experienced several dramatic recoveries, and doctors have more than once urged that family members be flown in to say good-bye before he died. While Heidi Baker was speaking at a U.S. conference in October 2008, Rolland was thousands of miles

Figure 6.1a–c. Medical file from Hoag Hospital, Newport Beach, California, for Heidi Baker, October 22, 2005. (a) Emergency room admission form. (b) Doctor's examination notes. (c) Laboratory results. Courtesy Heidi Baker.

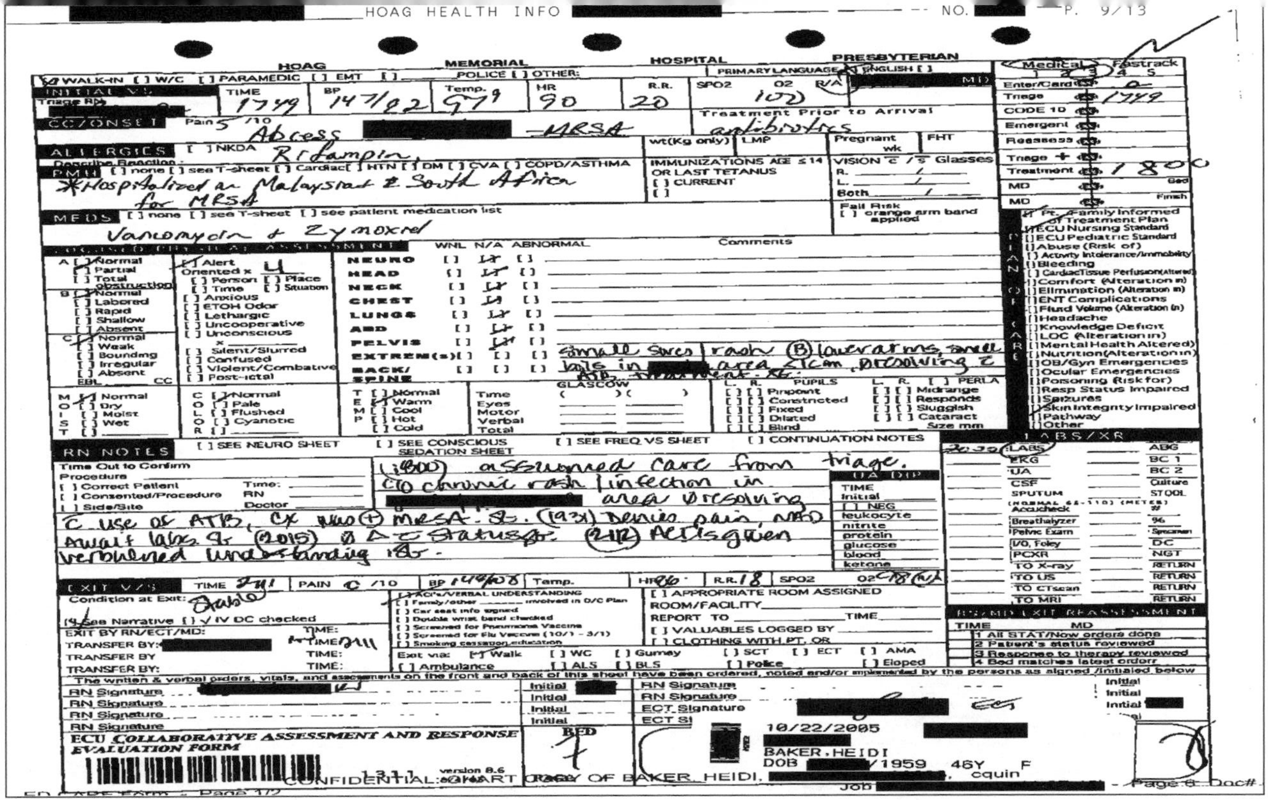

HOAG HEALTH INFO

B

PHYSICAL EXAM
Nursing Assessment Reviewed
VS / BP __ / __ Temp __ P __ R __
Vitals Reviewed

General Appearance
- Acute distress
  - mild / moderate / severe distress
- alert
- anxious / lethargic
- cyanotic / diaphoretic / pallid / jaundiced

SKIN
- warm, dry
- nml color
- skin rash / erythema / lesion / plaque

localized:
- generalized
- face, eye R/L
- neck / anterior / posterior
- trunk, chest / abdomen / back
- extremities

character:
- symmetric / asymmetric
- macular / papular / maculopapular
- fine / confluent / patchy
- linear / lacy / polycyclic
- vesicular / bullous
- rough texture like sand paper
- urticarial / erythematous / petechial
- skin-line distribution like pityriasis
- rosea

site:
- warmth / tenderness / swelling
- lymphangitis / thickening
- scaly / well defined border
- scaling / inflammation / crusting
- weeping / inflammation / crusting

EXTREMITIES
- nml inspection
- normal ROM
- joint tender
- no pedal edema
  - edema, hands / arms / legs / pedal

EENT
- eyes, nml inspection
- gums, nml
- pharynx nml
  - scleral icterus / injected conjunctiva
  - pharyngeal erythema / exudates

NECK
- trachea midline
- no swelling
  - stiff neck / meningismus
  - lymphadenopathy

RESP / CVS
- no resp. distress
- breath sounds nml
- reg. rate, rhythm
- heart sounds nml
  - rales / rhonchi
  - wheezing
  - tachycardia / bradycardia __/6 sys / dias
  - murmur grade __/6 sys / dias

ABDOMEN
- non-tender
- no organomegaly
  - tenderness
  - hepatomegaly / splenomegaly

RECTAL
- non-tender
- slide functional
  - rectal tenderness / mass / drainage

NEURO / PSYCH
- oriented x3
- mood / affect nml
- CN's nml as tested
- no motor / sensy deficit
  - disoriented to person / place / time
  - depressed affect
  - facial droop / EOM palsy / anisocoria
  - weakness / sensory loss

Skin Rash / Insect Bite / Abscess-43

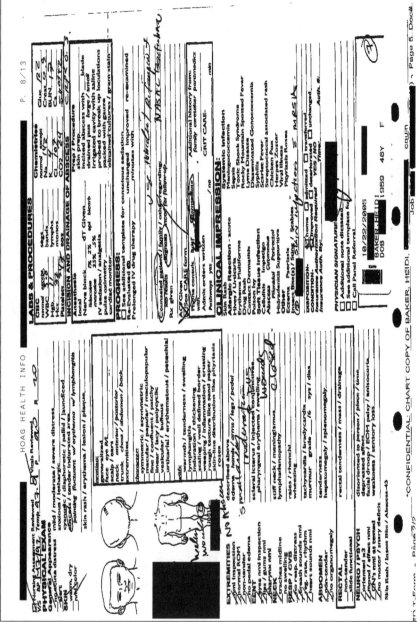

LABS & PROCEDURES

CBC
- WBC
- VBC
- Hgb
- Hct
- Platelets

segs
bands
lymphs
monos

Chemistries
- Na
- K
- Cl
- CO2
- Glu
- Creat
- BUN

INCISION AND DRAINAGE OF ABSCESS

Anesthesia dT Given
- local
- Nerve block
- % 2% .5% epi   lidocaine / bicarb
- mepivicaine 25% .5%
- IV sedation / analgesia
- pulse oximetry
- cardiac monitor

Prep / Procedure
- skin prep
- incised abscess with __ blade
- drained pus, large / small
- irrigated cavity with saline
- probed to break up loculations
- packed with gauze
- obtained cultures / gram stain

PROGRESS:
- See additional template for conscious sedation
- Re-Evaluated @
- Prolonged IV drug therapy ___ minutes with ___

unchanged   improved   re-examined

Counseled patient / family / other regarding
  diagnosis   prognosis   need for follow-up.
Rx given

CRIT CARE- ___ min

Additional history from:
family, caretaker, paramedics

CARE form

Phone consult. with

Admit orders yes / no

Pathway yes / no

CLINICAL IMPRESSION:
- Skin Rash
- Skin Reaction - acute
- Hives / Urticaria
- Erythema Multiforme
- Poison Ivy
- Contact Dermatitis
- Cellulitis
- Abscess
- Impetigo
- Hidradenitis Suppurativa
- Other
- Eczema
- Insect Bite(s) / Skin
- Systemic Infection
- Meningococcemia
- Sepsis
- Toxic Shock Syndrome
- Rocky Mountain Spotted Fever
- Lyme Disease
- Disseminated Gonococcemia
- Syphilis
- Scarlet Fever
- Strep Associated rash
- Chicken Pox
- Herpes Zoster
- Viral Illness
- Pityriasis Rosea
- Psoriasis
- Scabies

DISPOSITION-
- Additional note dictated
- See additional template for
- Call Panel Referral

CONDITION-
- home
- admitted
- transferred
- Improved
- deteriorated
- unchanged

Insurance Authorization Required YES / No
Insurance Auth. By: ___ Auth. #: ___

PHYSICIAN SIGNATURE

BAKER, HEIDI
DOB 1959 46Y F

Page 5. Doc#.

ED_T_Form - Page 7/2

C

HOAG MEMORIAL HOSPITAL PRESBYTERIAN
ONE HOAG DRIVE, PO BOX 6100 NEWPORT BEACH, CA 92658-6100
, MD   LABORATORY DIRECTOR

NAME: BAKER, HEIDI   AGE: 46Y SEX: F LOC: DIAG   ADMIT DATE: 10/24/2005

Page: 1

------------------------------ STOOL SPECIMENS ------------------------------

10/24/2005 STAPH ONLY CULTURE
           ACC.NO.:   TRANSPORT TIME: UNKNO Final report 10/27/2005
           SPECIMEN DESCRIPTION:
           SPECIAL REQUESTS: None

CULTURE RESULT: No Staphylococcus aureus isolated

END OF REPORT
                              NAME: BAKER, HEIDI   DISCH DATE: 10/24/2005
                              ACCT: V
                              DR :

LABORATORY REPORT
OUTPATIENT MEDICAL RECORDS -- FINAL
PRINT DATE: 10/29/2005 05:20   MR#:

away in a hospital intensive-care unit with cerebral malaria, and doctors had just called to say they did not know if he would make it. Again, while my research group was following Heidi Baker around to village outreaches in rural Mozambique in June 2009, the Bakers' children had been flown in to Africa just in time for Rolland to be flown out to Germany for a last-ditch effort at experimental medical treatment. Rolland, who had been diagnosed with dementia (he could not recognize most people) and posttraumatic stress disorder (after witnessing violent murders of African Christians), and could not walk or feed or dress himself, appeared to be dying for reasons that doctors could not fully pin down. Rolland surprised his doctors—but not his family—by again making a full recovery. A few months later he passed a flying test to renew his airplane pilot's license. When I interviewed him in December 2010, Baker appeared to have normal short- and long-term memory, seemed mentally sharp, and, indeed, gave more sophisticated and detailed answers to my questions than have most pentecostal leaders I have interviewed.[16]

Heidi Baker did not slacken her pace even at moments when doctors had given up her husband to die. As she explained in an interview conducted in 2008, during one such period when Rolland was critically ill, "So we have a few challenges, but God has given us a calling and our days are numbered by the Lord. We cannot live in fear. It has to be fearless love. What He tells you to do, you do. If you die, you die. If you live, you live. It's ok either way." So in a love that extended not only to her husband and immediate family but also to Mozambicans and westerners, Baker persevered in doing what she believed God had called her to do. She does not believe that God sends diseases, "but because He's God He just takes something the enemy means to destroy you or kill you . . . . God just turns it around and you get stronger and more compassionate." Baker calls Mozambique "home" and refers to the thousands of orphaned children IM cares for as her "children." Baker claims to love "being in the dirt with the poor on the field all the time," but, she explains, she also feels "very much aware, a third of my life I'm called to travel to the nations . . . . to the one-third world . . . to call laid down lovers to give their lives for passion and compassion . . . and mercy and power. I want to see a radical army of lovers of God that just go into the darkest places on the planet and live a life of selfless love. . . . It's about all of us stopping for one. It's about all of us loving and carrying His mercy and compassion every day—whether it be across the street or around the world." It is paradoxical that Baker's prescription for global revival is stopping to love one person.[17]

Baker does not appear the least self-conscious that her construction of "love" might be interpreted differently by some of those whom she envisions as her beneficiaries. A white woman who describes herself as a mother to thousands of impoverished African children as she goes selflessly into "the dirt" in the "darkest places" might be critically interpreted not as loving but as culturally arrogant and paternalistic. Indeed, Baker herself suggests that not all Mozambicans feel loved by her beneficent overtures. Some villagers, including traditional healers and Muslim leaders who understandably feel threatened by Baker, have thrown rocks and shot guns at her and taken out a contract on her life (for $20). Although claiming to love even those who oppose her, in Baker's worldview because she is an ambassador of God's love, opposition must have a demonic source. Referring to both sickness and resistance by Africans, "Satan tries everything he can to stop us, throwing at us crisis after crisis just when we feel we can't handle one more." From the perspective of certain Mozambicans, Baker herself may appear to be a source of crisis sent by less than benign spiritual forces.[18]

Yet Baker insists that hers is a mission of love, and love is the key to healing. She describes the relationship between "love" and healing "power" as "two wings" because "you can't fly with one." So

> power and love are very much connected. . . . If you have great compassion and concern for the dying and the sick and you have no power to see them healed, you end up a very sad person. But the merciful love of God is that His love has teeth. He doesn't give you this radical compassion so you just sob in the dirt and have no answer. He gives you radical compassion because he knows very well that any, any human being who would yield themselves to the power of the Holy Spirit would have the power to lay hands on the sick and they

would be healed. . . . He's a loving God and a powerful God and He
does not put love in your heart without any power. That would be
sick and sad. God is a powerful and loving God and He gives us
both. So we have two wings and now we soar.

Baker claims that, as love and power work together in Mozambique,
"we have amazing miracles here. The deaf hear and the blind see and
the crippled walk and the dead are raised." An estimated two hundred
fifty individuals have reportedly been raised from the dead through
the prayers of Mozambican IM leaders (but, it is interesting to note,
not through the prayers of Baker herself).[19]

Some western Christians have charged that the Bakers' focus on
miraculous healing is out of proportion. Rolland Baker responds
that "this movement does not chase health and wealth [indeed, Heidi
Baker is sharply critical of 'prosperity theology'] or manifestations,
or signs and wonders. . . . We don't chase miracles. They chase us.
We preach the straight gospel. We like miracles because we like
God. You know when you love somebody you like what they do.
Miracles by themselves don't thrill people with God. It didn't always
thrill people with Jesus when he was on earth. The fact is that a
miracle by itself does not accomplish what God is after. Miracles
demonstrate that God is real. People can see evidence that God is
here. His fingerprint is on us." Rolland argues that miracles serve a
very practical purpose: "We need and expect miracles of all kinds to
sustain us and confirm the Gospel in our ministry. . . . We don't
apologize for seeking and valuing power, because without it love is
incomplete and ineffectual. . . . We believe we experience miracles
because we value them and ask for them, understanding that He will
give them to us only if they will not take us further from Him. . . .
The engine behind the growth of IM in Mozambique has been a
marriage of love and power." This does not mean that the Bakers
experience triumph in every situation. As Rolland acknowledges,
"We understand that such great fruit also comes with the reality
of disappointments, attacks, personal struggles and tragic failures.
These will not keep us from being overjoyed with all that God has
done among us." In addition to the Bakers' own numerous battles

with sickness, some of IM's black African leaders and church members have been beaten and killed by Africans of other religions—and not resurrected.[20]

While driving away from a predominantly Muslim village where we had accompanied Heidi Baker to measure hearing and vision thresholds in 2009, she offhandedly commented that at least this time the villagers had not tried to poison them. When I pressed for an explanation, she said that during the previous visit, an IM staff member had noticed that the food looked too red, so they stopped eating it and took a sample to a city to have it analyzed; it contained poisonous snake venom. Baker nevertheless returned to this same village—taking researchers with her but without bothering to mention the incident until after we had left. She only added the precaution of also bringing along an IM cook. Such seemingly high-risk behavior scarcely raises an eyebrow in IM culture.[21]

The Bakers acknowledge that not every person for whom they pray is healed. They call themselves and others to a "tenacious love" that Heidi defines as "a kind of love that it never dies, you don't stop praying. We've seen hundreds of blind people see, but we also have a home for the blind. . . . We never ever stop believing. We just keep loving, loving, loving, loving. . . . Some healings that we have are instantaneous and some are taking place over a period of time." This perspective contextualizes such behaviors as when I observed Baker publicly praying for a blind woman at great length despite having previously prayed for the same woman on multiple occasions without apparent benefit.[22]

Baker emphasizes that healing is not limited to Mozambique—while implicitly confirming that healing does appear to be a more common experience where modernist worldviews are less entrenched. In Baker's assessment, "Westerners often think they'll have less healings, but that doesn't need to be the case at all." She likes to relate anecdotes like that of a man for whom she prayed in England. His spine had been severed, he was a paraplegic, and he had MS. He kept a notebook in which he had recorded every time someone prayed for his healing—a total of 1,138 times. He experienced healing the 1,139th time, after which he traveled around England giving his testimony. On another occasion, Baker was preaching in a Canadian city about

"God giving us bigger hearts and hearts of compassion and love." She saw a woman leaving the meeting and felt led to jump out from behind the pulpit to run and catch her, and "I heard the Lord say 'I'm giving her a new heart,' so I told her . . . and she collapsed on the floor, screaming, and yelling, and sobbing." A year later, Baker returned to the same church, and the woman approached carrying a manila envelope. She said that when Baker prayed for her she had heart disease and, because no hearts were available for transplant, she had been given less than six weeks to live. The manila envelope contained x-ray images of the new heart she received during Baker's prayer. Reflecting her lack of interest in medical documentation, Baker did not ask for the x-rays. Baker did take note of the woman's testimony that she had hated her husband so much before her healing that she was planning to divorce him even though she was about to die. When she received prayer, God "healed her physical heart, but also her emotional heart." She and her husband "forgave each other, fell in love, and then they quit their daytime jobs, moved into the inner city, and started working with prostitutes." Baker considered this woman's emotional and spiritual healing, which made forgiveness possible, as being comparable in significance to her physical healing.[23]

Indeed, forgiveness is a theme that recurs in many healing narratives, as in the following, also from IM.

Francis: Forgive Them

On the evening of September 23, 2003, Francis, a black South African man, was standing at the entrance to a church fellowship hall where IM was hosting a regional conference. It was 4:00 P.M., and Francis had gone outside to lock the gate and quiet a gang who had come to cause trouble. Four men approached and beat Francis, saying that "we want to kill you today." After the assailants had left, Francis was transported by car to a hospital where he was pronounced dead at 11:00 P.M. Everyone at the church continued praying from a distance while a handful of Christians gathered around Francis in the hospital morgue. At 12:15 A.M., Francis began to breathe. His eyes and lips were still swollen shut, and his extensive and still excruciatingly painful injuries made it appear that full recovery would be slow. That night, Francis could only croak out two words: "Forgive them." Early the next morning, the police found one of the attackers and called for someone from the church to come to the police station and press charges. Having learned of Francis's words the night before, the church refused, much to the chagrin of the police, who worried that the action would encourage more crime. Within minutes, the hospital also called—asking that someone come pick up Francis immediately since all of his wounds had inexplicably disappeared. Not a bruise or scratch was visible, and Francis could see and talk normally, and so there was no reason for him to keep taking up space in the hospital.[24]

Francis reportedly went directly from the hospital to the police station to request the release of his assailant. He says, "I asked them just to release that man because I've already forgiven him. The police officers firstly denied my request because they say [sic], 'How do you forgive someone who has beaten you to death like this?' Then I said to them, 'No, this guy doesn't know what he did.' Then the police accepted my request. Then they released him. Then I hugged him, and tell [sic] him that God loves him. And then I said to him, 'You know my brother, I'll urge you just to accept Jesus as your Lord and Savior and go back home happy.'" This man did reportedly become a Christian, attend Bible school, and, as of 2007, was active as an evangelist in the Iris network.[25]

It is of course possible that Francis was mistakenly pronounced dead, after which he revived and recovered from his wounds surprisingly rapidly through natural healing processes, rather than being supernaturally resurrected and miraculously restored to health as he believes. In one sense it does not matter whether Francis had in point of fact died, because he supposed this to be the case, and yet he forgave the men whom he understood to be his murderers. An interesting feature of this account is that the recovery was incomplete until just after Francis and his church—perceiving God's love to have been demonstrated concretely by resurrection—were motivated to forgive the men who had attempted, apparently successfully, to beat Francis to death. This act of forgiveness made such an impression on the assailant—who viewed himself as a murderer—that he changed his life course to become a Christian evangelist.

George: From Victim to Victor

Like Francis, George—whose narrative of healing from a terminal brain tumor opens chapter 4—believes that God rescued him from a death sentence. His story also illustrates the dense web of network connections that characterizes global pentecostal healing practices. George, who grew up a cessationist Baptist, was first influenced by the Toronto Blessing in 1994, while he was a foreign exchange student from the United States to Scotland, and visited a revival service led by a team visiting from Toronto. George was frankly skeptical of the phenomena he observed during the meetings and left apparently unaffected. A few days later, he was praying by himself in his college dormitory room when he had an unusually strong impression of God's love for him. As George described the experience, "I literally fell over out of my chair and laughed and cried the whole night. For the first time, I had not only known but also felt the love of God." Yet the team from Toronto left as abruptly as they came, leaving behind little teaching on what to do with such experiences. Nine years passed before George's health crisis led him to investigate what had become of the Toronto Blessing.[26]

George had never heard of Randy Clark until 2003, when a friend who lived several thousand miles away informed George via e-mail that Clark had been the one preaching when the Toronto Blessing began, and that he had gone on to establish Global Awakening. Learning that GA was hosting its annual Voice of the Apostles conference several weeks later, George boarded a plane to attend. While he was there, he received prayer from Clark, the Brazilian Davi Silva, and Dennis Balcombe, a missionary to China. This was one in a series of numerous pentecostal conferences George attended during the next five months—traveling an estimated fifty-thousand miles back and forth across the United States and Canada and to several other countries—in his search for healing. George received prayer from a number of prominent itinerant evangelists, including the Argentinian Pablo Bottari, the Canadian Todd Bentley, the Palestinian Canadian American Benny Hinn, and the Indian Kenyan American Mahesh Chavda, as well as the U.S. itinerants Bill Johnson, Gary Oates, James Maloney, and Dutch Sheets. George also received prayer from many lower-profile Christian pastors and laypersons at various healing rooms and church services around the country. George's practice of seeking prayer repeatedly reflects a theology that the effects of prayer are cumulative and that "faith" is exhibited by perseverance rather than by praying once and then "claiming" healing regardless of whether anything seems to change.[27]

George attests that he is glad he cannot pinpoint the exact moment of his healing. He does point to a series of moments "when the Holy Spirit ministered powerfully through the prayers of specific individuals. It is the Lord alone who gets the glory for my healing—but the Lord chose to work through the loving prayers of a number of his faithful servants." Even before George had any evidence of his healing, he began to take other people who needed healing with him to pentecostal conferences. He himself also prayed for others' healing as a volunteer in healing rooms and on ANGA-affiliated international ministry trips. Many of the people with whom George interacted in these settings also began to report healing experiences and to begin praying for other people's healing as well. As George looked back on his and his family's experiences in 2010, he reflected that "our lives are wonderfully full in ways that we wouldn't have imagined before I had the brain tumor and got healed. God took our worst nightmare, defeated the enemy, and turned the whole thing into the greatest blessing of our lives. 1 Cor. 15:57: 'But thanks be to God! He gives us the victory through our Lord Jesus Christ.'"[28]

Mahesh Chavda: Only Love Can Make a Miracle

While George was pursuing healing for himself, one of the many healing evangelists he sought ministry from was Mahesh Chavda. In 2004, George traveled to Chicago, after hearing that Chavda was to speak there at a conference hosted by HUB (His United Body) Ministries. HUB was founded by Nancy Magiera after she spent time at the Toronto Blessing (one of numerous stories that exceed the scope of this book). HUB regularly hosts visits by both Chavda and Heidi Baker. Magiera often mentions Toronto as she addresses her Chicago audiences. In the past decade she has hosted a series of Toronto- and ANGA-affiliated speakers who appear in this book, including Randy Clark, Georgian Banov, John and Carol Arnott, and Gary and Kathi Oates. While Chavda was speaking in 2004, he paused in the middle of his sermon to deliver a word of knowledge, or presumably divine revelation, concerning a woman whose husband had cancer. George's wife responded to the word, bringing George with her to the front of the crowded hotel meeting room. Chavda believed that a demon had wrapped itself around George like a python snake, so he commanded it to unwrap itself, and George fell down screaming. When George arose, Chavda told him that there was "much for you to do," which George interpreted as a *prophecy,* or divinely revealed insight, about the ministry that he would himself be called by God to do. A few months later, George again sought prayer from Chavda, this time in Charlotte, North Carolina, where Mahesh Chavda Ministries (now Chavda Ministries International) was hosting its annual conference. The ANGA-leader Bill Johnson (based out of Redding, California) is a regular speaker at these conferences—and George received prayer from Johnson as well as Chavda. This sequence of meeting connections illustrates how Toronto Blessing–ANGA network leaders often travel thousands of miles to speak at each other's conferences, sometimes praying repeatedly for the same individuals at multiple venues.[29]

Global travel—and healing—have indeed been significant themes in Chavda's life story. His father, born in 1893, was descended from India's royal Rajput ("sons of kings") caste and had migrated from India to Kenya (at that time, both part of the British empire) before Mahesh was born. Mahesh was the first person in his family lineage to convert from Hinduism to Christianity, which he did after being given a New Testament by a Baptist missionary from America and having had a vision of "heaven" in which he believes he met Jesus. One may ask whether Chavda's Hindu worldview made him more receptive to visionary experiences than would have been the case for someone whose worldview had space only for materialistic forces. With financial help from Baptists in America, Chavda left Kenya in 1964 to attend college and graduate school in Texas. There he began a Ph.D. program in English literature, although ultimately he instead completed a doctorate at Sacramento Theological Seminary in California.[30]

In 1972, while still in Texas and scraping together funds to pay for graduate courses a la carte, Chavda received a letter from his family, which now lived in London. The letter informed Chavda that his mother was terminally ill with bone cancer and relayed her request that he visit before she died. Unable to afford a plane ticket, Chavda avowedly wept off and on for three days, after which he had another visionary experience during which he found himself singing in a language he did not understand (he knew six languages). The next day, a Catholic nun interpreted his description of the experience as "baptism in the Holy Spirit" and introduced him to a local, nondenominational Charismatic prayer group. Chavda felt a renewed interest in reading the Bible—especially the parts about Jesus healing the sick and a verse in Hebrews: "Jesus Christ is the same yesterday and today and forever." This verse emboldened Chavda to ask God, if Jesus was still healing today, if he could even heal his mother. A voice seemed to respond, "Pray for her." Chavda rebutted, "How can I pray for her? She is in London, and I am in Texas." Again, Chavda believed he heard a response: "There is no distance in my Spirit. Pray for your mother. Ask me to heal her." Chavda did, and two weeks later he received a letter reporting his mother's surprising recovery. After Chavda told his mother about his prayers, she interpreted her healing as a response and became a Christian. Despite the emphasis pentecostals generally place on proximal prayer, in this instance distant intercession was credited for healing. Eighteen years later, when Chavda published his autobiography, his mother was a healthy woman in her seventies.[31]

Soon after his mother's healing, Chavda sensed God leading him, while still a graduate student, to take a part-time job at the nearby Lubbock State School for Retarded Children. He spent much time praying for the healing of these children and attributed improvements in a number of them to his prayers. This period of time, like his mother's healing, was formative for Chavda. As he describes the impact of the experience: "Now I was learning that the power of God was to be found in the love of God. When the Lord sent me to the State School, he did not say, 'I am sending you as my ambassador of power' or 'of miracles.' He said, 'I am sending you as my ambassador of love.' That was the way I saw myself and that was the way I prayed for the children: that the Lord would make his love real to them. The healings came almost as a by-product. I learned that only love can make a miracle." This theme, of the relationship between God's power and love, is one that recurs in a number of different healing narratives. The perception that love produces miracles motivated Chavda to lay aside his English studies to become a pastor and itinerant evangelist. He took his first pastorate in 1974, married his wife Bonnie in 1976, and by 1979 was receiving international ministry invitations as word spread of dramatic healings occurring at his meetings.[32]

This same year, 1979, Chavda's first son, Benjamin, was born. Two weeks after his birth, Benjamin was diagnosed with a congenital kidney defect; 97 percent of all children born with that condition die within weeks. The doctors did what they could, and the Chavdas and many others prayed. It was a six-month battle during which Benjamin, in the intensive-care unit, suffered obvious pain spasms. Then on one particular day, Chavda had an impression that God was telling him that the pain he felt in watching his son suffer was similar to the pain God had felt in watching his son Jesus die, and that "it is because my Son suffered in this way that your son need not suffer. This day I have healed your son." That same day the pain spasms seemed to stop and medical tests showed that Benjamin's kidneys had begun to function. At the time of Chavda's autobiography, Benjamin was a healthy eleven-year-old. Chavda recalls that:

> I was forever changed by the experience with Ben. I had prayed for healing for people many times in the past, but it would never be the same for me after that. Never would I be able to encounter someone who was sick without remembering the terrible anguish Bonnie and I had experienced. Never would I be able to minister to a sick person without identifying with the fear and confusion and heartache that were every bit as real to them as they had been to us. Never would I be able to pray for healing out of a selfish desire to impress people. . . . I would always carry in my heart the ache that I felt as I watched my son suffer, the ache that God the Father felt as he watched Jesus suffer, and the compassion with which he looks upon all his children who are afflicted. Because of the pain I had

carried in my heart for Ben, I would always have room in my heart for the pain of others.

Chavda did not believe that God had caused the suffering of his son or of the many other people for whom he prayed. On the contrary, "the tragedy and heartache all around me was the work of the evil one, of Satan, not of the Lord." But God, Chavda believed, had used suffering to teach him compassion.[33]

In 1984, twenty years after leaving Kenya, Chavda returned to Africa to conduct an evangelistic healing convention among the poor; in subsequent years, Africa became his most frequent ministry destination. Weeks before a greatly anticipated trip to Zambia and Zaire (now the Democratic Republic of Congo) in 1985, Bonnie Chavda, who had by this point delivered two normal daughters, gave birth prematurely to a son. Baby Aaron weighed in at one pound eight ounces and had numerous complications, which the doctors suspected included brain damage and cystic fibrosis. As the baby hovered between life and death, the Chavdas believed God was calling Mahesh to carry through his plans for a two-month trip to Africa. Not knowing whether his son was alive or dead (he had been able to call home only once), Chavda was speaking at around noon one day to thirty thousand people in Kinshasa, the capital of Zaire (as it was then called), when he believed the Holy Spirit was communicating an unusual word of knowledge: "There is a man here whose son died this morning. Invite him to come forward. I want to do something wonderful for him." A man ran to the front of the crowd, Chavda prayed for resurrection, and the man ran off.[34]

Chavda later heard what had happened. The man's name was Mulamba Manikai, and his six-year-old son, Katshinyi, had reportedly died at four o'clock that morning of cerebral malaria. Doctors at Kinshasa's Mikondo Clinic had pronounced him dead after administering an injection to revive him, sticking needles into his arms and chest, and holding an open flame against his legs. Katshinyi was transported to Mama Yemo Hospital where the staff wrote a notification of death (reproduced in chapter 3 of this book) and sent Manikai to borrow money to pay for a burial permit. Manikai's brother, Kuamba, stayed at the hospital holding the boy's apparently lifeless body. Manikai was one of the few people in his family or community who was a Christian, and he prayed, "I have told many people that you are the Good Shepherd. How will they believe me if my own son dies?" Manikai remembered the Bible story in which the woman Dorcas dies, but God's servant Peter has just arrived in the city and raises her from the dead. Manikai believes God said to him, "Why are you weeping? My servant is in this city. Go to him." Manikai went immediately to where he knew Chavda was preaching, and just as he arrived he heard Chavda call forward the man whose son had just died. Manikai ran to the front of the crowd, and as soon as Chavda finished praying for him, he ran back to the hospital. Kuamba takes up the story: "It was midday. I was sitting there holding the body of my brother's son in my arms. Suddenly, I felt his body move. Then he sneezed. He sat up in my arms and asked for something to eat." In response to this apparent resurrection, Munikai's entire family became Christians and started a church and a choir of seventy-five children. Chavda visited with the family whenever he returned to Kinshasa, and as of 1990, Katshinyi was still doing well. As in the case of Francis's alleged resurrection, whether or not Katshinyi was really dead his and his community's belief that he was raised from the dead exerted a profound social effect.[35]

Chavda's son Aaron also lived and regained mental and physical health, growing into a normal five-year-old as of the writing of Chavda's account. As of 2011, Chavda still conducts international conventions, but he also believes God has called him to be a "missionary to America." He spends much of his time pastoring congregations in Charlotte, North Carolina and Atlanta, Georgia, as well as hosting conferences that attract international crowds and itinerating to speak at ANGA-affiliated conferences across North America. Chavda still looks back on his mother's recovery from apparently terminal cancer nearly forty years ago as the turning point that oriented his life toward praying for other people's healing. That change has in turn influenced many others—including George, whose story introduced Chavda's—who have also given testimonies of experiencing healing through Chavda's prayers.[36]

Mimi: From Asthmatic to Track Scholar

Before he had ever heard of Mahesh Chavda, George attended GA's 2003 Voice of the Apostles conference in Pennsylvania. As a result, he decided to travel with GA to Cuba and then to Brazil in 2004. On George's return to the United States from Brazil, the pastor of the church he had recently started attending (a church planted by the same Vineyard networks that gave rise to ANGA) gave him a few minutes at the microphone on a Sunday morning to talk about the "miracles" he had avowedly seen through his own prayers. At the end of the service, several people asked George to pray for them to be healed of various conditions. The next Sunday, the pastor again gave up service time because several of the individuals for whom George had prayed during the previous Sunday's service wanted to testify to having been healed. This pattern continued for the next several years, with testimonies generating interest in prayer, which led to more testimonies. So many people began to request prayer that George could not pray for them all by himself. Drawing on what he had learned from his experiences with GA and similar pentecostal groups, George developed a prayer ministry training class (which he came to teach at regular intervals not only at his current church but also for various other interested groups). From this class emerged a prayer team that began to offer ministry every Sunday morning—typically remaining for an hour or more after each service as a line of people waited their turn for prayer.[37]

The prayer team membership included a family of four—a couple and their two teenage daughters—all of whom became interested in prayer ministry because of their own needs for healing. The mother, Lisa, suffered from temporomandibular joint disorder (TMJ)—a condition in her case caused by a failed chiropractic adjustment and not taken seriously by conventional medical doctors. The father, Sean, was bothered by knee pain. The elder daughter, Mimi, had severe asthma and allergies. And the younger daughter, Diana, felt constant pain in one rib. All four members of the Smith family requested prayer for themselves at every opportunity, but while they were waiting for their own healing they also began to pray for others.[38]

When in the summer of 2004 George announced that he was going to drive halfway across the country to a healing conference hosted by Mahesh Chavda Ministries in Charlotte, North Carolina, the Smiths were by then intrigued enough to ask to come along. Mimi, fourteen years old at the time, was the most determined: she resolved that she would not leave the conference until her asthma had been healed. Asthma and related allergies and infections had been a constant battle since Mimi was a small child. Despite the nebulizer machine and medications prescribed by her doctor, her reaction to atmospheric particles was so intense that she had to leave school because the chalk dust bothered her so much. She was, moreover, laid up for weeks at a time by frequent colds that predictably turned into pneumonia.[39]

In North Carolina, each member of the Smith family received prayer repeatedly, but without obvious effect, from each of the conference speakers—Mahesh and Bonnie Chavda, Bill Johnson, and Bobby Conner—as well as other lay prayer-team members. On the fourth and final night of the conference, the meeting was drawing to a close. Feeling discouraged and even angry at the lack of change in her condition, Mimi got in line shortly after midnight for one final prayer from a conference speaker, Bobby Conner, whose avowed gifting was prophecy rather than healing. Ten minutes later, as Mimi and a few other stragglers stood around talking in the meeting venue, her face started to turn red, and she began crying and seemed to be hyperventilating. As her parents tell the story, they were not sure whether Mimi was being healed or whether they should call 911.[40]

I was conducting field research at this event and, observing the commotion, spoke with Mimi's parents to find out what had happened. After the Smiths returned to their hotel room, Mimi seemed to be on the verge of hyperventilation throughout the night—in her mother's evaluation, because she was taking in more oxygen than she was accustomed to getting. By the next morning, Mimi sensed that she had been completely healed of asthma. She went home and threw away her nebulizer and medications, returned to school, and joined the track team. The recurrent colds and pneumonia ceased. Three years later, she won a track scholarship to college. She also began leading Bible studies and praying for healing for her friends, many of whom were nonpentecostal evangelicals, and several of whom had been unchurched until she persuaded them to become Christians. Mimi decided to pursue a nursing degree, because she thought it would be useful in overseas missions.[41]

In 2011, I followed up with Mimi—at this point a twenty-one-year old who had recently returned from one of several international ministry trips to Brazil as a prayer team member and apprentice preacher. By this time, each member of Mimi's family had also avowedly experienced healing through prayer: from the TMJ, the knee problems, and the rib pain—and as a bonus, from a chocolate allergy (even though the healing rooms team that prayed for this last condition had done so reluctantly, suggesting that it might be good to be allergic to chocolate, because it is fattening). The entire family continued to seek opportunities to pray for others, occasionally traveling with ANGA affiliates to Brazil and Colombia to minister. They also participated in evangelistic and charitable outreaches to economically disadvantaged members of their local community, a number of whom (from the Smiths' perspective) appeared to experience healing and decided to become Christians. It is not possible to know whether the recipients of such outreach overtures experienced these interactions as loving, paternalistic, or an uneasy combination.[42]

Donna: A Thorn in the Side Removed

Some time after moving away from the city where the Smiths lived, George met Donna in 2006 at a potluck hosted by a church George was visiting. As often happened when George was around, the conversation quickly turned to the topic of healing. Donna shared that she had been experiencing chronic pain in her right side since 1999. The pain was debilitating and excruciating. It hurt to drive, breathe, or write, and sleep was elusive. She had consulted numerous medical specialists and undergone a battery of tests and exploratory operations, none of which diagnosed or alleviated the pain. Donna, who at the time attended a nonpentecostal evangelical church, concluded that God must have given her the pain as a "thorn in my side" and resigned herself to "live with it."[43]

A few months before, Donna had stumbled on a book, *When Heaven Invades Earth* (2003), written by Bill Johnson. Reading this book convinced Donna that "the Lord did not give me this pain, and that it was from the enemy. I knew that my loving Heavenly Father would not treat me this way, but that he wanted me to be whole spiritually, emotionally and physically." When, after publishing his book, Johnson himself lost his father, age seventy-five, to cancer, he still insisted that "everyone who came to Jesus was healed. Not everyone who comes to me is and . . . . I don't want to lower the standard of Scripture to the level of my experience." He added, "I'm not looking for comfort to ease me that allows me to stay where I'm at. . . . Did we measure up [with my father]? No, but the answer isn't guilt and shame. The answer is just realizing that, no, we're not there yet. . . . I have the liberty to pursue [God] in private to close the gap between his level and mine." Donna was convinced by Johnson's reasoning but did not know where to go from there. Her pain persisted, even though she was taking narcotic pain relievers. Donna and her husband began praying for healing, but they felt the need for help.[44]

Soon after Donna met George, she and others who were planting the church that had facilitated the potluck meeting asked George to teach a class on healing ministry. George did so, and a Sunday morning prayer ministry team formed. Several years later, after George had moved on to another church, the team was still offering weekly prayer to individuals, a number of whom reported healing. George started healing rooms out of his home that were loosely based on the International Association of Healing Rooms model (which had in turn been shaped by both Bill Johnson and Randy Clark). Donna was one of the first to make an appointment for prayer ministry at George's healing rooms, which focused more on in-depth deliverance from demonic influences than the IAHR twenty-minute-ministry model.[45]

Donna's first multihour prayer appointment focused on emotional and spiritual hurts rather than physical pain. Donna felt a deep release from unforgiveness—which she perceived as coming from God toward herself and held by her against others and even against herself—and deep emotional wounds. Donna recalls, "I didn't have any sensation while they prayed for the physical healing, other than the pain 'moving' a bit around my body" (a phenomenon interpreted by pentecostals as evidence of a demonic source of the pain). The next morning, however, "I woke up and I could move my arm in a 360 degree circle. That was the first time I had been able to do that since the onset of the pain in 1999. It was incredible. It did not take me an hour to get out of bed, nor did I have to walk hunched over for the first hour I was awake. I was absolutely astonished and thankful that the Lord had worked in this way. The progress was remarkable." Donna was soon able to stop taking any pain medications. Although not yet healed completely, she felt encouraged to begin an aggressive, three-year-long journey of seeking prayer at every opportunity, even trekking coast to coast to ANGA-affiliated conferences and IAHR healing rooms in order to do so.[46]

Donna's case is interesting as an example of someone who experienced a "partial healing" on one occasion, not during but several hours after receiving prayer. She subsequently attended many healing events without experiencing any noticeable benefit at the time but was determined, as an expression of faith, to persevere in seeking prayer repeatedly. Memorable stops along the way included a GA School of Healing and Impartation in Cincinnati, Ohio, at which Randy Clark was a speaker and to which George took Donna and a number of others in January 2007. At the conference, Donna experienced a strange choking sensation—interpreted as a demonic force opposing her pursuit of healing—but no further pain relief. Donna and her husband also traveled to Johnson's church in Redding, California, where she was introduced to the "sozo," or saved, healed, and delivered, model of prayer ministry, which Donna later came to use extensively in praying for others.[47]

The final major episode in Donna's healing journey occurred anticlimactically in 2009 at a conference in Charlotte, North Carolina, hosted by Mahesh Chavda at which Bill Johnson was speaking. Ironically, Donna had attended this particular conference not for herself as she had so many others, but in order to drive a friend who also needed healing. Amid a flurry of other conference activities, Johnson paused briefly during a sermon to deliver a word of knowledge that someone had pain in the ride side and God wanted to heal it now. The conference DVD shows that the entire episode lasted about five seconds.

Johnson placed his hand on the same area of his own side where Donna's pain had been and asked whoever had the pain to poke that area to see if it hurt, saying "God is healing your pain." Donna—and only she, out of the twelve hundred persons present—stood up and poked the area. It happened to be her customary way of checking for pain. She found that at this moment it did not hurt for the first time in ten years. Donna, to all appearances, nonchalantly sat down, without any visible expression of happiness or surprise. The pain was simply gone.[48]

One of the striking features of Donna's account is how undramatic the entire episode appeared. Many such words of knowledge are delivered at pentecostal conferences. Often there is no way of knowing the outcome, especially when no obvious commotion ensues; this particular example is instructive in suggesting that more may happen in some cases than meets the eye. After initially hearing her story, I followed up with Donna on several occasions. A few months after the conference experience, the pain "tried to return"—a common trope in such narratives. But when this happened, Donna—who had been warned by pentecostal friends that this might occur (on the basis of biblical stories in which demons that have been cast out attempt to return)—briefly commanded the pain to leave in Jesus's name, which it did. After a few such occurrences, the pain stopped coming back, and Donna enjoyed sustained relief. A year later, Donna wrote, "It has been a year of incredible freedom. I have lived without the 'thorn in my side' of consistent, severe pain. Though it was a journey, it is a miracle." Two years after her healing experience, in 2011, Donna reported, "I'm still healed. Thank you, Jesus!" After experiencing healing for herself, Donna became active in praying for other people's healing and driving groups of people to GA healing conferences. Donna considers her entire life's focus to have shifted from being self-centered to kingdom oriented.[49]

Susan: Trading Sorrows for Joy

One of the people who traveled with George and Donna to GA's Cincinnati healing school in 2007 was Susan, a twenty-one-year-old college student, whom I first interviewed alongside others in her group in Cincinnati. Susan's unapologetic reason for attending was that she was tired of always feeling sick, sorrowful, and oppressed. Within the past two years, she had suffered two bouts of mononucleosis (even though one should be immune after contracting the disease once), on top of years of chronic fatigue; headaches; constipation; depression; and tormenting, suicidal thoughts. Susan dated the beginning of what she interpreted as "demonic" visitations back to when she still slept in a crib. (Her first memory was a vivid dream in which she was chased and strangled by blood-red snakes in a children's water park.) From that time forward, evil spirits had—"on a very regular basis," as Susan described her experience of liberation in an e-mail several weeks later— "temporarily paralyzed me, stricken me with fear and anxiety, taunted me, caused blackouts, put me under sleep spells, filled my thoughts so that I cannot hear or think, made it so that I cannot read, and plagued me with incessant nightmares." Susan had repeatedly tried to tell the demons to leave her alone "in Jesus' name . . . but that did not ever seem to work." In fact, things only got "progressively worse" after she became a Christian. The more she tried to read the Bible, "the worse the torment." As she sank into ever deeper sorrow and depression throughout her grade-school years, "thoughts of suicide were a regular for me" even as an eleven-year-old. During her third year of college, she succumbed to an even deeper depression. Susan had tried a few times to discuss her physical and spiritual problems with various pastors and ministry leaders, but no one had taken her concerns seriously.[50]

Susan had concluded that the best she could hope for was to manage her spiritually and physically distressing symptoms as best as she could. She never imagined that what she later called "deliverance," or complete freedom, was possible. During the Cincinnati conference, Susan drank in the encouraging teaching, but at the same time felt her whole body shaking and her teeth chattering, and experienced "unbelievable pain in my abdomen and head. I knew what was going on. The demons had been exposed and were not happy at all." As soon as the conference concluded, Susan made an appointment at the healing rooms that George directed. During the several days while she waited for her appointment, Susan experienced intense "migraines, frequent blackouts, and debilitating spells of sleep in which I couldn't wake for hours on end," all of which she interpreted as demonic resistance to her approaching deliverance.[51]

Susan's first healing rooms session stalled in mid-course. As a general practice, ministry teams consisted of two to three lay Christians, including at least one member of the same gender as the recipient, in a private room. The team that prayed for Susan asked her a battery of questions and instructed her to say aloud a series of printed, liturgical prayers. The prayers led Susan to forgive those who had wronged her, to repent of judgments she had made against others, and to renounce generational curses and dabbling with "occult" practices, all of which were deemed openings to demonic oppression—and "legal" justifications for the demons to refuse to leave despite Susan's repeated commands. During the session, Susan recounts that she found it difficult to speak or even to breathe. She felt her mind flooded with so much confusion that she had trouble reading the renunciation prayers. Periodically, the team leader paused to command these "manifestations" to stop, after which Susan felt able to continue. She sensed the leader place a hand gently on her shoulder and heard him calmly and quietly command the "unclean spirits to leave in the name and authority of Jesus of Nazareth." Susan felt some, but not all, of the oppression lift. For a few minutes, she felt an "awesome" joy, laughter, and peace—but the torment soon descended again. The leader reinterviewed Susan, looking for additional "open doors" to the enemy, and again commanded the spirits to leave. Susan still felt terrible—her body shook and her teeth chattered, and she felt overwhelmed by anxiety and grief. The hour was growing late and everyone seemed tired, so the leader "bound" the spirits and adjourned the evening's session, proposing that everyone in the room consider spending a few days in prayer and fasting before reconvening (drawing on Jesus's instruction that some kinds of demons can be driven out only through prayer and fasting).[52]

Susan, who had never fasted before, believed God was telling her to fast on nothing but water for the next ten days. During this period, Susan perceived an intense inner battle to be raging. She awoke from a nightmare with her arm paralyzed—more completely than having simply fallen asleep. She commanded the afflicting spirit to leave in

Jesus's name "AND IT DID. I instantly received full use of my arm again, just like that!" But she still fought sleep spells, headaches, and blackouts. Several times, she violently vomited a substance that appeared to her eerily green, and she heard voices tempting her that if she would only break the fast, everything would be better. Resisting the voices, Susan returned for further deliverance ministry, still fasting. On this occasion, the ministry team, which had also been fasting, prayed for just five or ten minutes before Susan perceived demonic presences begin lifting off her: "When you have been plagued by these spirits your whole life, you know when they are gone. They stop filling your thoughts. They stop speaking to you. It was like a weight had been lifted off of my shoulders." Within minutes, she began to experience "joy, peace, and laughter" as the ministry team prayed that she would be filled with the Holy Spirit. The team next prayed for healing of her colon: "Instantly, I felt fire in my side. It was the most overwhelming internal heat I had ever experienced. It was not like a painful burn, but a soothing, live fire that overcame me. During this time, I suddenly felt my circulation open up. I felt blood actually rushing into my constantly ice cold feet." As the team leader moved his hand over to Susan's painfully tensed-up shoulder, "I literally felt the knots in my shoulder untying!" Over the course of the subsequent days and weeks, Susan reported the disappearance of all of her former physical and spiritual problems.[53]

I interviewed and followed up with Susan over a period of five years after her healing experience. As of our most recent encounter in 2011, Susan appears happy and energetic. Although there are no empirical means of investigating whether she was ever really the victim of demonic influences, she says that her life has been totally different since she went through deliverance ministry. She has become active in telling friends and coworkers about her faith and in praying for those who are sick or believe themselves to be oppressed by demons. Several of her friends have perceived themselves healed through her prayers and as a result have decided to become Christians; Susan has publicly baptized three of them. Susan directs a "house of prayer" modeled on the 24/7 "IHOP," or International House of Prayer, headquartered in Kansas City, Missouri. She also feels that God is calling her to go strategically into what she considers "New Age" settings where she had formerly felt comfortable as a participant. Now she has the goal of persuading others to follow Jesus.[54]

Because of her healing experience, Susan claims to be newly aware that God loves her. She feels "loved not only by family and friends, but by the Creator Himself.... Before receiving physical/mental/emotional/spiritual healing, it felt like depression and other ailments clouded my vision so much so that I could only see myself and my own problems. Now that all the obstacles on the inside of me have been removed, my vision has naturally transitioned to looking towards the needs of others rather than just my own." This comment offers insight into how an experience of feeling loved by God through healing leads toward love for others—by removing obstacles to perceiving other people's needs. Susan's entire family, moreover, has attested to her having been changed. Susan's mother was at first skeptical regarding the healing-rooms group that had prayed for Susan's deliverance. Yet she later brought with her to a healing rooms training seminar half a dozen coworkers who share in her nonprofit ministry to abused women, so that they could all receive training in incorporating deliverance into their ministry. As of 2011, this group reports a higher success rate with their clients than before they learned about deliverance. Data are unavailable concerning how these clients perceived the new approach.[55]

A notable feature of Susan's narrative is that she decided to disseminate a written version of her testimony through ANGA networks in 2010 shortly after reading about how the Brazilian Davi Silva had falsified his dramatic testimony of healing from Down's syndrome. As Susan put it, "I read about Davi, and I instantly felt Holy Spirit speak in His still quiet way, 'but your testimony is true.'" So she decided to tell her story, in a sense, to counteract the influence exerted by Silva's falsification. This response illustrates the intertextuality of pentecostal culture—even across cultural, linguistic, and geographic boundaries—in which individuals read each other's stories and in turn make their own contributions to the body of largely informally circulated, identity-building texts that reflect and shape global pentecostalism.[56]

Fernando: Changing Bars

After traveling with GA and affiliated groups on several international ministry trips as a prayer team member and occasional preacher, George began accepting invitations to travel on his own as a conference speaker, both around the U.S. and internationally. Such invitations emerged out of a dense web of relational connections, as the following sequence of interactions illustrates. One of the many people who had played a role in George's healing and deliverance was James Maloney. Maloney is a healing evangelist who speaks at ANGA conferences (Bill Johnson wrote the foreword for Maloney's first book) as well as frequently traveling to the Middle East. His ministry grew out of his own experience of healing from physical and emotional wounds after being neglected and abused as an infant. George joined Maloney's team for a ministry trip to Honduras in 2009 (just weeks after a military coup). On that trip, several of the Honduran pastors reportedly articulated their desire not only to have healing evangelists visit and minister healing, but also to equip local pastors and laity to minister more effectively to their own people after the evangelists had left.[57]

At the invitation of the Honduran pastors, George and another couple returned the following year to preach at equipping conferences for pastors. Two weeks after the conclusion of the 2010 conferences, one Honduran pastor reported that he had gone back to his church and prayed for a woman using the method he had just learned. This woman had had an enlarged womb for eighteen years, which was, the pastor claimed, instantly healed. A long-term Honduran missionary wrote several weeks after the conference: "I know here everyone was thrilled with the meetings and the ACTIVATION. Not just someone coming to do miracles, but someone activating them to do them." Another of the pastors, Fernando, who attended the Honduras 2010 meetings, had traveled all the way from Nicaragua for the event.[58]

Fernando attests that he was once a "powerful" Sandinista fighter and a drug addict. He had had a dramatic, instantaneous experience of conversion and deliverance from addiction through the ministry of Ernesto, a long-term Latino missionary from Los Angeles. Fifteen years earlier, Ernesto, already in Nicaragua, had visited the Toronto Blessing. When he returned home, the same kinds of phenomena (for instance, healings and laughter) that he had experienced in Toronto began to happen in his own churches in Nicaragua. Ernesto now works with the Bulgarian ANGA Revival Alliance member Georgian Banov to minister in the most impoverished areas of Nicaragua. After Fernando converted, he began to work alongside Ernesto in planting churches. Having "found the joy of the Lord," he had "changed bars (*cambié de bar*)" and now "drinks from the Holy Spirit."[59]

Fernando is considered by other Nicaraguan pentecostals to be an "apostle." He oversees a network of churches throughout the country, and he attests to having once raised the dead. As Fernando tells this story, the five-year-old son of a neighbor had been sick. In an effort to heal him, someone had tied around his neck a thick cord intended as a shamanic amulet (*brujería*). The boy nevertheless died, and his mother, frantically screaming, carried his body into the street. Fernando cut the cord off his neck and then bent over the dead body to pray and—here Fernando added a detail that he and his auditors considered humorous—the first indication that life had returned to the boy's body was that he urinated on Fernando's face.[60]

Despite such memorable personal experiences and the phenomena that Ernesto had brought back from Toronto, Fernando felt "like a stranger" in Nicaraguan evangelical culture. From Fernando's perspective, few churches were regularly experiencing the level of spiritual power that he had come to expect. Fernando felt "right at home" at the Honduras 2010 meetings, which were characterized by numerous testimonies of healing, joyous laughter, and appearances of golden "glory dust" (interpreted by pentecostals as a supernatural phenomenon). He wanted all of that for Nicaragua, which is why he invited George to hold the same kinds of meetings there that he had led in Honduras.[61]

Antonio: Putting a Challenging Teaching into Practice

Later in 2010, George went to Nicaragua to lead conferences designed to equip pastors to pray for healing and deliverance. Although there are well-established evangelical churches in Nicaragua, some of which have been influenced by the Toronto Blessing, few have heard much teaching on how to pray for healing. The pastor of one of the churches that hosted George's visit, Antonio, said that this new teaching was very challenging, because the members of his church had faith for forgiveness of sins, but they did not have the same faith for healing. George, like many ANGA-network pentecostals, teaches that, through the atoning death and resurrection of Jesus of Nazareth, God provided both forgiveness from sin and healing from disease, because according to the prophet Isaiah: "by his wounds we are healed."[62]

As George preached on the first night of the conference, Fernando's wife, Gabriela, attested to healing from pain in her throat and kidney. Antonio also experienced healing from pain in his molar teeth and ear (and when George returned to Nicaragua a year later, in 2011, Antonio reported that he was still healed). Grateful and encouraged by the healings, later that first evening in 2010 Antonio visited his mother in the hospital—wanting to put into practice what he had just learned about prayer for healing. Antonio's mother experienced instant healing from heart pains and left the hospital. The next day, Antonio applied the new teaching to pray for Geovany, a member of his church, after which Geovany attested to being healed from three months of pain in the right shin due to poor circulation and surgery. Having just experienced healing for himself, Geovany immediately prayed for his wife, Hazel, who had not been able to sing on account of a tumor in her throat; after prayer, her throat opened up so that she could sing. Geovany next prayed for another woman with a baby who had a fever. Not only the did the baby's skin feel palpably cooler after the prayer, but the mother—whose broken toe was bandaged—reported (crying, she was so moved by the experience) that while Geovany was praying for her baby the pain left her toe and she was now able to move it, even though Geovany had not prayed for her toe. This sequence of anecdotes illustrates the networked quality of pentecostal healing practices. One person's healing experience frequently exerts an impact on many others through complex, often transgeographic and cross-cultural, relational patterns.[63]

Conclusion

The narratives that have formed the bulk of this chapter do not constitute proof that any of the attested healings have occurred, let alone
that there is a divine or suprahuman explanation. What this chapter
has illustrated is how *perceived* divine healing experiences have the
potential to exert lasting effects—not only on the person claiming
healing but also on family members, friends, and even on individuals
with whom network connections are strikingly weak, indirect, or transitory. Although not every perceived healing experience has an enduring impact, the interlocking case studies presented here show that ripple effects sometimes travel like waves of increasing magnitude across
global pentecostal networks as one perceived healing generates many
others. The final task of this book is to propose an interpretive framework to bring together the diverse approaches taken in the preceding
chapters and assess what happens when people pray for other people's
healing.

Conclusion

What Science Can Show
about Prayer

*

This book began by asking about the relationship between science and religion, affirming the importance of respecting their distinct magisteria but also suggesting the advantages of bringing scientific perspectives to bear on religious practices in a manner that is not simplistically reductionist. Although science can never prove nor disprove the so-called healing power of prayer, empirical perspectives can reveal a great deal about prayer for healing—just as attunement to religious perceptions can illumine much about the nature and practice of science. The preceding chapters presented a series of views of how scientists and religious practitioners construct healing prayer, and of the empirical outcomes of praying for healing. The first assignment of this conclusion is to bring the images reflected by each chapter into focus in order to evaluate intersections between perceptions and measurements of healing. This assessment lays the groundwork for a second charge—developing a theoretical model for interpreting the effects of healing prayer practices.

Studying Healing Prayer in the Context of Global Pentecostal Networks

The prevalence of expectant prayer for healing among Pentecostal and Charismatic Christians makes these groups a logical focus for exploring questions about prayer and healing. In particular, as the Apostolic Network of Global Awakening and Iris Ministries grew out of the Toronto Blessing, they made prayer for healing a prominent feature of conferences and international ministry trips, coincidentally providing convenient settings for empirical research. Participants in such pentecostal networks identify as members of a global Christian community that apparently transcends markers of ethnicity, language, and social class, as healing prayer functions as a defining ritual. Healing practices spread as the global North imports a supernatural worldview in which God, angels, and demons intervene in natural affairs, whereas the global South imports a democratized model in which ordinary Christians act as agents of healing.

The effects of globalization, including the globalization of pentecostal networks and healing practices, are not uniformly benign. Pentecostal approaches to healing can obscure or even intensify the pathogenic effects of systemic economic and political inequities. But participation in healing practices can also provide a strategy for social and political empowerment and produce tangible physical and emotional benefits. Early critics of the Toronto Blessing charged that the event failed to produce global revival or to benefit economically poor people. From the vantage of 2011, it appears that Toronto became less significant as a pilgrimage destination as its influences diffused, and other locations, prominently including some of the poorest areas of the world—places such as the *favelas* of urban Brazil, ostracized gypsy communities in Bulgaria, and mud-hut villages in rural Mozambique—became hosts to Toronto-influenced revivals in which prayer for healing is a characteristic practice.

Why Scientific Methods Should Be Used to Study Prayer and How to Do It

To ask the question of whether science can prove or disprove the healing power of prayer points toward the unparalleled cultural authority of "science" in the modern Western world. Yet science in its current form is itself a culturally constructed category, simultaneously incorporating both scientific approaches and a variety of core sensibilities about the nature of the material world. Indeed, the arguments wielded in debates over prayer studies illustrate that scientists do not always behave dispassionately but can be just as driven by doctrinaire philosophical and theological agendas as can adherents of religious communities. Debates over whether prayer should be the subject of scientific study began as an intramural argument between European Protestant and Catholic Christians, with the latter finding support from mainstream scientists. In the nineteenth century, scientific naturalists took the lead in urging empirical studies, whereas Protestant Christians resisted. A century later, both sets of cultural players switched sides. Scientific naturalists opposed the study of prayer, while Protestant and Catholic Christians could be found among the supporters (and opponents) of prayer studies. Strangest of all, the dictum of separating the magisteria of science and religion has sometimes devolved into dogmatic insistence that religious practices are off limits for scientific study, coupled with an assertion of the absence of empirical effects from practices that lack scientific validation.

Despite the controversies generated by empirical studies of prayer, such studies should be undertaken. Given global health crises that conventional medicine has not adequately addressed, people everywhere pray for healing, expecting it may help and assuming it will not hurt. It is an empirical question whether prayer for healing does, under certain circumstances, produce empirical effects. If prayer is demonstrably bad for one's health, then the widespread application of intercessory prayer as a complementary therapy may be ethically problematic. If, conversely, prayer directly or indirectly produces health benefits, then studying prayer practices may provide insights that can be used to improve global health. Prayer can be studied empirically without any inappropriate blurring of science and religion. Although the mechanisms by which prayer may affect health are so far poorly understood, a growing body of empirical evidence points toward plausible physiological and psychosocial mechanisms by which thoughts, emotions, and social interactions influence health—without resorting to "supernatural" explanations.

This book has argued that an appropriate role for theology in empirical research on prayer is as an analytic tool to design studies with construct validity and ecological validity. In other words, studies should be designed to take into account beliefs and practices involved in praying for healing in specific, natural contexts—such as Toronto-influenced pentecostal networks. Theologically attuned studies are more likely to find any effects that exist while reducing the likelihood of seeming to find effects that are not really there. Empirical findings, even of a therapeutic benefit from prayer, do *not* justify the theological conclusion that scientists should promote pentecostal prayer, just as neuroscientific studies of Buddhist meditation do not justify the corollary that doctors should endorse Buddhism.

In designing empirical studies of prayer, it is important to use types of data and methods suited to the particular questions considered. As the scientific theorist Peter Lipton advises, "variety in the data" is an "evidential virtue." The goal of comprehensive explanation can tempt the best researchers to stretch findings further than they naturally extend. Researchers have, for example, been susceptible to relying on a single data pool—such as medical records or survey responses—to answer such a complex question as whether prayer really results in healing. Not finding compelling evidence based on one data set or method, researchers may prematurely conclude that there is no effect, in violation of the rationalist astronomer Carl Sagan's dictum that the "absence of evidence is not evidence of absence." Such findings may reveal more about the limitations of relying too heavily on any one form of evidence or research method than they do about the empirical effects of prayer.[1]

Using a Variety of Data to Ask and Answer Appropriate Questions

Medical Records: Are Healing Claims Documented?

Medical evidence provides one index of whether someone claiming healing exhibits improved health. Medical records can indicate that a problem was at one point diagnosed by a credentialed professional and that on subsequent examination the condition appeared better or resolved, and that there is no obvious medical or natural explanation. Despite the apparent objectivity of x-rays, laboratory reports, and doctors' notes, the significance of such documents requires subjective interpretation. Medical documentation cannot prove that prayer accounts for a recovery or that a divine or other suprahuman agent or force is responsible, or even that a condition has been permanently cured. Nor does the absence or incompleteness of medical documentation constitute evidence of the absence of healing.

As with controversies surrounding clinical tests, there is a cultural history to how scientists and religious practitioners construct medical documentation and how medical records have been used in debates over religious healing. In the early twentieth century, those interested in discrediting religious healing claims were the first to propose using medical records as the standard for determining whether healings had occurred and how claims should be explained. Between the 1960s and the early 1990s, North American Charismatics took the initiative in collecting before-and-after medical documentation of attested healings. Since the 1990s, North American pentecostals have largely backed away from collecting medical records, focusing instead on testimonies of subjectively experienced improvements. Reflecting a long-standing ambivalence toward modern medicine and a developing, postmodern esteem for narrative, spiritual experience, and physical sensation, some pentecostals view interest in medical documentation as the antipode of faith. Indifference to medical validation of healing testimonies encourages exaggeration of the numbers of healings reported, and in some instances the intentional falsification of healings that never occurred.

Despite the challenges of collecting medical records and the inherent limitations to what such records can reveal, data collected between the 1960s and 2011 do indicate that some, though not all, individuals attesting to religious healing exhibited medically surprising recoveries. Medical records point to resolution of a wide variety of diseases and disabilities, including severe auditory and visual impairments and metastasized cancers. This evidence does not, however, by itself explain these recoveries. There are also cases in which the medical evidence reveals inflated and even fraudulent claims.

Surveys: How Do Sufferers Perceive Healing Prayer?

Surveys of participants in GA and IM healing conferences provide a cross-sectional gauge of certain people's perceptions of the meanings and outcomes of prayer practices at one moment in time. The survey conducted for this project was not designed to assess any cumulative effects of participating in multiple healing conferences. Survey data cannot confirm the accuracy of perceived changes in physical health or attributions of divine causation. Nor can surveys reflect how perceptions may differ at another point in time. Nevertheless, how people experience and interpret their participation in healing rituals constitutes one important dimension of understanding the effects of prayer practices.

Most of the Brazilians and North Americans surveyed attested to past experiences of divine healing of physical ailments. Past healings, even of relatively minor conditions, elicited commentary years or decades later. Respondents interpreted healings that had stood the test of time as evidence of divine superintendence over their lives. Past healing experiences, even if only partial, encouraged respondents to seek future prayer for the same or additional problems. Most conference attendees reported a current need for healing of a physical problem, although relatively few conditions appeared to be life threatening.

Many, but far from all, conference attendees reported experiencing healing at the current conference. Demographic factors (including race, nationality, education, income, age, gender, and pentecostal identity) did not predict healing needs, expectations, or experiences. Respondents were more likely to report healing of a physical than an emotional or spiritual problem, just as they were more likely to have reported needing a physical healing; the most common problem noted was pain. People were no more likely to report healing of conditions with less severe symptoms, of shorter duration, or of a less life-threatening nature than the conditions they had reported needing healed. Most respondents based their assessment of healing on the alleviation of physical symptoms and, consequently, did not report healing of conditions that produced no or inconsistent symptoms.

Respondents did not understand healing as an all-or-nothing phenomenon but as a process that often takes time and repeated prayers to complete, especially for more serious conditions; even dramatic improvements are understood as the result of previously laid groundwork. Most respondents had already sought medical help, possibly alongside alternative remedies. Most had also prayed for healing of the same condition before the current conference, and most planned to continue praying, and possibly seeking medical treatment, if they were not healed during this event. It is interesting that those who reported a high expectation of healing during the surveyed event were no more likely to experience healing than those who admitted to not expecting healing.

The typical respondent claiming healing reported being "almost completely" healed from pain related to the same physical problem she came to the conference wanting to have healed. Respondents attributed sicknesses to natural and spiritual causes, but they credited healing following prayer to divine activity, possibly mixed with human faith. Those reporting healing often explained the experience as tangible evidence of God's love and power.

Prospective Trials: Can Health Outcomes of Prayer be Measured?

Prospective clinical trials of proximal intercessory prayer (PIP) are well suited to answering the question of whether prayer practices result in measurable health changes. (Indeed, they are better suited than the more common approach of studying distant intercessory prayer.) As with any form of data, there are limits to the information about healing experiences that quantifiable measurements can provide. Scientific equipment cannot measure qualitative effects, such as the physical sensations and avowedly spiritual phenomena that people sometimes claim to experience during prayer for healing. The study we conducted, which focused on measuring auditory and visual thresholds before and after PIP, was designed to determine whether PIP results in any measurable effects; the study did not seek to isolate responsible mechanisms or to assess whether changes were long term.

We began with the null hypothesis that PIP would have no significant effect. In rural Mozambique, we measured highly significant improvements in hearing and statistically significant improvements in vision across the tested populations. Two auditory subjects exhibited hearing thresholds reduced by over 50 dBHL (on a 0–100 scale from perfect hearing to deafness). Three visual subjects improved from being unable to read the top line of an eye chart (20/400) to being able to read relatively fine print (20/80 or better); one visual subject who could not count fingers from 1′ away before PIP afterward read the 20/125 line of a vision chart. Potential confounds such as inadvertent hypnosis or suggestion do not obviously account for these findings. Much as survey respondents typically perceived improvement along a continuum, we measured improved hearing and vision thresholds rather than generally finding a change from total deafness or blindness to a clinical standard of perfection. We partially replicated these results in a follow-up study in urban Brazil. We found statistically significant improvements in visual thresholds; hearing thresholds also improved significantly, but this result must be viewed with caution, due to post-PIP reduction in ambient noise in the Brazil data. In the few cases where we could conduct retests the following day, we measured further improvements—supporting the perception that post-PIP improvements are sometimes progressive. We attempted similar tests in the United States, but found the field conditions surprisingly more challenging, because fewer people actively seek prayer for healing of impaired vision or hearing, and testing procedures proved more disruptive to natural prayer practices.

Follow-up: Do Healing Experiences Produce Lasting Effects?

Longitudinal follow-up observations and interviews of subjects reporting healing help to answer the question of whether healing experiences lead to any long-term changes. As with every other class of data, there are limits to what follow-up, even when conducted over as many as eight years as in this study, can demonstrate. The case study approach is not well suited to statistical analysis, nor is it easy to demonstrate that selected examples are representative. The claim that a healing has been maintained over time does not in itself constitute proof. There is often no way to verify informants' claims—for instance that someone was dead and then resurrected, or oppressed by demons and then liberated—but it is sometimes possible, through repeated observations, to note changes in a person's demeanor and behavior after a perceived healing and to trace lines of influence on other people.

The interlocking set of case studies analyzed indicate that, in certain instances, healing experiences reshape the attitudes and behaviors of those who perceive themselves to have been healed. There is also evidence that the effects multiply as influences extend to family, friends, and other people in the healed individual's social network with whom relational ties may be weak, indirect, or transitory. Through a complex web of social interactions that bridge distinct geographic and social groups and mediate cultural and linguistic differences, a single healing experience can generate a domino effect that reverberates through global pentecostal networks. One individual who experiences healing prays for another, who also experiences healing, who prays for another, and so on as the effects branch outward. Healings set off chain reactions. For instance, they may inspire forgiveness of those who caused an affliction, which is understood to release more healing for the one who forgave, and prompt the one forgiven to express love, possibly by praying for others to be healed. Those who convert to pentecostal Christianity typically point to successful healing interactions, often following unsuccessful attempts to experience healing through other medical and religious practices, as motivating their decisions. Indeed, there is evidence that the global expansion of pentecostalism occurs primarily through the repetition of many such healing exchanges.

Individuals interviewed recalled past healing experiences as defining life events through which they personally experienced God's love and power. Healing experiences attributed to divine love motivated informants to forgive those who had wronged them; to pray for other people's healing, both close to home and by traveling to other countries; to participate in acts of social benevolence intended to benefit economically poor people; and to engage in high-risk behavior for the purpose of helping others. Not all such efforts achieved their intended effects; examples can be cited in which the same actions that socially powerful agents constructed as "loving" may have been constructed by recipients as paternalistic, coercive, and harmful. But where sickness tended toward self-focus, healing removed obstacles to seeing the needs of others, and the experience of relief from suffering heightened compassion for other people's suffering. Informants understood love as a key to releasing power for healing. Although informants acknowledged delays and failure in seeking healing for themselves and for others, many refused to stop believing, loving, or praying for a fuller release of love and power to heal.

Toward a Theory of the Effects of Healing Prayer

None of the empirical perspectives presented, alone or in combination, proves that prayer results in healing for the reasons given by practitioners. Nevertheless, the widespread perception that prayer releases divine healing has demonstrably real social effects, and in some cases the social interactions involved in healing rituals produce measurable health effects. Many pentecostals practice prayer for healing in the context of globalized social networks. Theories of pentecostal prayer should therefore involve a social networks perspective.

The frequency with which the pentecostals studied correlate healing experiences with expressions of love suggests that a study of pentecostal healing is in part a study of the emotions, particularly social exchanges of love, including altruistic behavior. Here it is useful to build on the sociological theories of social constructionism, social networks, interaction ritual chains, love energy, and Godly Love that were outlined in the introduction. The Godly Love model posits a *perceived* "dynamic interaction between divine and human love that enlivens and expands benevolence." The model does not imply ontological claims about whether or not divine or suprahuman agents or forces actually exist or intervene in human affairs. The crucial theoretical question is how socially mediated perceptions affect the behaviors of individuals and interdependent social units. Using the labels *exemplars* (akin to my term *leaders*), *collaborators* (akin to *partners*), *beneficiaries* (akin to *recipients*), and *God* (akin to *suprahuman source/object*), Lee and Poloma depict Godly Love as a "diamond model" of interactions among occupants of four social roles (figure 7.1).[2]

The diamond model accentuates the theoretical claim that "Godly Love is ultimately about interactions in a network, not character traits of individuals." By implication, altruism may be explained less as a

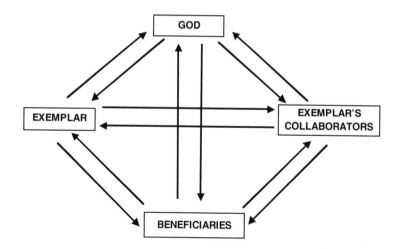

Figure 7.1. The diamond model of Godly Love. Reprinted with permission from Matthew T. Lee and Margaret M. Poloma, *A Sociological Study of the Great Commandment in Pentecostalism: The Practice of Godly Love as Benevolent Service* (Lewiston, N.Y.: Edwin Mellen, 2009), 29.

product of exceptional personality traits or biological dispositions than as a result of social interactions that generate love energy. The effects may multiply as they spread because, as Lee and Poloma explain, a "flame can light many torches." Thus, one Godly Love interaction can produce offshoots that diffuse widely through interrelated social networks.[3]

My study suggests that social interactions focused on healing rituals create an effervescence or augmentation of morally suffused emotional energy. To put it simply, individuals who experience healing through pentecostal prayer rituals credit divine love and power for their recoveries, and they consequently feel motivated to express greater love for God and other people. As motivational energy empowers benevolent actions, the effects snowball. Even one dramatic healing experience can position an individual in the social role of a leader in pentecostal networks, someone who models healing practices for partners and recipients. Leaders function as brokers of social capital as the widespread, even global, dissemination of exemplary healing testimonies bridges otherwise separate social networks and spurs others to express love within and across networks. As leaders and partners direct their energy toward recipients—by praying for healing or seeking to meet other practical needs—leaders and partners both disburse and draw energy from these interactions; as a result, the net volume of energy available to do benevolent work increases. Sometimes efforts to extend love misfire, as when inequitable power relations allow leaders—intentionally or not—to coerce partners and recipients to respond to initiatives in particular ways. Yet the willingness of pentecostals to expend energy is sustained by the perception that theirs is not a closed system in which the total value of energy must be conserved. Rather, pentecostals perceive themselves to be continually receiving additional energy input from a hypothesized divine source. This perception of the ongoing entry of unlimited love—regardless of whether any such inflow actually occurs—facilitates the productive social interactions that generate new energy as leaders, partners, and recipients all experience love through their mutual exchanges.

Any diagram of the healing exchanges that cement and proliferate pentecostal networks must necessarily be highly selective and incomplete. Figure 7.2 uses some of the individuals who populate this book to represent a single sector of a much wider, decentralized network system. Repositioning the camera would bring different individuals into the center of view. As narrated in chapter 6, Randy Clark's healing at age eighteen generated ripples that augmented into surging currents to expand the reach of pentecostal networks. Just as concentric circles surround Clark—with the closest embracing members of the Revival Alliance, the next encompassing other ministry partners, and the final circle denoting recipients—a similar set of circles could be drawn around other individuals in this network. Double arrows indicate mutual relationships; single arrows suggest primarily unidirectional influences. Certain individuals exhibit thicker network connections, whereas others are more peripheral to the hubs selected here—but many of these apparently minor figures play major leadership roles in different spheres of influence. Even individuals figured here as recipients become partners and leaders when interacting with other recipients. The outer ring represents a kind of expanding universe of love energy,

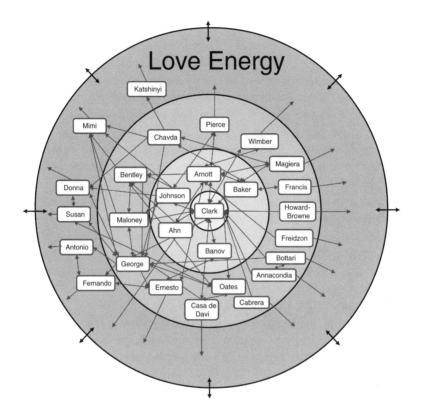

Figure 7.2. A network model of love energy flows.

with participants in healing rituals envisioning themselves as receiving love as they extend love to other people and back toward the presumed energy source.

Although not numerically quantifiable, the love energy generated by participating in healing rituals can be measured qualitatively, drawing on the five measures proposed by the sociologist Pitirim Sorokin: intensity, extensity, duration, purity, and adequacy. Informants reporting healing experiences commonly report subsequent changes in their behavior that can be interpreted as exhibiting increases in both the intensity and extensity of their expressions of love, although sometimes there appears to be a tradeoff between these qualities. Those who become pentecostal network leaders after themselves receiving healing may give more sacrificially, or intensely, of their time, money, or energy to meet other people's needs. For instance, they may spend many hours praying for others; fast from food while praying for breakthrough; or provide homes for orphaned children. Leaders may not only show concern for family, friends, or in-group members but, more extensively, undertake grueling international travel schedules to benefit those in other countries. There is a tension here between extensity and intensity, because service to others, particularly when it involves time-consuming or high-risk behaviors, can take away from time and energy available for investing in immediate relationships with family and friends. For some individuals, there is evidence that the effects of a single healing experience endure over a period of years or decades, prompting continual exertion on behalf of others. It seems though that those individuals who respond to healing experiences primarily by undertaking international ministry trips may exhibit love energy of shorter duration than those who engage in longer-term forms of service. Evidence suggests that those who perceive themselves to be the recipients of intense experiences of divine love—expressed through healing of a condition that is especially severe or long term, or that has a poor prognosis—may express qualitatively higher degrees of love energy compared with those who experienced more minor healings. It seems also that healing experienced after persistent prayers over a longer period of time may make a deeper, more enduring impression on recipients than healing that is rapidly and easily experienced.[4]

The final two measures, purity and adequacy, are more difficult to gauge, because they involve more complex considerations. There is clear evidence of the impurity of motives of those individuals who can be demonstrated to have falsified their healing claims or dehumanized those for whom they prayed while seeking to add to pseudostatistical tallies of healings; such actions appear self-promoting rather than benevolent. Certain pentecostals, perhaps unconsciously, may use healing rituals to bolster their own political and economic positions at the expense of other members of their social networks. Most of those active in praying for others do seem concerned with the well-being of recipients, although those praying may at times exhibit condescending attitudes and engage in controlling behaviors. Leaders and partners in healing rituals may also hope to reap immaterial benefits, such as increased faith, the privilege of witnessing apparent miracles, and future-oriented heavenly rewards, from participating in global revivals. There is suggestive evidence that participation in healing rituals in the context of pentecostal networks builds social capital and indirectly exerts largely positive health effects on all participants, regardless of whether their role is that of leader, partner, or recipient.

Such interactions map uneasily onto predominant understandings of altruism, which require that truly altruistic actors must not be motivated by even immaterial self-interest. Such a restrictive definition of altruism may, however, miss the dynamics of the production of love energy and in effect define out of existence a significant social phenomenon. Leaders and partners *need* recipients as targets of their benevolence and draw emotional energy from their interactions with them. But it is significant that the result is a net increase in the love energy available to be spread throughout and beyond involved social networks. Moreover, because individuals and larger social units can simultaneously occupy multiple network roles, bestowal of benevolence does not necessarily imply patronizing attitudes or a hierarchical relationship among those occupying various roles. Indeed, in the pentecostal worldview, those positioned as recipients—in other words, those who need help from other network members and especially those who lack worldly power and status—are accorded higher spiritual status and envisioned as potential partners and leaders. Thus, a range of motives seems to be involved in healing rituals, and the presence of immaterial forms of self-interest does not seem inherently opposed to the expression of altruism.[5]

The question of adequacy seems particularly germane to evaluating whether prayer for healing should be classed as a form of benevolence. One way to evaluate adequacy is to ask whether prayer for healing results in healing or cure. There is evidence that many, though by no means all, recipients of prayer perceive themselves to have been healed; medical records confirm that some of those reporting healing exhibited medically surprising recoveries; and data indicate that proximal intercessory prayer sometimes produces measurable health effects. There are also clear instances of failure, as when people remain blind or deaf or die of cancer despite repeated prayers for healing. Some of those for whom a cure remains elusive doubtless experience disappointment, frustration, and intensified suffering. Yet some of those who fail to experience a cure indicate that they feel loved because of the social support of having someone pray for them or that they feel benefited by a partial improvement in symptoms. When successful, the performance of healing rituals motivates recipients to act as partners and leaders who seek to express love for others, for instance, by praying for other people's healing or by seeking to meet the practical needs of economically poor people. There is reason to suspect, however, that privileging divine healing as a particularly valuable embodiment of love may also lead to myopia regarding systemic social and political causes of suffering, thereby promoting disinterest in using natural tools to meet people's needs. If, moreover, prayer exerts its benefits through natural mechanisms, but practitioners inaccurately attribute healing to divine activity, even inadvertent deception may undermine the adequacy of the ritual as an expression of love. Conversely, the argument can be forwarded that practices are adequate as long as they result in healing, whether or not the causes are fully understood. To add further complexity, perception of a divine process, whether or not accurate, may activate therapeutic mindbody interactions. There may also be a tension between adequacy of effects and purity of motives, because the practices most effective in producing healing may yield the greatest benefits for leaders and partners as well as recipients.

The five measures of love energy assessed here provide one, but certainly not the only, tool for interpreting the social significance of healing prayer rituals. In actual practice, most prayer for healing occurs in the fluid context of relationships, often under the pressure of intense human suffering. Mortal humans, faced with needs that appear to be more than a match for their material resources, call out for divine or suprahuman assistance. When help seems to come, people respond in gratitude by doing what their ritual participation has taught them how to do: pray for themselves and for others, often in the context of pentecostal social networks.

Future Research

This book has not answered all the questions it raised, and this has not been the intention. My hope is that other researchers will build in various ways on the foundations laid here and accept an invitation to bring science and religion into dialogue to examine empirical effects of prayer for healing. I, too, am continuing to build—with plans for at least two related books about spiritual healing practices, both within and beyond Christian cultures. I would also like to see larger-scale, more refined clinical trials of the effects of proximal intercessory prayer on subjects in such countries as Mozambique, Brazil, India, and the United States. Perhaps the most obvious conclusion to draw from findings collected to date is that, regardless of what researchers have to say, people from around the world will continue to pray for healing and perceive healing, and many of them will do so in the context of expanding global pentecostal networks. Given this empirical fact, it seems prudent to draw on as many perspectives and methods as possible to understand the implications for how people will experience the twenty-first-century world.

Appendix

Healing Survey

Study # 06-11383

Indiana University – Bloomington
Study Information Sheet
Healing Survey

You are invited to participate in a research study. My name is Dr. Candy Gunther Brown, and I am an associate professor of religious studies at Indiana University. After receiving my Ph.D. from Harvard University, I published *The Word in the World: Evangelical Writing, Publishing, and Reading in America, 1789-1880* (Chapel Hill: University of North Carolina Press, 2004). I am writing a book about divine healing and hope that you can help. The purpose of this study is to learn about any healing that you may experience during this conference.

INFORMATION

I am asking you to complete a survey on divine healing that consists of a "pre-conference" and a "post-conference" questionnaire. Please fill out the survey even if you do not need healing, and even if you do not experience a manifestation of healing. Completing each questionnaire should take about 10 minutes. You must be at least 18 years old to participate. All of your answers are anonymous. Please do not write your name on the survey.

BEFORE or EARLY in the conference, please answer the questions on BOTH sides of the PINK "Pre-Conference Healing Survey." Circle the answers that BEST describe you, or fill in the blanks that apply to you. Please wait until the END of the conference or you are READY TO LEAVE to complete the "Post-Conference Healing Survey." After completing the pink and blue forms, please return both forms still stapled together (even if they are blank) to the box marked "Healing Surveys."

If you would be willing to talk with me about any healing that you may experience, please complete a "Testimony Contact Card." Return this card to the box marked "Testimony Contact Cards" at the END of the conference or when you are READY TO LEAVE. I am most interested in receiving a contact card from you if you have a significant healing experience at this conference. Please DO NOT RETURN the card if you do not want me to contact you. If you do return the card, I will call you in about six weeks. At this time, I will confirm that you understand the purposes of my research and any risks or benefits to you, and that you still wish to participate. I will ask you questions about the healing you experienced. Our conversation will last from five to thirty minutes. You may end the conversation at any time. I will tape record our conversation for research purposes only. No one else will have access to the recording. I will destroy the recording and your "Testimony Contact Card" after transcribing the interview.

If, during a follow-up interview, you indicate that you have medical records to document your healing, I will invite you to de-identify copies of your records and send them to me. I will explain to you how to de-identify your medical records, for instance, by blotting out any names, addresses, numbers, or dates; this would take you about twenty minutes.

BENEFITS

Participation in this study will not benefit you directly. Your participation may benefit others by helping them to experience healing.

CONFIDENTIALITY

I will make every effort to maintain confidentiality of all records that may in any way identify you. If you participate in a follow-up interview, I will not include your name in my tape recording or transcription of our conversation, and I will destroy your "Testimony Contact Card" after completing your interview. Prior to being destroyed, testimony contact cards will be stored in a locked file cabinet in a locked office, to which no one besides me has access. If you choose to send me de-identified medical records, I will destroy any envelopes, cover letters, or other materials that might identify you. The results of this research may be published, but your name and identity will not be revealed and your record will remain anonymous.

CONTACT

If you have questions at any time about the study or the procedures, you may contact me: Dr. Candy Gunther Brown, Department of Religious Studies, Sycamore Hall 230, Indiana University, Bloomington, IN 47405, (812) 855-8929, browncg@indiana.edu.

If you feel you have not been treated according to the descriptions in this form, or your rights as a participant in research have not been honored during the course of this project, you may contact the office for the Indiana University Bloomington Human Subjects Committee, Carmichael Center L03, 530 E. Kirkwood Ave., Bloomington, IN 47408, (812) 855-3067, iub_hsc@indiana.edu.

PARTICIPATION

Your participation in this study is voluntary, and you may refuse to participate without penalty. If you decide to participate, you may withdraw from the study at any time without penalty and without loss of benefits to which you are otherwise entitled. If you withdraw from the study before data collection is completed any data identifying you will be destroyed.

English-language, conference version
Information Sheet Date: 14 October 2006.

Pre-Conference Healing Survey
(Please fill out at BEGINNING of conference)

Please circle any or all of the following that apply to you, and/or fill in the applicable blanks:

nder: Female   Male

:e: 18-29   30-39   40-49   50-59   60-69   70-79   80+

ce/Ethnicity: Caucasian   Black   Latino/a   Asian   Native American   Other: _____

ucation: Eighth grade or less   High School Diploma   College Degree   Post-Graduate Degree

come: $20,000 or less $20-39,000 $40-59,000 $60-79,000 $80-99,000 $100,000 or more

ligion: Protestant   Catholic   Other: _____

If you circled "Protestant" or "Catholic," list any denomination(s) or order(s) to which you feel connected, and/or specify "nondenominational": _____

Circle any or all of the following with which you identify: Charismatic Pentecostal Evangelical Liberal

Have you ever received divine or spiritual healing of an illness, pain, or disability?

YES   NO   NOT SURE

) If "yes," please describe your most significant healing experience:

_____
_____
_____
_____

Do you need healing for any illness, pain, or disability?

YES   NO   NOT SURE

) If "No," THANK YOU for your help! Please skip the rest of this pink form, but AFTER the conference has
ded, do not forget to answer the questions on the blue form and to return BOTH the pink and blue forms.

"Yes," please describe the ONE illness, pain, or disability that you MOST want healed:

_____
_____

How do you explain the cause of the condition you described?

_____
_____

How likely do you think it is that you will receive healing of the condition during this conference?

0   1   2   3   4   5   6   7   8   9   10

(**0**=Not at all likely; **5**=Not sure; **10**=Completely certain.)

(continued on back)

6) <u>In the past 7 days</u>, how much has this condition affected your life?

0   1   2   3   4   5   6   7   8   9   10

(**0**=I have been unaware of it; **1**=Only slightly bothered me; **5**=Bothered me quite a bit, but I can still perform daily activities; **10**=Bothered me as much as it ever has, and I have not been able to perform daily activities.)

7) How long have you had this condition?

ALL MY LIFE   MORE THAN 5 YEARS   1-5 YEARS   6 MONTHS TO 1 YEAR   LESS THAN 6 MONTHS

8) Before this conference, have you or another person ever prayed for healing of this condition?

YES, MORE THAN 5 TIMES   YES, 2-5 TIMES   YES, ONCE   NO, NEVER   NOT SURE

8b) If "Yes," how much did your symptoms improve?

| NOT AT ALL | LESS THAN HALF | ABOUT HALF | MORE THAN HALF | PARTIALLY, BUT SYMPTOMS RETURNED | COMPLETELY, BUT SYMPTOMS RETURNED |

9) Other than prayer, have you ever tried alternative medical or spiritual remedies for healing of this condition? Please circle one or more of the following:

CHIROPRACTIC   MASSAGE   MEDITATION   ACUPUNCTURE   HERBAL   YOGA   REIKI

NATUROPATHY   HOMEOPATHY   THERAPEUTIC TOUCH   CHRISTIAN SCIENCE   NATIVE AMERICAN

UNITY   SANTERIA   CURANDEROS/AS   PSYCHIC   OTHER: _____   NOT SURE   NONE

9b) If "Yes," how much did your symptoms improve?

| NOT AT ALL | LESS THAN HALF | ABOUT HALF | MORE THAN HALF | PARTIALLY, BUT SYMPTOMS RETURNED | COMPLETELY, BUT SYMPTOMS RETURNED |

10) Have you ever been to a physician or other health-care professional about your condition?

YES, MORE THAN 5 TIMES   YES, 2-5 TIMES   YES, ONCE   NO, NEVER   NOT SURE

10b) If "Yes," how much did your symptoms improve?

| NOT AT ALL | LESS THAN HALF | ABOUT HALF | MORE THAN HALF | PARTIALLY, BUT SYMPTOMS RETURNED | COMPLETELY, BUT SYMPTOMS RETURNED |

11) How did the doctor describe the cause of your pain, illness, or disability? (What <u>diagnosis</u> was given?)

_____

_____

12) How much healing does the doctor expect for you? (What <u>prognosis</u> was given?)

| TERMINAL | NO IMPROVEMENT, BUT NOT TERMINAL | SOME IMPROVEMENT, BUT CHRONIC PROBLEM | FULL RECOVERY WITHIN 1 YEAR | FULL RECOVERY WITHIN 1 MONTH |

13) Circle any/all of the following from which you might seek aid if you still need healing after this conference:

PRAYER   PHYSICIAN OR OTHER HEALTH-CARE PROFESSIONAL   ALTERNATIVE MEDICAL OR SPIRITUAL REMEDIES (see question 9)—please specify which: _____

Post-Conference Healing Survey
(Please fill out at END of conference)

1) Did you receive healing (complete or partial) for any pain, illness, or disability at this conference?

      YES   NO   NOT SURE

1b) If "No," THANK YOU for your help! Please skip the rest of this form, but do not forget to return BOTH the pink and blue forms (still stapled together) to the box marked "Healing Surveys," even if you left sections blank.

If "Yes," please list all of the pains, illnesses, or disabilities that were healed over the last few days.

_____

_____

1c) If you were healed of more than one pain, illness, or disability, please CIRCLE the ONE most significant condition you listed above. For the rest of the questions, please think about that ONE pain, illness, or disability.

2) How much have your symptoms improved?

NOT AT ALL	LESS THAN HALF	ABOUT HALF	MORE THAN HALF	ALMOST COMPLETELY	COMPLETELY

3) How do you know that your condition has been healed?

_____

_____

4) How do you explain your healing?

_____

_____

5) <u>Right now</u>, how much does your pain, illness, or disability affect you?

    0   1   2   3   4   5   6   7   8   9   10

    (**0**=I have been unaware of it; **1**=Only slightly bothered me; **5**=Bothered me quite a bit, but I can still perform daily activities; **10**=Bothered me as much as it ever has, and I have not been able to perform daily activities.)

6) Circle any/all of the following from which you might seek aid if you ever need another condition healed:

    PRAYER   PHYSICIAN OR OTHER   ALTERNATIVE MEDICAL OR SPIRITUAL REMEDIES
                    HEALTH-CARE PROFESSIONAL   (see question 11)—please specify which: _____

If your most significant healing was of the SAME condition you described on the pre-conference survey, you may skip the rest of the questions. Otherwise, please continue with your most significant healing still in mind:

7) Did you come to this conference expecting healing of the condition you circled?

YES	NO, I DID NOT KNOW I NEEDED HEALING	NO, I DID NOT THINK I WOULD BE HEALED	NO, I WANTED SOMETHING ELSE HEALED (AND IT WAS NOT HEALED)	NO, I WANTED SOMETHING ELSE HEALED (AND IT WAS HEALED, TOO)	NOT SURE

(continued on back)

8) <u>In the past 7 days</u>, how much has this condition affected your life?

0   1   2   3   4   5   6   7   8   9   10

9) How long have you had this condition?

ALL MY LIFE   MORE THAN 5 YEARS   1-5 YEARS   6 MONTHS TO 1 YEAR   LESS THAN 6 MONTHS

10) Before this conference, had you or another person ever prayed for healing of this condition?

YES, MORE THAN 5 TIMES   YES, 2-5 TIMES   YES, ONCE   NO, NEVER   NOT SURE

10b) If "Yes," how much did your symptoms improve?

| NOT AT ALL | LESS THAN HALF | ABOUT HALF | MORE THAN HALF | PARTIALLY, BUT SYMPTOMS RETURNED | COMPLETELY, BUT SYMPTOMS RETURNED |

11) Other than prayer, had you ever tried alternative medical or spiritual remedies for healing of this condition? Please circle one or more of the following, and/or fill in the blank if "other":

CHIROPRACTIC   MASSAGE   MEDITATION   ACUPUNCTURE   HERBAL   YOGA   REIKI

NATUROPATHY   HOMEOPATHY   THERAPEUTIC TOUCH   CHRISTIAN SCIENCE   NATIVE AMERICAN

UNITY   SANTERIA   CURANDEROS/AS   PSYCHIC   OTHER: _____   NOT SURE   NONE

11b) If "Yes," how much did your symptoms improve?

| NOT AT ALL | LESS THAN HALF | ABOUT HALF | MORE THAN HALF | PARTIALLY, BUT SYMPTOMS RETURNED | COMPLETELY, BUT SYMPTOMS RETURNED |

12) Had you ever been to a physician or other health-care professional about your condition?

YES, MORE THAN 5 TIMES   YES, 2-5 TIMES   YES, ONCE   NO, NEVER   NOT SURE

12b) If "Yes," how much did your symptoms improve?

| NOT AT ALL | LESS THAN HALF | ABOUT HALF | MORE THAN HALF | PARTIALLY, BUT SYMPTOMS RETURNED | COMPLETELY, BUT SYMPTOMS RETURNED |

13) How did the doctor describe the cause of your pain, illness, or disability? (What <u>diagnosis</u> was given?)

_____

_____

14) How much healing did the doctor expect for you? (What <u>prognosis</u> was given?)

TERMINAL   NO IMPROVEMENT, BUT NOT TERMINAL   SOME IMPROVEMENT, BUT CHRONIC PROBLEM   FULL RECOVERY WITHIN 1 YEAR   FULL RECOVERY WITHIN 1 MONTH

Please return BOTH the pink and blue forms (still stapled together) to the box marked "Healing Surveys." Also, please consider returning a "Testimony Contact Card" to the box marked for it. THANK YOU for your help!

Notes

Introduction

1. Claudia Wallis, "Faith and Healing," *Time*, June 24, 1996, 63, quoted in Ronald L. Numbers, "Science Without God: Natural Laws and Christian Beliefs," in *When Science and Christianity Meet,* ed. David C. Lindberg and Numbers (Chicago: University of Chicago Press, 2003), 284; John Cole, "Gallup Poll Again Shows Confusion," *NCSE Reports* (Spring 1996): 9; General Social Survey, 1997, data extracted from indices for 1983–87, University of Michigan Institute for Social Research, www.icpsr.umich.edu/icpsrweb/ICPSR/access/index.jsp (accessed 9/26/11), cited in Michael S. Goldstein, *Alternative Health Care: Medicine, Miracle, or Mirage?* (Philadelphia: Temple University Press, 1999), 80; Claudia Kalb et al., "Faith and Healing," *Newsweek*, November 10, 2003, 44–56; Robert Bruce Mullin, *Miracles and the Modern Religious Imagination* (New Haven: Yale University Press, 1996), 262; Stephen J. Pullum, *"Foul Demons, Come Out!": The Rhetoric of Twentieth-Century American Faith Healing* (Westport, CT: Praeger, 1999), 150; Rodney Stark, *What Americans Really Believe: New Findings from the Baylor Surveys of Religion* (Waco, TX: Baylor University Press, 2008), 57; John Templeton Foundation, "Survey Reveals HMO Executives Overwhelmingly Recognize Role of Spirituality in Health Care," 1997, cited in Goldstein, *Alternative Health Care*, 7. The Louis Finkelstein Institute for Religious and Social Studies of the Jewish Theological Seminary in New York City conducted a national survey of 1,100 physicians in 2004, cited in Robert D. Orr, "Responding to Patient Beliefs in Miracles," *Southern Medical Journal* 100 (December 2007): 1263.

2. Anne M. McCaffrey et al., "Prayer for Health Concerns: Results of a National Survey on Prevalence and Patterns of Use," *Archives of Internal Medicine* 164 (2004): 858–862; David M. Eisenberg et al., "Trends in Alternative Medicine Use in the United States, 1990–1997: Results of a Follow-Up National Survey," *Journal of the American Medical Association* 280 (November 11, 1998): 1569–1575; Patricia M. Barnes et al., "Complementary and Alternative Medicine Use among Adults: United States, 2002," *Advance Data from Vital and Health Statistics* 343

(May 27, 2004): 1–20; Dietland L. Wahner-Roedler et al., "Use of Complementary and Alternative Medical Therapies by Patients Referred to a Fibromyalgia Treatment Program at a Tertiary Care Center," *Mayo Clinic Proceedings* 80 (2005): 55–60.

3. Herbert Benson et al., "Study of the Therapeutic Effects of Intercessory Prayer (STEP) in Cardiac Bypass Patients: A Multicenter Randomized Trial of Uncertainty and Certainty of Receiving Intercessory Prayer," *American Heart Journal* 151 (2006): 934.

4. Candy Gunther Brown, Ph.D., Stephen C. Mory, M.D., Rebecca Williams, M.B. BChir., DTM&H, and Michael J. McClymond, Ph.D., "Study of the Therapeutic Effects of Proximal Intercessory Prayer (STEPP) on Auditory and Visual Impairments in Rural Mozambique," *Southern Medical Journal* 103.9 (September 2010): 864–869; Shari Roan, "Prayer for Healing Works at Close Range," *Los Angeles Times*, August 4, 2010, articles.latimes.com/2010/aug/04/news/la-heb-prayer-20100804 (accessed 9/26/11); NBC News, August 5, 2010.

5. P. Z. Meyers, "Templeton Prayer Study Meets Expectations," *Pharyngula*, August 4, 2010, scienceblogs.com/pharyngula/2010/08/templeton_prayer_study _meets_e.php (accessed 9/16/11); comment posted in response to Meyers, "Templeton Prayer Study."

6. Norman Gevitz, ed., *Other Healers: Unorthodox Medicine in America* (Baltimore: Johns Hopkins University Press, 1988). For one influential effort to define science, see Karl R. Popper, *Conjectures and Refutations* (London: Routledge and Keagan Paul, 1963), 33–39. There is no one, consensual definition of religion, whether understood in substantive, formal, or functionalist terms; for examples, see Thomas Tweed, *Crossing and Dwelling: A Theory of Religion* (Cambridge, MA: Harvard University Press, 2006), 73; Seth D. Kunin, *Religion: The Modern Theories* (Baltimore: Johns Hopkins University Press, 2003). For the usefulness of the term *suprahuman* in encompassing nontheistic religious beliefs, see Émile Durkheim, *The Division of Labor in Society*, trans. W. D. Halls, rev. ed. (New York: Free, 1984), 131. Ian G. Barbour, *When Science Meets Religion: Enemies, Strangers, or Partners?* (San Francisco: HarperSanFrancisco, 2000), xii, 2–3, offers insight into several possible ways of viewing the relationship between science and religion.

7. Herbert Leventhal, *In the Shadow of the Enlightenment: Occultism and Renaissance Science in Eighteenth-Century America* (New York: New York University Press, 1976); Brian Vickers, *Occult and Scientific Mentalities in the Renaissance* (Cambridge: Cambridge University Press, 1984); Allen G. Debus, ed., *Science, Medicine and Society in the Renaissance: Essays to Honor Walter Pagel*, 2 vols. (New York: Neale Watson Academic Publications, 1972); Thomas S. Kuhn, *The*

Structure of Scientific Revolutions, 3rd ed. (Chicago: Chicago University Press, 1996), 12–13.

8. Donald Kennedy, "Twilight for the Enlightenment?" *Science* 308.5719 (April 8, 2005): 165.

9. Stephen Jay Gould, "Nonoverlapping Magisteria," *Natural History* 106 (March 1997): 19, 62.

10. Lee J. Cronbach and Paul E. Meehl, "Construct Validity in Psychological Tests," *Psychological Bulletin* 52 (1955): 281–302; Robert J. Sbordone and Charles J. Long, eds., *Ecological Validity of Neuropsychological Testing* (Delray Beach, FL: GR/St. Lucie, 1996).

11. "Society Will Proceed with Dalai Lama Lecture at Neuroscience 2005 in Washington, D.C.," *Neuroscience Quarterly* (2011), www.sfn.org/index.aspx?pagename=neuroscienceQuarterly_05fall_dalai (accessed 9/26/11); Anne Harrington and Arthur Zajonc, eds., *The Dalai Lama at MIT* (Cambridge, MA: Harvard University Press, 2006).

12. W. I. Thomas and D. S. Thomas, *The Child in America: Behavior Problems and Programs* (New York: Knopf, 1928), 571–572.

13. William James, *The Varieties of Religious Experience: A Study in Human Nature* (1902; New York: Modern Library, 1929), 14–15; Peter L. Berger, *The Sacred Canopy: Elements of a Sociological Theory of Religion* (Garden City, NY: Doubleday, 1967); Berger, *The Social Reality of Religion* (London: Faber & Faber, 1969), 106, 182; Douglas V. Porpora, "Methodological Atheism, Methodological Agnosticism and Religious Experience," *Journal for the Theory of Social Behavior* 36 (2006): 58.

14. Candy Gunther Brown, *The Word in the World: Evangelical Writing, Publishing, and Reading in America, 1789–1880* (Chapel Hill: University of North Carolina Press, 2004). Many American studies programs are highly attuned to globalization.

15. For a fuller discussion of the terms *Pentecostal, Charismatic,* and *pentecostal,* see chapter 1. All research received appropriate Institutional Review Board approvals: Saint Louis University IRB #13946, and Indiana University IRB #06-11383.

16. Charles Bennett, "*Science* Title Misstep," and Collin Norman, "Response," *Science* 232 (June 10, 2011): 1263.

17. Kuhn, *Structure of Scientific Revolutions,* 64, 148; Elliot G. Mishler et al., *Social Contexts of Health, Illness, and Patient Care* (New York: Cambridge University Press, 1981), 1; Robert A. Hahn, *Sickness and Healing: An Anthropological Perspective* (New Haven: Yale University Press, 1995), 132; Meredith B. McGuire and Debra Kantor, *Ritual Healing in Suburban America* (New Brunswick, NJ: Rutgers University Press, 1988), 5.

18. Norman Gevitz, "Three Perspectives on Unorthodox Medicine," and David J. Hufford, "Contemporary Folk Medicine," in *Other Healers,* ed. Gevitz, 16, 256.

19. Andrew Weil, *Health and Healing* (Boston: Houghton Mifflin, 1988), 28.

20. Estimates of pentecostal membership vary widely, the most conservative ranging from a quarter to over a half billion people; see Luis Lugo et al., *Spirit and Power: A 10-Country Survey of Pentecostals* (Washington, DC: Pew Forum on Religion & Public Life, October 2006), pewforum.org/Christian/Evangelical-Protestant-Churches/Spirit-and-Power.aspx (accessed 9/26/11); David B. Barrett, George Thomas Kurian, and Todd M. Johnson, *World Christian Encyclopedia: A Comparative Survey of Churches and Religion in the Modern World,* 2nd ed., 2 vols. (New York: Oxford University Press, 2001); Philip Jenkins, *The Next Christendom: The Coming of Global Christianity* (New York: Oxford University Press, 2002), 2–5, 8; David Martin, *Pentecostalism: The World Their Parish* (Malden, MA: Blackwell, 2002), xvii; Barna Group, "Is American Christianity Turning Charismatic?" January 7, 2008, reports the results of a nationwide telephone survey conducted in December 2007 among a random sample of 1,005 adults, www .barna.org/barna-update/article/18-congregations/52-is-american-christianity -turning-charismatic (accessed 9/26/11), although the study has been criticized as overestimating the number of U.S. pentecostals; Candy Gunther Brown, ed., *Global Pentecostal and Charismatic Healing* [hereafter *GPCH*] (New York: Oxford University Press, 2011).

21. John Corrigan, ed., *Religion and Emotion: Approaches and Interpretations* (New York: Oxford University Press, 2004); Emmanuel Levinas, "Substitution," in *Emmanuel Levinas: Basic Philosophical Writings,* trans. and ed. Adriaan T. Peperzak, Simon Critchley, and Robert Bernasconi (Bloomington: Indiana University Press, 1996), 79–95; Immanuel Kant, *The Moral Law,* trans. and ed. H. J. Paton (London: Hutchinson, 1964); 66–68; Robert Wuthnow, "Altruism and Sociological Theory," *Social Service Review* 67 (1993): 356; David D. Hall, ed., *Lived Religion in America: Toward a History of Practice* (Princeton, NJ: Princeton University Press, 1997); Laurie F. Maffly-Kipp, Leigh Eric Schmidt, and Mark R. Valeri, *Practicing Protestants: Histories of Christian Life in America, 1630–1965* (Baltimore: Johns Hopkins University Press, 2006); Meredith B. McGuire, *Lived Religion: Faith and Practice in Everyday Life* (New York: Oxford University Press, 2008); R. Marie Griffith, *Born Again Bodies: Flesh and Spirit in American Christianity* (Berkeley: University of California Press, 2004); Peter L. Berger and Thomas Luckmann, *The Social Construction of Reality: A Treatise in the Sociology of Knowledge* (Garden City, NY: Doubleday, 1966); Andrew Pickering, *Constructing Quarks: A Sociological History of Particle Physics* (Chicago: University of Chicago Press, 1984).

22. David D. Hall, *A History of the Book in America: The Colonial Book in the Atlantic World* (Cambridge: Cambridge University Press, 2000); James K. Honeyford, "No Religion, But Social: Religious Societies, Social Religion, and the Creation of the Social Category in England and America, 1580–1750," (Ph.D. diss., Indiana University, 2010); Susan O'Brien, "A Transatlantic Community of Saints: The Great Awakening and the First Evangelical Network, 1735–1755," *American Historical Review* 91 (October 1986): 811–832; Heather D. Curtis, "The Global Character of Nineteenth-Century Divine Healing," in *GPCH*, 29–45; Manuel A. Vásquez and Marie Friedmann Marquardt, *Globalizing the Sacred: Religion across the Americas* (New Brunswick, NJ: Rutgers University Press, 2003); 227–228; André Corten and Ruth Marshall-Fratani, introduction to *Between Babel and Pentecost: Transnational Pentecostalism in Africa and Latin America* (Bloomington: Indiana University Press, 2001), 3, 6; John Joseph Page, "Brasil Para Christo: The Cultural Construction of Pentecostal Networks in Brazil," (Ph.D. diss., New York University, 1984), i.

23. Linton C. Freeman, *The Development of Social Network Analysis: A Study in the Sociology of Science* (Vancouver, BC: Empirical, 2004), 1; Mark Granovetter, "The Strength of Weak Ties: A Network Theory Revisited," *Sociological Theory* 1 (1983): 202; Stanley Wasserman and Katherine Faust, *Social Network Analysis: Methods and Applications* (New York: Cambridge University Press, 1994), 4; Nan Lin, Karen Cook, and Donald S. Burt, eds., *Social Capital: Theory and Research* (New Brunswick, NJ: Transaction, 2001), viii; Nan Lin, "Building a Network Theory of Social Capital," in *Social Capital*, eds. Lin, Cook, and Burt, 6. The religious studies scholar Thomas Tweed, *Crossing and Dwelling*, 54, considers "flow" to be a "better metaphor than network for cultural analysis," but there need not be a rigid distinction since cultural flows often travel through social networks.

24. Randall Collins, *Interaction Ritual Chains* (Princeton, NJ: Princeton University Press, 2004), 6, 38–39; Émile Durkheim, *The Elementary Forms of Religious Life*, rev. ed. (New York: Simon & Schuster, 1995), 220; Stephen Post and Jill Neimark, *Why Good Things Happen to Good People: The Exciting New Research That Proves the Link between Doing Good and Living a Longer, Healthier, Happier Life* (New York: Random House, 2007). Potential health benefits notwithstanding, sociologists have observed a tendency of North Americans to withdraw from social involvement—a phenomenon epitomized by the title of Robert D. Putnam's book, *Bowling Alone: The Collapse and Revival of American Community* (New York: Simon & Schuster, 2000).

25. Pitirim A. Sorokin, *The Ways and Power of Love: Types, Factors, and Techniques of Moral Transformation*, rev. ed. (Philadelphia: Templeton Foundation Press, 2002), 15, 26, 36–37.

26. Matthew T. Lee and Margaret M. Poloma, *A Sociological Study of the Great Commandment in Pentecostalism: The Practice of Godly Love as Benevolent Service* (Lewiston, NY: Edwin Mellen, 2009), 7, 10; Margaret M. Poloma and Ralph W. Hood, Jr., *Blood and Fire: Godly Love in a Pentecostal Emerging Church* (New York: New York University Press, 2008), 4; Matthew T. Lee, Margaret M. Poloma, and Stephen G. Post, *The Heart of Religion* (New York: Oxford University Press, forthcoming).

27. The church is described as the body of Christ in biblical passages such as 1 Corinthians 12:27; the gifts and fruits of the Holy Spirit are listed in 1 Corinthians 12:8 and Galatians 5:22–23.

1. From Toronto Blessing to Global Awakening

1. Randy Clark, *Lighting Fires: Keeping the Spirit of Revival Alive in Your Heart and the Hearts of Others Around You* (Lake Mary, FL: Creation House, 1998), 87–88. I privilege the term *deliverance* over *exorcism* to refer to the practice of expelling "demons." *Deliverance* is the term generally preferred by the pentecostals studied and reflects their priority on freeing people from "oppression" rather than conversing with or seeking sensationalized encounters with "evil spirits."

2. Ruth Gledhill, in "Spread of Hysteria Fad Worries Church," *London Times,* June 18, 1994, 12, is credited as the first published writer to use the label "Toronto Blessing"; David Hilborn, ed., introduction to *'Toronto' in Perspective: Papers on the New Charismatic Wave of the Mid-1990's* (Waynesboro, GA: Acute, 2001), 4, 7; Global Awakening, "About Us," www.globalawakening.com/Groups/1000014260 /Global_Awakening/Global/Global.aspx (accessed 10/7/11); Margaret Poloma, *Main Street Mystics: The Toronto Blessing and Reviving Pentecostalism* (New York: Rowman & Littlefield, 2003), 91. Although Protestants have frequently voiced suspicions of pilgrimages as superstitious, the practice has persisted throughout the history of Christianity, and has arguably become more prevalent in the past century. Indeed, tourism and pilgrimage serve some of the same purposes, as described by John F. Sears, *Sacred Places: American Tourist Attractions in the Nineteenth Century* (New York: Oxford University Press, 1989), 5–6; David Chidester and Edward T. Linenthal, eds., introduction to *American Sacred Space* (Bloomington: Indiana University Press, 1995), 6. I made research trips to Toronto in January 1995 and August 2005.

3. Nader Mikhaiel, *The Toronto Blessing and Slaying in the Spirit: The Telling Wonder; A Compelling New Approach to the Pentecostal Charismatic Signs and Wonders Debate* (Earlwood, NSW, Australia: Nader Mikhaiel, 1992), 20, 29, 44,

84; Hank Hanegraaff, *Counterfeit Revival* (Nashville: Word, 1997); Clark, *Lighting Fires*, 100; Donald R. Kantel, "The 'Toronto Blessing' Revival and Its Continuing Impact on Mission in Mozambique" (D.Min. diss., Regent University, 2007), 106; John Arnott, *The Father's Blessing* (Orlando: Creation House, 1995); John Wimber, interview by Margaret M. Poloma, cited in Kantel, "'Toronto Blessing,'" 104. I thank Michael McClymond for bringing Kantel's dissertation to my notice.

4. Randy Clark, interview by author, Harrisburg, Pennsylvania, November 4, 2005.

5. Martyn Percy, "The City on a Beach: Future Prospects for Charismatic Movements at the End of the Twentieth Century," in *Charismatic Christianity: Sociological Perspectives*, ed. Stephen Hunt, Malcolm Hamilton, and Tony Walter (New York: St. Martin's, 1997), 216; Percy, *Power and the Church: Ecclesiology in an Age of Transition* (London: Cassell, 1998), 207.

6. Luis Lugo et al., *Spirit and Power: A 10-Country Survey of Pentecostals* (Washington, DC: The Pew Forum on Religion & Public Life, October 2006), pewforum.org/Christian/Evangelical-Protestant-Churches/Spirit-and-Power .aspx (accessed 10/7/11).

7. Margaret M. Poloma and George Gallup, *Varieties of Prayer: A Survey Report* (Philadelphia: Trinity Press International, 1991), 6; Poloma and B. F. Pendleton, "The Effects of Prayer and Prayer Experience on Measures of General Wellbeing," *Journal of Psychology and Theology* 19 (1991): 71–83; Kevin L. Ladd and Bernard Spilka, "Inward, Outward, Upward Prayer: Scale Reliability and Validation," *Journal for the Scientific Study of Religion* 45, no. 2 (2006): 233–251.

8. This book avoids the term *faith healing* as analytically confusing, given the caricatured images of flamboyant, money-grubbing charlatanry it so readily evokes. The term *divine healing* better corresponds with the specific beliefs of the pentecostals studied, who generally attribute medically unexpected recoveries to God's power and love, rather than to merely human faith or an impersonal spiritual force, and expect that God can use anyone filled by the Holy Spirit—not just an unusually gifted individual—to heal the sick. For distinctions between healing and cure, see Pamela E. Klassen, "Textual Healing: Mainstream Protestants and the Therapeutic Text, 1900–1925," *Church History* 75, no. 4 (2006): 809–810; Susan S. Sered and Linda L. Barnes, introduction to *Religion and Healing in America*, ed. Barnes and Sered (New York: Oxford University Press, 2005), 10. On differentiating healings and miracles, see Robert Bruce Mullin, *Miracles and the Modern Religious Imagination* (New Haven: Yale University Press, 1996), 95. In practice, pentecostals rarely make a rigid distinction among the terms *healing*, *cure*, and *miracle*.

9. Global Awakening, "History of the Apostolic Network," www.globalawak ening.com/Group/Group.aspx?ID=1000022042 (accessed 10/7/11); Iris Ministries, "About Us," www.irismin.org/about (accessed 10/7/11); Kantel, "'Toronto Blessing,'" 13.

10. National Center for Complementary and Alternative Medicine, "Backgrounder: Energy Medicine; An Overview," NCCAM Publication No. D235 (Bethesda, MD: NIH, 2004, 2007), 1.

11. Amanda Porterfield, *Healing in the History of Christianity* (New York: Oxford University Press, 2005), 3; Luke 4:40, Matthew 4:34, Matthew 10:8, James 5: 13–15 (NIV). This is a simplified account of a multifaceted history that exceeds the scope of this book. Many excellent treatments of this history are available, including Ramsay MacMullen, *Christianizing the Roman Empire* (A.D. 100–400) (New Haven: Yale University Press, 1984); Morton T. Kelsey, *Psychology, Medicine and Christian Healing* (San Francisco: Harper & Row, 1988); and Francis MacNutt, *The Healing Reawakening: Reclaiming Our Lost Inheritance* (Grand Rapids, MI: Chosen, 2006).

12. Donald W. Dayton, *Theological Roots of Pentecostalism* (Grand Rapids, MI: Francis Asbury, 1987), 115–118; Mark A. Noll, David W. Bebbington, and George A. Rawlyk, eds., *Evangelicalism: Comparative Studies of Popular Protestantism in North America, the British Isles, and Beyond, 1700–1990* (New York: Oxford University Press, 1994); Pamela Klassen, "Radio Mind: Protestant Experimentalists on the Frontiers of Healing," *Journal of the American Academy of Religion* 75, no. 3 (2007): 651–683; Donald M. Lewis, ed., introduction to *Christianity Reborn: The Global Expansion of Evangelicalism in the Twentieth Century* (Grand Rapids, MI: Eerdmans, 2004), 1; Walter J. Hollenweger, "An Introduction to Pentecostalisms," *Journal of Beliefs and Values* 25 (2004): 129; Candy Gunther Brown, "Healing and Revivals," *Encyclopedia of Religious Revivals in America,* ed. Michael J. McClymond (Westport, CT: Greenwood, 2007), 201–204; Heather D. Curtis, "The Global Character of Nineteenth-Century Divine Healing," in *Global Pentecostal and Charismatic Healing* [hereafter *GPCH*], ed. Candy Gunther Brown (New York: Oxford University Press, 2011), 31 .

13. Curtis, *Faith in the Great Physician: Suffering and Divine Healing in American Culture, 1860–1900* (Baltimore: Johns Hopkins University Press, 2007); James Robinson, *Divine Healing: The Formative Years, 1825–1880s; Theological Roots in the Transatlantic World* (Eugene, OR: Pickwick, 2011); Paul Gale Chappell, "The Divine Healing Movement in America," (Ph.D. diss., Drew University, 1983).

14. Brown, introduction to *GPCH,* 6–9; Murray W. Dempster, Byron D. Klaus, and Douglas Petersen, *The Globalization of Pentecostalism: A Religion Made to Travel* (Irvine, CA: Regnum, 1999); Karla O. Poewe, *Charismatic Chris-*

tianity as a Global Culture (Columbia: University of South Carolina Press, 1994); Roland Robertson, *Globalization: Social Theory and Global Culture* (London: Sage, 1992), 8, 184; David Martin, "Evangelical Expansion in Global Society," in *Christianity Reborn,* ed. Lewis, 273; Ulf Hannerz, *Transnational Connections: Culture, People, Places* (New York: Routledge, 1996), 102; Peter Geschiere and Birgit Meyer, "Globalization and Identity: Dialectics of Flow and Closure," *Development and Change* 29, no. 4 (1998): 602; Simon Coleman, *The Globalisation of Charismatic Christianity: Spreading the Gospel of Prosperity* (Cambridge: Cambridge University Press, 2000), 55; Thomas A. Tweed, *Crossing and Dwelling: A Theory of Religion* (Cambridge, MA: Harvard University Press, 2006), 127; Martin Riesebrodt, "Religion in Global Perspective," 607, in *The Oxford Handbook of Global Religions,* ed. Mark Juergensmeyer (New York: Oxford University Press, 2006), 599–600; Arjun Appadurai, *Modernity at Large: Cultural Dimensions of Globalization* (Minneapolis: University of Minnesota Press, 1996), 5.

15. 1 Corinthians 12:8 (AV); Paul's letter to the Galatians 5:22–23 (NAS) gives a parallel list of nine "fruits" of the Spirit, namely love, joy, peace, patience, kindness, goodness, faithfulness, gentleness, and self-control. In quoting Bible verses, I have selected the translations that I most often see used by the pentecostals studied, even though this means using different versions from verse to verse. The lower-case term *charismatic* connotes broader meanings, which are informed by the sociologist Max Weber's influential theory of leadership; Weber, "The Sociology of Charismatic Authority," in *Max Weber: Essays in Sociology,* ed. and trans. H. H. Gerth and C. Wright Mills (New York: Oxford University Press, 1946), 245–252.

16. Allan Anderson, *Spreading Fires: The Missionary Nature of Early Pentecostalism* (Maryknoll, NY: Orbis, 2007); Walter J. Hollenweger, *Pentecostalism: Origins and Developments Worldwide* (Peabody, MA: Hendrickson, 1997); David Martin, *Pentecostalism: The World Their Parish* (Malden, MA: Blackwell, 2002); Edith L. Blumhofer, Russell P. Spittler, and Grant A. Wacker, eds., *Pentecostal Currents in American Protestantism* (Urbana: University of Illinois Press, 1999); Mary Jo Neitz, *Charisma and Community: A Study of Religious Commitment within the Charismatic Renewal* (New Brunswick, NJ: Transaction, 1987).

17. Cecil M. Robeck, Jr., *The Azusa Street Mission and Revival: The Birth of the Global Pentecostal Movement* (Nashville: Nelson, 2006); Gastón Espinosa, "Latino Pentecostal Healing in the North American Borderlands," in *GPCH,* 130–131; Harvey Cox, *Fire from Heaven: The Rise of Pentecostal Spirituality and the Reshaping of Religion in the Twenty-first Century* (Reading, MA: Addison-Wesley, 1995), 68.

18. Minnie F. Abrams, *The Baptism of the Holy Ghost and Fire, Matt. 3:11* (Kedgaon, India: Mukti Mission Press, 1906); Candy Gunther Brown, "From Tent

Meetings and Store-front Healing Rooms to Walmarts and the Internet: Healing Spaces in the United States, the Americas, and the World, 1906–2006," *Church History* (September 2006): 643.

19. See *GPCH*; David Edwin Harrell, Jr., *All Things Are Possible: The Healing and Charismatic Revivals in Modern America* (Bloomington: Indiana University Press, 1975), 166; Hollenweger, *Pentecostalism*, 243; John Wimber and Kevin Springer, *Power Evangelism* (San Francisco: Harper & Row, 1986; Ventura, CA: Gospel Light, 2009), 79.

20. Candy Gunther Brown, "Healing Words: Narratives of Spiritual Healing and Kathryn Kuhlman's Uses of Print Culture, 1947–1976," in *Religion and the Culture of Print in Modern America,* ed. Charles L. Cohen and Paul S. Boyer (Madison: University of Wisconsin Press, 2008), 271–297; Thomas J. Csordas, "Catholic Charismatic Healing in Global Perspective: The Cases of India, Brazil, and Nigeria," in *GPCH*, 331–332, 334, 344; Simon Coleman, "Why Health *and* Wealth? Dimensions of Prosperity among Swedish Charismatics," in *GPCH*, 59; Arlene Sánchez Walsh, "Santidad, Salvación, Sanidad, Liberación: The Word of Faith Movement among Twenty-First-Century Latina/o Pentecostals," in *GPCH*, 152; Catherine Bowler, "Blessed Bodies: Healing within the African American Faith Movement," in *GPCH*, 86; Claudia Währisch-Oblau, "Material Salvation: Healing, Deliverance, and 'Breakthrough' in African Migrant Churches in Germany," in *GPCH*, 64; Paul Gifford, "Healing in African Pentecostalism: The 'Victorious Living' of David Oyedepo," in *GPCH*, 251–266; Matthew Marostica, "Learning from the Master: Carlos Annacondia and the Standardization of Pentecostal Practices in and beyond Argentina," in *GPCH*, 207–227.

21. Mullin, *Miracles,* 263–265; Candy Gunther Brown, "Vineyard Christian Fellowships," in *The Encyclopedia of Christianity*, ed. Craig Noll (Grand Rapids, MI: Eerdmans, 2008), 5:680–682.

22. Brown, "Vineyard Christian Fellowships"; editorial, *Christianity Today,* February 9, 1998, quoted in Vineyard USA, "Vineyard History," www.vineyard usa.org/site/about/vineyard-history (accessed 10/7/11); Kevin Springer, preface to *Power Evangelism*, by Wimber and Springer, 8.

23. John Wimber and Kevin Springer, *Power Healing* (San Francisco: Harper & Row, 1987), 193–94; 1 Corinthians 12:8 (AV). For a psychological interpretation of "hearing God" in the Vineyard movement, see Tanya M. Luhrmann, "The Art of Hearing God: Absorption, Dissociation, and Contemporary American Spirituality," *Spiritus: A Journal of Christian Spirituality* 5, no. 2 (Fall 2005): 133–157.

24. Wimber and Springer, *Power Evangelism*, 84; Don Williams, "Friend and Encourager," 56, in *John Wimber: His Influence and Legacy* (Guildford, Surrey: Eagle, 1998), 56. The phrase *signs and wonders* is borrowed from various references

in the Bible, e.g., Exodus 7:3, Acts 4:30 (AV); Wimber and Springer, *Power Healing*, 14; Brown, "Vineyard Christian Fellowships"; Bill Jackson, *The Quest for the Radical Middle: A History of the Vineyard* (Cape Town: Vineyard International, 1999); Paul Kennedy, "Satisfied Customers: Miracles at the Vineyard Christian Fellowship," *Mental Health, Religion & Culture* 1, no. 2 (November 1998): 135–152; Donald Miller, *Reinventing American Protestantism: Christianity in the New Millennium* (Berkeley: University of California Press, 1997); Miller, "Routinizing Charisma: The Vineyard Christian Fellowship in the Post-Wimber Era," *Pneuma* 25, no. 2 (Fall 2003): 216–239; Robin Dale Perrin, "Signs and Wonders: The Growth of the Vineyard Christian Fellowship" (Ph.D. diss., Washington State University, 1989); Perrin and Armand L. Mauss, "Saints and Seekers: Sources of Recruitment to the Vineyard Christian Fellowship," *Review of Religious Research* 33, no. 2 (December 1991): 97–111; Vineyard USA, "Vineyard History," www.vineyardusa.org/site/about/vineyard-history (accessed 10/7/11).

25. Vineyard USA, "Vineyard Core Values," www.vineyardusa.org/site/about/vineyard-values (accessed 10/7/11); Max Weber, *The Theory of Social and Economic Organizations,* trans. A. M. Henderson and Talcott Parsons (New York: Simon & Schuster, 1947), 358–392; Wimber and Springer, *Power Healing,* 157; Randy Clark, sermon in Carmi, Illinois, April 17, 2010; Doug (a leader in the Vineyard Community Fellowship–St. Louis), personal communication to author, September 2001; field notes from School of Healing and Impartation, St. Louis, Missouri, February 28–March 3, 2006. In speaking of living between the "already and the not yet," Wimber explicitly borrowed from Professor George Ladd of Fuller Seminary. Throughout this book, I have used pseudonyms (recognizable by the use of a first name only) to protect the identities of informants; I use real names when quoting from written statements by public figures or published authors.

26. "Toronto's Racial Diversity," www.toronto.ca/toronto_facts/diversity.htm (accessed 10/7/11); John Arnott, "When It All Began," *Spread the Fire*, February 1999, 6, quoted in Poloma, *Main Street Mystics*, 153; Marostica, "Learning from the Master," 222; Benny Hinn, *Welcome, Holy Spirit: How You Can Experience the Dynamic Work of the Holy Spirit in Your Life* (Nashville: Thomas Nelson, 1995), 11; Wayne E. Warner, *Kathryn Kuhlman: The Woman Behind the Miracles* (Ann Arbor: Servant, 1993), 32; Candy Gunther Brown, "Maria Woodworth-Etter," in *Encyclopedia of Religious Revivals,* ed. McClymond, 471–472; Julia Duin, "Praise the Lord and Pass the New Wine," *Charisma,* August 1994, 22; I thank Michael McClymond for pointing out the ironic imagery.

27. Clark, *Lighting Fires,* 95, 127; Clark, interview by Margaret M. Poloma and Matthew T. Lee, tape recording, Mechanicsburg, Pennsylvania, August 28, 2008;

Clark, *Lighting Fires*, 127; Global Awakening, "International Ministry Trip Reports from the Nations," www.globalawakening.com/Groups/1000013724/Global _Awakening/Global/International/Reports/Reports.aspx (accessed 10/7/11).

28. Global Awakening, "Vision and Mission Statements," www.globalawak ening.com/Group/Group.aspx?ID=1000014270 (accessed 10/7/11); Clark, interview by Poloma and Lee.; Global Awakening, "Organization Directory," www .globalawakening.com/Groups/1000014268/Global_Awakening/Global/Direc tory/Apostolic_Network/Apostolic_Network.aspx (accessed 10/7/11); Randy Clark, *God Can Use Little Ole Me: Remarkable Stories of Ordinary Christians* (Shippensburg, PA: Revival, 1998).

29. Benny Hinn Ministries, "Pastor Benny Holds Historic Healing Services in India!" www.bennyhinn.org/dnld/india.pdf (accessed 10/7/11); UCKG Help Centre, "History of UCKG," www.uckg.org/show_details.php?tbl_content_id=CNT -03 (accessed 10/7/11). Prosperity theology has become a popular topic among researchers, for instance Coleman, "Why Health *and* Wealth?," Bowler, "Blessed Bodies," Sánchez Walsh, "Santidad, Salvación, Sanidad, Liberación," and Gifford, "Healing in African Pentecostalism," all in *GPCH*.

30. Field notes, e.g., Harrisburg, Pennsylvania, November 4, 2005, and October 30, 2008; Randy Clark, "Benefits of Partnership," sermon delivered to GA team in Imperatriz, Maranhão, Brazil, September 24, 2007.

31. Clark, "Benefits of Partnership." For a discussion of Mensa Otabil, the pastor of Ghana's International Central Gospel Church, see Paul Gifford, "The Complex Provenance of Some Elements of African Pentecostal Theology," in *Between Babel and Pentecost: Transnational Pentecostalism in Africa and Latin America,* ed. André Corten and Ruth Marshall-Fratani (Bloomington: Indiana University Press, 2001), 73. On Reinhard Bonnke, a German evangelist who itinerates across Africa, see Marko Kuhn, *Prophetic Christianity in Western Kenya: Political, Cultural and Theological Aspects of African Independent Churches* (Frankfurt am Main: Peter Lang, 2008), 244; Währisch-Oblau, "Material Salvation," 70; Marostica, "Learning from the Master," 221. For treatments of David Yonggi Cho, the pastor of South Korea's Yoido Full Gospel Church, see Wonsuk Ma, "Asian (Classical) Pentecostal Theology in Context," in *Asian and Pentecostal: The Charismatic Face of Christianity in Asia,* ed. Allan Anderson and Edmond Tang (Costa Mesa, CA: Regnum, 2005), 66; Allan Anderson, *An Introduction to Pentecostalism: Global Charismatic Christianity* (Cambridge: Cambridge University Press, 2004), 222; Sean Kim, "Reenchanted: Divine Healing in Korean Protestantism," in *GPCH*. Brazil's Universal Church of the Kingdom of God, under the leadership of Sérgio Von Helder, is discussed by R. Andrew Chesnut, *Born Again in Brazil: The Pentecostal Boom and the Pathogens of Poverty* (New Brunswick, NJ: Rutgers University Press, 1997), 45; Chesnut, "Exorcising the

Demons of Deprivation: Divine Healing and Conversion in Brazilian Pentecostalism," in *GPCH*, 174. There has been relatively little academic research on Mahesh Chavda, an internationally prominent itinerant evangelist of Indian descent born in Kenya and currently based out of All Nations Church in Fort Mill, South Carolina; or on David Hogan, a North American who has reputedly planted hundreds of churches among indigenous peoples in rural Mexico; both are discussed by John Crowder, *Miracle Workers, Reformers and the New Mystics* (Shippensburg, PA: Destiny Image, 2006), 74, 143. Little has been written on the Norwegian Leif Hetland, founder of Global Mission Awareness, which is active in twenty-two countries, most influentially Pakistan; Leif Hetland Ministries, www.leifhetlandministries.com/ (accessed 10/7/11); or Dennis Balcombe, U.S. missionary to China and founder of Revival Chinese Ministries International; Revival Chinese Ministries International, "Dennis Balcombe," rcmi.ac/eng.htm (accessed 10/7/11).

32. Global Awakening, "Voice of the Apostles," events.globalawakening.com/topics-voa (accessed 10/7/11).

33. The Arnotts handed over pastoral leadership of TACF to Steve and Sandra Long in 2006 when John retired at age sixty-five, allowing the Arnotts to accept increasing international responsibilities. Catch the Fire Toronto! "Dear Friends," www.ctftoronto.com/about/name-change (accessed 10/7/11); Weber, *Theory of Social and Economic Organizations.* For the argument that routinization alternates with revival, see Margaret M. Poloma and John C. Green, *The Assemblies of God: Godly Love and the Revitalization of American Pentecostalism* (New York: New York University Press, 2010), 17; Partners in Harvest: Spreading the Fire, "A Little Bit About Us," partnersinharvest.org/about (accessed 10/25

34. Bethel Church, "Dear Friends," www.ibethel.org/site/bethel-and-the-assemblies-of-god (accessed 10/7/11); Bill Johnson, interview by Margaret M. Poloma, video recording, Harrisburg, Pennsylvania, October 30, 2008.

35. Bethel Church, www.ibethel.org/site/ (accessed 10/7/11); Ministry of Bethel Church, "Sozo: Saved, Healed, Delivered," www.bethelsozo.com/ (accessed 10/7/11). *Sozo* is a Greek word that, according to pentecostal counts, appears 110 times in the New Testament and is variously translated as "saved," "healed," and "delivered"; the model emphasizes renunciation of the "lies" that God possesses the same characteristics as people, especially parents, who have caused emotional wounds. Bethel International, "Brazil," www.ibethelinternational.org/brazil/ (accessed 10/7/11); Bethel International, "Heroes of the Nation," www.ibethelinternational.org/kenya/ (accessed 10/7/11).

36. Kantel, "'Toronto Blessing,'" 67; HROCK Church, "Our Story," www.hrockchurch.com/our_story.html (accessed 10/7/11); Global Celebration, "History," www.globalcelebration.com/about-us/history/ (accessed 10/7/11).

37. Heidi Baker, interview by Margaret M. Poloma, video recording (made by author), Harrisburg, Pennsylvania, October 30, 2008; H. Baker, interview by Donald Kantel, Pemba, Cabo Delgado, Mozambique, March 27, 2006, transcription in Kantel, "'Toronto Blessing,'" 195; Rolland Baker, "Core Values at Iris: Simple, Controversial and Not Optional!" e-mail newsletter, September 17, 2010; Iris Ministries, www.irismin.org/ (accessed 11/24/10); R. Baker and H. Baker, *There Is Always Enough: God's Miraculous Provision among the Poorest Children on Earth* (Grand Rapids, MI: Chosen, 2003); H. Baker and R. Baker, *Expecting Miracles: True Stories of God's Supernatural Power and How You Can Experience It* (Grand Rapids, MI: Chosen, 2007); H. Baker with Shara Pradhan, *Compelled by Love: How to Change the World through the Simple Power of Love in Action* (Lake Mary, FL: Charisma House, 2008).

38. Johnson, interview by Poloma.

39. Stephen Hunt, "The Florida 'Outpouring' Revival," *PentecoStudies* 8, no. 1 (2009): 37–57; Todd Bentley, *Journey into the Miraculous: An Ordinary Man Touched by a Supernatural God* (Ladysmith, BC: Sound of Fire, 2003), 29–38.

40. Global Awakening, "Public Statement on Todd Bentley from Revival Alliance," October 23, 2008, www.globalawakening.com/Mobile/default.aspx?group_id=1000014260&article_id=1000041374 (accessed 10/7/11); Johnson, interview by Poloma; Rick Joyner, "Todd Bentley's Phase 2 Release," www.freshfireusa.com/index.php/media/index/0/157 (accessed 10/7/11); Bill Johnson, "Update from Bill Johnson on Todd Bentley," www.freshfireusa.com/index.php/articles/view/216 (accessed 10/25/11).

41. Pablo Deiros, endorsement for *God Can Use,* by Clark, ii; Randy Clark, ed., introduction to *Power, Holiness, and Evangelism: Rediscovering God's Purity, Power, and Passion for the Lost* (Shippensburg, PA: Destiny Image, 1999), xxiv.

42. Randy Clark, interview by author, Imperatriz, Maranhão, Brazil, September 22, 2007; Marostica, "Learning from the Master," in *GPCH*, 215; Clark, *Ministry Training Manual* (Mechanicsburg, PA: Global Awakening, 2002), M1–42; Pablo Bottari, *Free in Christ: Your Complete Handbook on the Ministry of Deliverance* [*Libres in Christo: La Importancia del Ministerio de Liberación*] (Lake Mary, FL: Creation House, 2000); Heidi Baker, interview by Clark, video recording, Pemba, Cabo Delgado, Mozambique, June 4, 2009; Omar Cabrera, *Lo Positivo del "No"* ["The Positive of 'No'"] (Miami, FL: Vida, 2002); Carlos Annacondia, *Listen to Me, Satan!* ["¡Oíme Bien, Satanás!"] (Lake Mary, FL: Charisma House, 2008). A Casa de Davi band, for instance, flew to Harrisburg, Pennsylvania, to lead worship and speak at GA's fifteen-hundred-person Voice of the Apostles conference, November 5–8, 2003; Casa de Davi, www.casadedavi.com.br/ws/, maintained an English-language website until sometime between June 21, 2011 and October 7, 2011.

43. Clark, "Benefits of Partnership"; "prophetic words" circulate informally in GA networks via word of mouth, e-mails, newsletters, and sermons; H. Baker, quoted by Clark in interview by Poloma; Clark, interview by Poloma.

44. Benedict Anderson, *Imagined Communities: Reflections on the Origin and Spread of Nationalism* (London: Verso, 1983).

45. Catherine Bowler, "Searching for Faith on Benny Hinn's Holy Land Tour," paper presented at the American Society of Church History, New York, January 2009. Compare the greater emphasis on taking personal responsibility for one's own healing in the Word of Faith churches described by Bowler, "Blessed Bodies," and Sánchez Walsh, "Santidad, Salvación, Sanidad, Liberación," in *GPCH*.

46. Victor and Edith Turner, *Image and Pilgrimage in Christian Culture* (New York: Columbia University Press, 1978); Catherine Bell, *Ritual Theory, Ritual Practice* (New York: Oxford University Press, 1992); Mircea Eliade, *The Sacred and the Profane: The Nature of Religion,* trans. Willard R. Trask (San Diego: Harcourt Brace, 1987), 20–65; Chidester and Linenthal, introduction to *American Sacred Space,* 10.

47. Lamin Sanneh, "Mission and the Modern Imperative—Retrospect and Prospect: Charting a Course," in *Earthen Vessels American Evangelicals and Foreign Missions, 1880–1980,* ed. Joel A. Carpenter and Wilbert R. Shenk (Grand Rapids, MI: Eerdmans, 1990), 301; Angela Tarango, "Jesus as the Great Physician: Pentecostal Native North Americans within the Assemblies of God and New Understandings of Pentecostal Healing," in *GPCH,* 107–126; John C. Rowe, ed., *Post-Nationalist American Studies* (Berkeley: University of California Press, 2000), 23; Michel Foucault, *The Birth of the Clinic: An Archaeology of Medical Perception,* trans. A. M. Sheridan Smith (New York: Vintage, 1994), xi; Susan Sontag, *Illness as Metaphor and AIDS and Its Metaphors* (New York: Farrar, Straus & Giroux, 1988), 6; Elaine Scarry, *The Body in Pain: The Making and Unmaking of the World* (New York: Oxford University Press, 1985), 6; Walter Hollenweger, "Evangelism and Brazilian Pentecostals," *Ecumenical Review* 20 (April 1968): 166; Robert A. Orsi, *Between Heaven and Earth: The Religious Worlds People Make and the Scholars Who Study Them* (Princeton: Princeton University Press, 2005), 28.

48. Field notes, Rio de Janeiro, Rio de Janeiro, Brazil, September 15, 2007.

49. A. F. Droogers, "Globalization and Pentecostal Success," in *Between Babel and Pentecost,* ed. Corten and Marshall-Fratani, 55. Postcolonial theorists have exposed how imposition of the English language can reinforce relations of dominance, a pattern that can be resisted when cross-cultural communication is conducted in local languages; Philip Jenkins, *The Next Christendom: the Coming of Global Christianity* (New York: Oxford University Press, 2002), 113.

50. Clark, sermon to Assemblies of God churches in Imperatriz, Maranhão, Brazil, September 24, 2007.

51. Mark, sermon to GA team in Londrina, Paraná, Brazil, June 11, 2008. Two years later, on June 18, 2010, Mark, an expatriate American with Brazilian citizenship, similarly called members of Casa de Davi to repentance, publishing a public retraction of claims made by a Brazilian leader that were discovered to be false (see chapter 3); the retraction was removed from Casa de Davi's website sometime between June 21, 2011 and October 7, 2011. Pablo Deiros and Pablo Bottari, "Deliverance From Dark Strongholds," in *Power, Holiness, and Evangelism*, ed. Clark, 111; for example, speaking at a conference in St. Louis, Missouri on September 25, 2003, Bottari denounced U.S. participation in certain sectors of alternative healthcare.

52. David Martin, *Tongues of Fire: The Explosion of Protestantism in Latin America* (Cambridge, MA: Blackwell, 1990), 107; André F. Droogers, "Globalization and Pentecostal Success," in *Between Babel and Pentecost*, ed. Corten and Marshall-Fratani, 4.

53. Clark, interview by author, 2007; Margaret M. Poloma, *The Assemblies of God at the Crossroads: Charisma and Institutional Dilemmas* (Knoxville: University of Tennessee Press, 1989), 85, has found in her sociological research that even many U.S. Assemblies of God pastors have "played down the significance of 'deliverance'"; Harvey Cox, *Fire From Heaven*, 109–10, has argued, moreover, that many middle-class pentecostal churches in the United States "have begun to soft-pedal healing, as they become more 'respectable.'" Disputes among GA team members (September 19, 2007) and between GA team members and Brazilian pastors (September 25, 2007) over how deliverance should be practiced arose at least twice during a single two-week GA trip. There are even disagreements over who needs deliverance. Some pentecostals, for instance, teach that Christians—at least "Spirit-filled" Christians—cannot be troubled by demons. Others will perform deliverance only on Christians on the premise that demons can too easily return to non-Christians because doors to their entrance will not have been closed. For the importance and controversial nature of deliverance among Brazilian Pentecostals, see André Corten, *Pentecostalism in Brazil: Emotion of the Poor and Theological Romanticism* (New York: St. Martin's, 1999), 35; Chesnut, *Born Again in Brazil*, 45-46; Stephen Selka "Morality in the Religious Marketplace: Evangelical Christianity, Candomblé and the Struggle for Moral Distinction in Brazil," *American Ethnologist* 37, no. 2 (2010): 291–307.

54. Poloma, *Main Street Mystics*, 87, argues that the Toronto Blessing reflects a "democratization of healing practices"; Chesnut, *Born Again in Brazil*, 80, 98; Chesnut, "Exorcising the Demons of Deprivation," 361; Poloma and Green, *Assem-*

blies of God, 127; Poloma, "Inspecting the Fruit of the 'Toronto Blessing': A Sociological Assessment," *Pneuma* 20 (1998): 43–70.

55. Wimber and Springer, *Power Healing,* 169–235; Bottari, *Libres en Christo.* To contextualize GA's dissemination of American-authored training materials translated into Portuguese, an estimated 70 percent of evangelical books published in Brazil in 1991 were translations; Paul Freston, "Contours of Latin American Pentecostalism," in *Christianity Reborn: The Global Expansion of Evangelicalism in the Twentieth Century,* ed. Donald M. Lewis (Grand Rapids, MI: Eerdmans, 2004), 249. See Gifford, "Complex Provenance," 68, for a similar observation that Ghanaian Christians have been more accepting of deliverance teachings when presented by Americans like Derek Prince rather than by fellow Africans. As the Ghanaian sociology professor Max Assimeng aptly put it in an interview by Gifford, May 26, 1995, "Things are truer if un-African, so we quote Americans"; see also Max Assimeng, *Salvation, Social Crisis and the Human Condition* (Accra: Ghana University Press, 1995).

56. Randy Clark, *There is More! Reclaiming the Power of Impartation* (Mechanicsburg, PA: Global Awakening, 2006); 1 Timothy 4:14–15. Illustrating the rapid emergence of leaders, two of Clark's associate preachers began as ordinary GA team members but became widely known in GA networks (and one of them subsequently branched off to form his own ANGA affiliate, Gary Oates Ministries) after they self-published books about avowed "impartation" experiences: Gary Oates, *Open My Eyes, Lord: A Practical Guide to Angelic Visitations and Heavenly Experiences* (Dallas, GA: Open Heaven Publications, 2004); Lucas Sherraden, *When Heaven Opens: Discovering the Power of Divine Encounters* (Stafford, TX: Sherraden, 2006). An additional wrinkle to this story is that by 2009 Sherraden had retired as a conference speaker and pastor and, as announced by a new website, had embarked on a career as a realtor.

57. George, trip journal, Belém, Pará, Brazil, September 12, 2004.

58. This anecdote is based primarily on a single evening's meeting in Imperatriz, Maranhão, Brazil, September 24, 2007, although some details were borrowed from similar services.

59. For misdiagnosis and placebo explanations, see Chesnut, *Born Again in Brazil,* 86–87; Sidney M. Greenfield, *Pilgrimage, Therapy, and the Relationship Between Healing and Imagination,* Discussion Paper No. 82 (Milwaukee: Department of Anthropology, University of Wisconsin-Milwaukee, 1989), 20; Corten, *Pentecostalism in Brazil,* 50. Miroslav Volf, "Materiality of Salvation: An Investigation in the Soteriologies of Liberation and Pentecostal Theologies," *Journal of Ecumenical Studies* 26, no. 3 (1989): 447–467.

60. George, trip journal, Belém, Brazil, September 12, 2004.

61. Leif Hetland, lecture, Global Awakening School of Healing and Impartation, Toronto, ON, August 20, 2005; Claude Lévi-Strauss, *Structural Anthropology* (Garden City, NJ: Doubleday, 1967), 206; Chidester and Linenthal, introduction to *American Sacred Space*, 10; Brown," Tent Meetings," 638–639; Global Awakening, "GodSquad," www.globalawakening.com/Groups/1000035814/Global _Awakening/Global/GFS/godsquadshow_com/godsquadshow_com.aspx (accessed 10/7/11).

62. Scott Lash and John Urry, *Economies of Signs and Space* (London: Sage, 1994); Martin Albrow, *The Global Age: State and Society Beyond Modernity* (Cambridge: Polity, 1996), 95; Jean Comaroff and John L. Comaroff, eds., *Modernity and Its Malcontents: Ritual and Power in Postcolonial Africa* (Chicago: University of Chicago Press, 1993), xxix.

2. Why Are Biomedical Tests of Prayer Controversial?

1. Herbert Benson et al., "Study of the Therapeutic Effects of Intercessory Prayer (STEP) in Cardiac Bypass Patients: a Multicenter Randomized Trial of Uncertainty and Certainty of Receiving Intercessory Prayer," *American Heart Journal* 151 (2006): 934; M. V. Gumede, *Traditional Healers: A Medical Practitioner's Perspective* (Braamfontein, South Africa: Skotaville, 1990), 38, 203.

2. Martin Luther, *Sermons on the Gospel of St. John, Chapters 14–16,* in *Luther's Works* (St. Louis: Concordia, 1961), 24:367; John Calvin, *Institutes of the Christian Religion* IV.18 (Grand Rapids: Eerdmans, 1953), 2:636, quoted in Morton T. Kelsey, *Psychology, Medicine and Christian Healing* (San Francisco: Harper & Row, 1988), 17; Robert Bruce Mullin, *Miracles and the Modern Religious Imagination* (New Haven: Yale University Press, 1996), 265.

3. Jaclyn Duffin, *Medical Miracles: Doctors, Saints, and Healing in the Modern World* (New York: Oxford University Press, 2009), 7–8; Paolo Zacchia, *Quaestiones medico-legales* (1657), cited in Duffin, *Medical Miracles,* 24; Ruth Harris, *Lourdes: Body and Spirit in the Secular Age* (New York: Viking, 1999), 18, 323–333; "List of Approved Lourdes Miracles," 1986, www.miraclehunter.com/marian_apparitions /approved_apparitions/lourdes/miracles4.html (accessed 10/8/11).

4. John Corrigan, *Business of the Heart: Religion and Emotion in the Nineteenth Century* (Berkeley: University of California Press, 2002), 207; Archibald Alexander, *Practical Truths* (New York: American Tract Society, 1852), 37, quoted in Rick Ostrander, *The Life of Prayer in a World of Science: Protestants, Prayer, and American Culture, 1870–1930* (New York: Oxford University Press, 2000), 7; Charles Albert Blanchard, *Getting Things from God: A Study of the Prayer Life*

(Chicago: Bible Institute Colportage Association, 1915), 53–60, quoted in Ostrander, *Life of Prayer,* 39; Andrew Murray, *The School of Obedience* (Chicago: Bible Institute Colportage Association, 1899), 62; Greg Johnson, "From Morning Watch to Quiet Time: The Historical and Theological Development of Private Prayer in Anglo-American Protestant Instruction, 1870–1950," (Ph.D. diss., Saint Louis University, 2007); Heather D. Curtis, *Faith in the Great Physician: Suffering and Divine Healing in American Culture, 1860–1900* (Baltimore: Johns Hopkins University Press, 2007), 1; "Office of the Visitation of the Sick," *Book of Common Prayer and Administration of the Sacraments and Other Rites and Ceremonies of the Church,* quoted in Kelsey, *Psychology,* 11–15. This service, although seldom used, is still found in the English Book of Common Prayer (with essentially the same wording preserved from the first, 1549, edition, to the 2011 edition), though an American revision of 1928 and a Canadian revision of 1959 modified the service in a more comforting direction; Church of England, "The Book of Common Prayer," justus.anglican.org/resources/bcp/england.htm (accessed 10/26/11); Mullin, *Miracles,* 98.

5. James C. Whorton, *Nature Cures: The History of Alternative Medicine in America* (New York: Oxford University Press, 2002), 247; Mullin, *Miracles,* 42, 189; Numbers, "Science Without God," 266.

6. Ostrander, *Life of Prayer,* 18–21. The American Congregationalist John O. Means published a compendium of British newspaper articles for American readers, *The Prayer-Gauge Debate* (Boston: Congregational Publishing Society, 1876); John Tyndall, "On Prayer as a Physical Force," *Contemporary Review* (October 1872), quoted in Means, *Prayer-Gauge Debate,* 111, 114–115; Robert Bruce Mullin, "Science, Miracles, and the Prayer-Gauge Debate," in *When Science and Christianity Meet,* ed. Lindberg and Numbers, 211, 213.

7. Mullin, "Science, Miracles," 214, 218.

8. James Monroe Buckley, *Faith-Healing, Christian Science, and Kindred Phenomena* (New York: Century Company, 1892), 46.

9. Francis Galton, "Statistical Inquiries into the Efficacy of Prayer," *Fortnightly Review* 12 (1872): 125, quoted in Wendy Cadge, "Saying Your Prayers, Constructing Your Religions: Medical Studies of Intercessory Prayer," *Journal of Religion* (2009): 303; Ostrander, *Life of Prayer,* 22.

10. Mullin, "Science, Miracles, and the Prayer-Gauge Debate," 18.

11. David Lindberg, *The Beginnings of Western Science: The European Scientific Tradition in Philosophical, Religious, and Institutional Context, Prehistory to* A.D. *1450* (Chicago: University of Chicago Press, 2007), 1–2; John Corrigan, formal response to conference paper by Candy Gunther Brown, "'God's Medicine

Bottle': The Cultural Uses of Printed Texts in American Divine Healing Movements, 1872–2007" (American Studies Association, Philadelphia, October 2007).

12. John G. Lake, *Adventures in God*, ed. Wilford H. Reidt (Tulsa: Harrison House, 1981), 37, 73–75, 81; Lake, *The John G. Lake Sermons on Dominion Over Demons, Disease and Death*, ed. Gordon Lindsay (Dallas: Christ for the Nations, 1980), 24; Lake, *John G. Lake: The Complete Collection of His Life Teachings*, ed. Roberts Liardon (Tulsa: Albury Publishing, 1999), 120, 179; Mullin, *Miracles*, 89; Paul Gale Chappell, "The Divine Healing Movement in America," (Ph.D. diss., Drew University, 1983), 56. Dowie was an exceptionally controversial figure who intentionally provoked medical ire with his infamous sermon "Doctors, Drugs, and Devils, Or the Foes of Christ the Healer," *Physical Culture*, April 1905, 81–86. Lake's seeming ambivalence fits Grant Wacker's characterization in *Heaven Below: Early Pentecostals and American Culture* (Cambridge, MA: Harvard University Press, 2001), 10, of early Pentecostals as intermingling the "primitive" and the "pragmatic."

13. Lake was not the first, nor the last, theologian to use the term *pneumatology* (popular among late-twentieth-century neurotheologians), although he did not discuss precedents. Lake referred instead to specific biblical passages, including James 5:14–15, Matthew 18:19, Mark 6:13, Luke 4:40, and Acts 28:8. Although apparently Lake never received a college or seminary degree, he enrolled at Garrett Bible Institute in Evanston, Illinois in 1897, and, under an exchange agreement, took science classes at Northwestern University. Lake, *Collection*, 285, 294, 410–411, 494; Lake, *Fire of God: John G. Lake in Spokane* (Spokane: Riley Christian Media, 2002), 57, 62; Lake, *John G. Lake: His Life, His Sermons, His Boldness of Faith* (Ft. Worth: Kenneth Copeland Ministries, 1994), 23, 304–305, 342; Lake, *Dominion*, 56, 133; Lake, *Adventures*, 18, 31, 101–102; Lake, *Spiritual Hunger, The God-men, and Other Sermons*, ed. Gordon Lindsay (Dallas: Christ for the Nations, 1978), 68, 83; Kemp Pendleton Burpeau, *God's Showman: A Historical Study of John G. Lake and South African–American Pentecostalism* (Oslo: Refleks, 2004), 27; James K. A. Smith and Amos Yong, eds., *Science and the Spirit: A Pentecostal Engagement with the Sciences* (Bloomington: Indiana University Press, 2010). James William Opp, *The Lord for the Body: Religion, Medicine, and Protestant Faith Healing in Canada, 1880–1930* (Ithaca, NY: McGill–Queen's University Press, 2005), 145, contrasts the nineteenth-century idea of prayer cloths as a means of encouraging faith with the Pentecostal emphasis on transferable power.

14. Ronald L. Numbers, "The Fall and Rise of the American Medical Profession," in *Sickness and Health in America: Readings in the History of Medicine and Public Health*, 3rd ed. (Madison: University of Wisconsin Press, 1978), 233; Lake, *Adventures*, 29–30, 101; Lake, *Fire of God*, 133, 142, 174–175; Lake, *Dominion*,

105, 108. It is strange that, given such examples, Burpeau, in *God's Showman,* 155, 175, characterizes Lake as uninterested in "quantitative proof or other corroborative objective evidence," instead relying on "subjective narrative accounts as definite proof of the 'power of God to work miracles.'" Whether or not Lake's assessments of these experiments corresponded with the evaluations of the involved doctors, whose reports have not survived, Lake's desire for medical verification is apparent. In noting Pentecostal resentment of the higher status of physicians, Grant Wacker, "The Pentecostal Tradition," in *Caring and Curing: Health and Medicine in the Western Religious Traditions,* ed. Ronald L. Numbers and Darrel W. Amundsen (New York: Macmillan, 1986), 524, suggests one possible motive for Lake's repeated efforts to gain scientific validation.

15. See, for example, John Crowder, *Miracle Workers, Reformers and the New Mystics* (Shippensburg, PA: Destiny Image, 2006), 286; John Lake III, foreword to Lake, *Collection,* 9; Cal Pierce, *Preparing the Way: The Reopening of the John G. Lake Healing Rooms in Spokane, Washington* (Hagerstown, MD: McDougal, 2001), 15, 105; Healing Rooms Ministries: International Headquarters, healingrooms.com/ (accessed 10/8/11). Mark Ogilbee and Jana Riess, *American Pilgrimage: Sacred Journeys and Spiritual Destinations* (Brewster, MA: Paraclete, 2006), includes a chapter on the Healing Rooms of the Santa Maria Valley; Margaret M. Poloma, "Old Wine, New Wineskins: The Rise of Healing Rooms in Revival Pentecostalism" *Pneuma* 28, no. 1 (2006): 59–71; Cal Pierce, interview by author, Lancaster, Pennsylvania, October 20, 2011.

16. Ann Taves, *Fits, Trances, and Visions: Experiencing Religion and Explaining Experience from Wesley to James* (Princeton, NJ: Princeton University Press, 1999), 261; Kenneth R. Livingston, "Religious Practice, Brain, and Belief," *Journal of Cognition and Culture* 5 (2005): 79; Walter B. Cannon, "'Voodoo' Death,'" *American Anthropologist* 44 (1942): 169–181, quoted in Otniel E. Dror, "'Voodoo Death': Fantasy, Excitement, and the Untenable Boundaries of Biomedical Science," in *The Politics of Healing: Histories of Alternative Medicine in Twentieth-Century North America,* ed. Robert D. Johnston (New York: Routledge, 2004), 79; Allan Young, "Walter Cannon and the Psychophysiology of Fear," in *Greater than the Parts: Holism in Biomedicine, 1920–1950,* ed. Christopher Lawrence and George Weisz (New York: Oxford University Press, 1998), 243–244.

17. Jack D. Pressman, "Human Understanding: Psychosomatic Medicine and the Mission of the Rockefeller Foundation," in *Greater than the Parts,* ed. Lawrence and Weisz, 193.

18. William R. Parker and Elaine St. Johns Dare, *Prayer Can Change Your Life: Experiments and Techniques in Prayer Therapy* (Englewood Cliffs, NJ: Prentice-Hall, 1957), cited in John R. Finney and H. Newton Maloney, Jr., "Empirical Studies of

Christian Prayer: A Review of the Literature," *Journal of Psychology and Theology* 13, no. 2 (1985): 108. For additional early clinical studies, see C. R. B. Joyce and R. M. C. Welldon, "The Efficacy of Prayer: A Double-Blind Clinical Trial," *Journal of Chronic Diseases* 18 (1965): 367–377; and P. J. Collipp, "The Efficacy of Prayer: A Triple Blind Study," *Medical Times* 97 (1969): 201–204, cited in Fred Rosner, "The Efficacy of Prayer: Scientific vs. Religious Evidence," *Journal of Religion and Health* 14, no. 4 (1975): 294–298.

19. See, for example, British Medical Association, *Divine Healing and Co-operation between Doctors and Clergy* (London: British Medical Association, 1956), 15. For a review article concluding that earlier suggestion studies had failed to demonstrate significant effects, see Amir Raz et al., "Critique of Claims of Improved Visual Acuity after Hypnotic Suggestion," *Optometry and Vision Science* 81 (2004): 872–879; Jerome D. Frank and Julia Frank, *Persuasion and Healing: A Comparative Study of Psychotherapy,* 3rd ed. (Baltimore: Johns Hopkins University Press, 1991), 105.

20. Mary Jo Meadow and Richard D. Kahoe, *Psychology of Religion: Religion in Individual Lives* (New York: Harper & Row, 1984), 120. For a theoretical discussion of "magic" and "religion," see the classic work of Émile Durkheim, *The Elementary Forms of Religious Life,* trans. and with an introduction by Karen E. Fields (New York: Simon & Schuster, 1995), 39.

21. Meadow and Kahoe, *Psychology of Religion,* 125.

22. Thomas Csordas, *The Sacred Self: A Cultural Phenomenology of Charismatic Healing* (Berkeley: University of California Press, 1994), xiii; Amanda Porterfield, *Healing in the History of Christianity* (New York: Oxford University Press, 2005), 17. For recent scholarship attributing the efficacy of prayer to a placebo effect, see Robert A. Scott, *Miracle Cures: Saints, Pilgrimage, and the Healing Powers of Belief* (Berkeley: University of California Press, 2010). On the efficacy of placebos, see Asbjørn Hróbjartsson and Peter C. Gøtzsche, "Placebo Interventions for All Clinical Conditions," *Cochrane Database Systematic Reviews* 1 (2010), art. no. CD003974, doi: 10.1002/14651858.CD003974.pub3; Anne Harrington, ed., *The Placebo Effect: An Interdisciplinary Exploration* (Cambridge, MA: Harvard University Press, 1997); Harrington, *The Cure Within: A History of Mind-Body Medicine* (New York: Norton, 2008), 250.

23. Herbert Benson, *The Relaxation Response* (New York: Morrow, 1975). After being featured in *Healing and the Mind,* a Bill Moyers television series (1993), Candace Pert published a book explaining her "bodymind" research to lay audiences: *Molecules of Emotion: Why You Feel the Way You Feel* (New York: Scribner, 1997). Everett L. Worthington, Jr., "Unforgiveness, Forgiveness, Religion, and Health During Aging," in *Religious Influences on Health and Well-Being in*

the Elderly, ed. K. Warner Schaie, Neal Krause, and Alan Booth (New York: Springer Publishing, 2004), 194, 195–196; Larry Dossey, *Prayer Is Good Medicine: How to Reap the Healing Benefits of Prayer* (San Francisco: HarperSanFrancisco, 1996), 66; Mario Beauregard and Vincent Paquette, "Neural Correlates of a Mystical Experience in Carmelite Nuns," *Neuroscience Letters* 405 (2006): 186–190.

24. Giacomo Bono and Michael E. McCullough, "Religion, Forgiveness, and Adjustment in Older Adulthood," in *Religious Influences,* ed. Schai, Krause, and Booth, 173; Harold G. Koenig, *Is Religion Good for Your Health? The Effects of Religion on Physical and Mental Health* (New York: Haworth Pastoral, 1997); Kenneth I. Pargament, *The Psychology of Religion and Coping: Theory, Research, Practice* (New York: Guilford, 1997).

25. Martin Marty, "Proof-Shroud," *Christian Century* 92 (April 2, 1980): 391.

26. Randolph C. Byrd, "Positive Therapeutic Effects of Intercessory Prayer in a Coronary Care Unit Population," *Southern Medical Journal* 81 (1988): 827, 829; Cadge, "Saying Your Prayers," 314; Richard P. Sloan, *Blind Faith: The Unholy Alliance of Religion and Medicine* (New York: St. Martin's Griffin, 2006), 160–161.

27. Kimberly A. Sherrill and David B. Larson, "Adult Burn Patients: The Role of Religion in Recovery," *Southern Medical Journal* 81 (1988): 821–825; William P. Wilson, "Religion and Healing," *Southern Medical Journal* 81 (1988): 819–829. In pursuing similar lines of reasoning in other publications, Wilson himself had previously provoked controversy among Christian as well as secular psychiatrists who objected to his apparent blurring of religion and science.

28. Steven Kreisman, letter to the editor, *Southern Medical Journal* 81 (1988): 1598.

29. "Editor's Note," *Southern Medical Journal* 81 (1988): 1598.

30. William S. Harris, et al., "A Randomized, Controlled Trial of the Effects of Remote, Intercessory Prayer on Outcomes in Patients Admitted to the Coronary Care Unit," *Archives of Internal Medicine* 159 (1999): 2274; Claire Badaracco, *Prescribing Faith: Medicine, Media, and Religion in American Culture* (Waco, TX: Baylor University Press, 2007), 104–105.

31. Julie Goldstein, "Waiving Informed Consent for Research on Spiritual Matters?" *Archives of Internal Medicine* 160 (2000): 1870–71; Prakash Pande, "Does Prayer Need Testing?" *Archives of Internal Medicine* 160 (2000): 1873–74; Richard Sloan and Emilia Bagiella, "Data without a Prayer," *Archives of Internal Medicine* 160 (2000): 1870; Donald Sandweiss, "P Value Out of Control," *Archives of Internal Medicine* 160 (2000): 1872; Mitchel Galishoff et al., "God, Prayer, and Coronary Unit Outcomes: Faith and Works," *Archives of Internal Medicine* 160 (2000): 1877. See also equally critical letters in the same journal section by Willem van der Does, "A Randomized, Controlled Trial of Prayer?" 1871–72; Dale

Hammerschmidt, "Ethical and Practical Problems in Studying Prayer," 1874–1875; Fred Rosner, "Therapeutic Efficacy of Prayer," 1875; Donald Hoover and Joseph Margolick, "Questions on the Design and Findings of a Randomized, Controlled Trial of the Effects of Remote, Intercessory Prayer on Outcomes in Patients Admitted to the Coronary Care Unit," 1875–1876; and Jennifer Smith, "The Effect of Remote Intercessory Prayer on Clinical Outcomes," 1876. Harris, "Randomized, Controlled Trial," 2278.

32. John T. Chibnall, Joseph M. Jeral, and Michael A. Cerullo, "Experiments on Distant Intercessory Prayer: God, Science, and the Lesson of Massah," *Archives of Internal Medicine* 161 (2001): 2529.

33. Kwang Y. Cha, Daniel P. Wirth, and Rogerio A. Lobo, "Does Prayer Influence the Success of *in Vitro* Fertilization-Embryo Transfer: Report of a Masked, Randomized Trial," *Journal of Reproductive Medicine* 46 (2001): 781–787; E. Roem, "The Columbia University 'Miracle' Story" (January 2005), and Dr. Bruce L. Flamm, "'Miracle' Study: Flawed and Fraud," 2004, www.improvingmedicalstatistics.com /Columbia%20Miracle%20Study1.htm (accessed 10/8/11); letter from Michael Carome, Division of Compliance Oversight, Office for Human Research Protections, Department of Health and Human Services, to Thomas Morris, Columbia University Health Sciences Division, December 21, 2001, www.hhs.gov/ohrp /detrm_letrs/dec01f.pdf (accessed 10/8/11).

34. Flamm, "'Miracle' Study."

35. Ibid.

36. Cha filed suit in the Los Angeles Superior Court in August 2007; the California Appellate Court reached a final judgment in 2009; "Court Vindicates Doctor Who Questioned Pregnancy 'Miracle' Report, Throws Out Kwang Yul Cha's Lawsuit," *24-7 Press Release,* October 25, 2009, www.24-7pressrelease.com /press-release/court-vindicates-doctor-who-questioned-pregnancy-miracle -report-throws-out-kwang-yul-chas-lawsuit-121781.php (accessed 10/8/11); Trudy Sassaman, "California's Highest Court Puts an End to Suit Against Critic of Prayer Study," *Riverside Atheism Examiner,* February 9, 2010, www.examiner .com/atheism-in-riverside/california-s-highest-court-puts-an-end-to-suit -against-critic-of-prayer-study (accessed 10/8/11). The disputed paper appeared in the journal *Fertility and Sterility* in 2005. A Korean-language journal had published a substantially similar article a year before, listing two of the same authors; the complex argument over authorship is described by Jonathan Gornall, "Duplicate Publication: A Bitter Dispute," *British Medical Journal* 334, no. 7596 (April 7, 2007): 717–720; the articles were originally published as J. H. Kim, S. H. Lee, S. W. Cho, et al., "The Quantitative Analysis of Mitochondrial DNA Copy Number in Premature Ovarian Failure Patients Using the Real-time Polymerase

Chain Reaction," *Korean Journal of Obstetrics and Gynecology* 47 (2004): 16–24; and K. Y. Cha, S. H. Lee, H. M. Chung, K. H. Baek, S. W. Cho, et al., "Quantification of Mitochondrial DNA Using Real-time Polymerase Chain Reaction in Patients with Premature Ovarian Failure," *Fertility and Sterility* 84 (2005): 1712–1718. "Indictment of Josepf Horvath and Daniel Wirth," www.quackwatch.org/11Ind /wirthindictment.html (accessed 10/8/11).

37. Leanne Roberts et al., "Intercessory Prayer for the Alleviation of Ill Health," *Cochrane Database of Systematic Reviews* 2 (2009), art no. CD000368, doi:10.1002/14651858.CD000368.pub3: 15.

38. Benedict Carey, "Long-Awaited Medical Study Questions the Power of Prayer," *New York Times*, March 31, 2006, www.nytimes.com/2006/03/31/health /31pray.html (accessed 10/8/11); Benson, "Study of the Therapeutic Effects of Intercessory Prayer (STEP)," 934; Badaracco, *Prescribing Faith*, 110.

39. Myrtle Fillmore, *Myrtle Fillmore's Healing Letters* (Unity Village, MO: Unity Books, 1988), 106, quoted in Jeremy Rapport, "Becoming Unity: The Making of an American Religion," (Ph.D. diss., Indiana University, 2010), 178; May Rowland, quoted in Neal Vahle, *The Unity Movement: Its Evolution and Spiritual Teachings* (Philadelphia: Templeton Foundation Press, 2002), 246–247; Rapport, "Becoming Unity," 294.

40. Candy Gunther Brown, "From Tent Meetings and Store-front Healing Rooms to Walmarts and the Internet: Healing Spaces in the United States, the Americas, and the World, 1906–2006," *Church History* (September 2006): 631–647; Francis MacNutt, *The Power to Heal* (Notre Dame, IN: Ave Maria Press, 1977), 40; Heidi Baker, interview by author, Impiri, Cabo Delgado, Mozambique, June 4, 2009.

41. Francis MacNutt, *Healing* (Notre Dame, IN: Ave Maria Press, 1974), 206; John Wimber and Kevin Springer, *Power Healing* (San Francisco: Harper & Row, 1987), 14.

42. MacNutt, *Power to Heal*, 33; MacNutt, formerly a Dominican priest with a B.A. from Harvard University and a Ph.D. in theology from the Aquinas Institute, was laicized when he married Judith Sewell in 1980. In 1976, he founded the Association of Christian Therapists, which had the goal of bringing prayer into the medical profession. In 1980, the MacNutts founded Christian Healing Ministries in Florida, with headquarters in Jacksonville by invitation of the Episcopal Diocese of Florida. The MacNutts have influenced Protestants as well as Catholics through their books and audiovisual materials on praying for healing.

43. Randy Clark, sermon in Imperatriz, Maranhão, Brazil, September 22, 2007; Margaret Poloma, e-mail communication to author, November 3, 2009, repeating the story as narrated to her by Baker's chauffeur.

44. Whorton, *Nature Cures,* 277; Candy Gunther Brown, "Practice," in "Part IV Global Reach (1898–present)," in *Religion in American History,* ed. Amanda Porterfield and John Corrigan (Malden, MA: Blackwell, 2010), 315; John A. Astin, Elaine Harkness, and Edzard Ernst, "The Efficacy of 'Distant Healing': A Systematic Review of Randomized Trials," *Annals of Internal Medicine* 132 (2000): 903–910; Leanne Roberts et al., "Intercessory Prayer for Ill Health: A Systematic Review," *Forschende Komplementärmedizin: Research in Complementary Medicine* 5 Suppl (1998): 82–86; Roberts, "Intercessory Prayer for the Alleviation of Ill Health."

45. Mitchell W. Krucoff et al., "Integrative Noetic Therapies as Adjuncts to Percutaneous Intervention During Unstable Coronary Syndromes: Monitoring and Actualization of Noetic Training (MANTRA) Feasibility Pilot," *American Heart Journal* 142 (2001): 760–769.

46. Roberts, "Intercessory Prayer for the Alleviation of Ill Health," 15, 2, 16.

47. Karsten Juhl Jørgensen, Asbjørn Hróbjartsson, and Peter C Gøtzsche, "Divine Intervention? A Cochrane Review on Intercessory Prayer Gone Beyond Science and Reason," *Journal of Negative Results in Biomedicine* 8, no. 7 (2009), www.jnrbm.com/content/8/1/7 (accessed 6/10/10); see also "Feedback" from Jørgensen, Hróbjartsson and Gøtzsche, April 16, 2008, in Roberts, "Intercessory Prayer for the Alleviation of Ill Health," 56–57.

48. "Feedback" from Chris Jackson, March 24, 2009, in Roberts, "Intercessory Prayer for the Alleviation of Ill Health," 58.

49. Roberts, "Intercessory Prayer for the Alleviation of Ill Health," 58.

50. Henry A. Guess, et al., *The Science of the Placebo: Toward an Interdisciplinary Research Agenda* (London: BMJ Books, 2002); Mariangela Di Lillo et al., "The Jefferson Scale of Physician Empathy: Preliminary Psychometrics and Group Comparisons in Italian Physicians," *Academic Medicine* 84 (2009): 1198–1202; Roberts, "Intercessory Prayer for the Alleviation of Ill Health," 8; Rob McCarney et al., "The Hawthorne Effect: A Randomized Controlled Trial," *BMC Medical Research Methodology* 7, no. 30 (2007), www.biomedcentral.com/1471-2288/7/30 (accessed 10/8/11); Harold S. Zamansky, Bertram Scharf, and Roger Brightbill, "The Effect of Expectancy for Hypnosis on Prehypnotic Performance," *Journal of Personality* 32 (1964): 236–248; Raz, "Critique of Claims"; John H. Taylor, "Practice Effects in a Simple Visual Detection Taks [sic]," *Nature* 201 (1964): 691–692.

51. Roberts, "Intercessory Prayer for the Alleviation of Ill Health," 16; David B. Larson and James P. Swyers, introduction to *Scientific Research on Spirituality and Health: A Report Based on the Scientific Progress in Spirituality Conferences,* ed. Larson, Swyers, and Michael E. McCullough (Rockville, MD: National Institute for Health Research, 1998), 5.

52. Dale A. Matthews, Sally M. Marlowe, and Francis MacNutt, "Effects of Intercessory Prayer on Patients with Rheumatoid Arthritis," *Southern Medical Journal* 93 (December 2000): 1177–1186. Leaders of the IAHR suggest that prayer sessions should be kept within twenty minutes in order to avoid devolving into counseling.

53. Matthews, Marlowe, MacNutt, "Effects of Intercessory Prayer," 1184–1185; Caryn E. Lerman, "Rheumatoid Arthritis: Psychological Factors in the Etiology, Course, and Treatment," *Clinical Psychology Review* 7 (1987): 413–425.

3. Are Healing Claims Documented?

1. British Medical Association, *Divine Healing and Co-operation between Doctors and Clergy* (London: British Medical Association, 1956), 15, 17, 30.

2. Ibid., 16, 19, 21, 23.

3. Ibid., 16.

4. Jaclyn Duffin, in her study of Catholic canonization miracles, argues that "miracles are not holdovers of magical superstition from an early age. They are modern." Duffin, *Medical Miracles: Doctors, Saints, and Healing in the Modern World* (New York: Oxford University Press, 2009), 11.

5. For a longer discussion of Catholic medical documentation and Lourdes, see chapter 2; D. Sackett et al., "Evidence-based Medicine: What It Is and What It Isn't," *British Medical Journal* 312 (1996): 71–72; Evan Willis and Kevin White, "Evidence-based Medicine and CAM," in *The Mainstreaming of Complementary and Alternative Medicine: Studies in Social Context,* ed. Philip Tovey, Gary Easthope, and Jon Adams (New York: Routledge, 2004), 53.

6. Grant Wacker, *Heaven Below: Early Pentecostals and American Culture* (Cambridge, MA: Harvard University Press, 2001); Eric Patterson and Edmund Rybarczyk, *The Future of Pentecostalism in the United States* (New York: Rowman & Littlefield, 2007).

7. James William Opp, *The Lord for the Body: Religion, Medicine, and Protestant Faith Healing in Canada, 1880–1930* (Ithaca, N.Y.: McGill–Queen's University Press, 2005), 177–195.

8. Ibid., 179, 183.

9. Ibid., 186.

10. Ibid., 187, 189–190; *Report on a Faith-Healing Campaign held by Rev. C. S. Price in Vancouver, B.C., May 1923*, Vancouver General Ministerial Association fonds, file 3, box 1, p. 9; Timothy Lenoir, "Inscription Practices and Materialities of Communication," in *Inscribing Science: Scientific Texts and the Materiality of Communication* (Stanford: Stanford University Press, 1998), 18.

11. Opp, *The Lord for the Body*, 193.

12. Pentecostals stepped up efforts to publish before-and-after medical records during the Voice of Healing revivals of the 1940s and the 1950s; David Edwin Harrell, Jr., *All Things Are Possible: The Healing and Charismatic Revivals in Modern America* (Bloomington: Indiana University Press, 1975), 90; Oral Roberts, quoted in David Edwin Harrell, *Oral Roberts: An American Life* (San Francisco: Harper & Row, 1985), 333.

13. Kathryn Kuhlman, *I Believe in Miracles: Streams of Healing from the Heart of a Woman of Faith*, rev. ed. (Gainesville, FL: Bridge-Logos, 1992), 3; Kuhlman, *I Believe in Miracles*, xiv; Wayne Warner, *Kathryn Kuhlman: The Woman Behind the Miracles* (Ann Arbor: Servant, 1993), 20; Jamie Buckingham, *Daughter of Destiny: Kathryn Kuhlman . . . Her Story* (Plainfield, NJ: Logos, 1999), 122; Emily Gardiner Neal, *A Reporter Finds God Through Spiritual Healing* (New York: Morehouse-Gorham, 1956), 185; Neal, *Where There's Smoke: The Mystery of Christian Healing* (New York: Morehouse-Barlow, 1967), 15; Neal, *The Healing Ministry: A Personal Journal* (New York: Crossroad, 1982), ix. For a fuller discussion of Kuhlman, see Candy Gunther Brown, "Healing Words: Narratives of Spiritual Healing and Kathryn Kuhlman's Uses of Print Culture, 1947–1976," in *Religion and the Culture of Print in Modern America*, ed. Charles L. Cohen and Paul S. Boyer (Madison: University of Wisconsin Press, 2008), 271–297.

14. Kuhlman, *I Believe in Miracles*, xiv; Buckingham, *Daughter of Destiny*, 179; Kuhlman, *God Can Do It Again: Amazing Testimonies Wrought by God's Extraordinary Servant*, rev. ed. (Gainesville, FL: Bridge-Logos, 1993); Kuhlman, *Nothing is Impossible with God: Modern-Day Miracles in the Ministry of a Daughter of Destiny*, rev. ed. (Gainesville, FL: Bridge-Logos, 1999).

15. Kuhlman, *I Believe in Miracles*, 38, 177; Warner, *Kathryn Kuhlman*, 269.

16. Kuhlman, *Nothing is Impossible with God*, 71.

17. "Religion: Miracle Woman," *Time*, September 14, 1970, quoted in Warner, *Kathryn Kuhlman*, 203; William A. Nolen, *Healing: A Doctor in Search of a Miracle* (New York: Random House, 1974), 42, 75, 101, 301. Nolen practiced surgery in the five-thousand-person town of Litchfield, Minnesota, while pursuing a second career as an author for the popular press. He wrote a monthly syndicated medical advice column for *McCall's* magazine and, within a span of fourteen years, published eight semi-autobiographical trade books, one of which, *The Making of a Surgeon* (New York: Random House, 1970), became an international bestseller.

18. H. Richard Casdorph, *The Miracles* (Plainfield, NJ: Logos International, 1976), 16.

19. Quackwatch, a generally respected website, provides a revealing window onto the close association between spiritual healing and alternative medicine in

the view of many conventional medical practitioners. See Saul Green, Ph.D., "Chelation Therapy: Unproven Claims and Unsound Theories," www.quackwatch .org/01QuackeryRelatedTopics/chelation.html; and Stephen Barrett, M.D., "Some Thoughts about Faith Healing," www.quackwatch.org/01QuackeryRelatedTopics /faith.html (both accessed 10/11/11); Colin Brown, *That You May Believe: Miracles and Faith Then and Now* (Grand Rapids, MI: Eerdmans, 1985), 183; Kuhlman, *Nothing is Impossible with God,* 39; Buckingham, *Daughter of Destiny,* 212.

20. Benny Hinn, *Lord, I Need a Miracle* (Nashville: Thomas Nelson, 1993), 1–2, 155–161.

21. Mahesh Chavda, *Only Love Can Make a Miracle* (Charlotte, NC: Mahesh Chavda Ministries, 2002), 80–81 photograph insert; Daniel Ekechukwu and Reinhard Bonnke, *Raised From the Dead: A 21st-Century Miracle Resurrection Story!* DVD (Orlando: Christ for All Nations, 2003).

22. World Christian Doctors Network: Searching for Evidence of Divine Healing, www.wcdn.org/wcdn_eng/main_e.htm (accessed 10/11/11).

23. Hearing loss of 91 dBHL or greater is considered "profound"; hearing loss of 71 to 90 dBHL is deemed "severe." This type of change in BERA and PTA measurements is unusual, especially if sensorineural hearing loss (which is generally permanent) was involved; it is not, however, unusual for infections or wax blockages to clear; e-mail communication from Mark Reinke, M.D., otolaryngologist, August 27, 2011.

24. The highly charged politico-religious climate of Korean evangelicalism makes it difficult even for the Korean-speaking pentecostal scholars consulted to cut through the controversy over Manmin Central Church. For an example of charges that the Manmin Church is a cult, see "World Christian Doctors Network [WCDN]—An Arm of the Manmin Cult," manmincult.com/world-christian -doctors-network-wcdn-an-arm-of-the-manmin-cult/ (accessed 10/11/11). Certain Korean Christians have, however, made similar accusations against various other large Korean pentecostal churches with which they disagree theologically and with which they compete for members. In contrast, the U.S.-based pentecostal ASSIST News Service has run a number of favorable articles on Manmin; the church's pastor, Jaerock Lee; and the WCDN; see, e.g., "Essence Author, Dr. Jaerock Lee, Appearing on the Miracle Channel, Canada," www.assistnews.net /Stories/2010/s10060082.htm (accessed 10/11/11).

25. "It's a Miracle: Reporting on Religion; A Primer on Journalism's Best Beat," Religion Writers: Religion Story Ideas & Sources, www.religionwriters.com/tools -resources/reporting-on-religion-a-primer-on-journalisms-best-beat/best-prac tices/miracle (accessed 10/11/11); "Raised from the Dead—Dr. Chauncey Crandall," video.google.com/videoplay?docid=-2334132798216105638&q=Raise+from

+the+Dead&total=1772&start=0&num=10&so=0&type=search&plindex=4# (accessed 10/11/11). Fox News New York aired a follow-up story for its 2007 Christmas special.

26. Chauncey Crandall, *Raising the Dead: A Doctor Encounters the Supernatural* (Nashville: FaithWords, 2010), 174–184; Chauncey Crandall, e-mail to author, April 14, 2009.

27. Kimberly Ervin Alexander, *Pentecostal Healing: Models in Theology and Practice* (Blandford Forum, Dorset: Deo, 2006), 228.

28. David C. Lewis, "Signs and Wonders in Sheffield: A Social Anthropologist's Analysis of Words of Knowledge, Manifestations of the Spirit, and the Effectiveness of Divine Healing," in *Power Healing*, ed. John Wimber and Kevin Springer (New York: Harper & Row, 1987), 248–269; David C. Lewis, *Healing: Fiction, Fantasy or Fact?* (London: Hodder & Stoughton, 1989). I thank Michael McClymond for drawing my attention to this book.

29. Lewis, *Healing*, 21–22; Paul Kennedy, "Satisfied Customers: Miracles at the Vineyard Christian Fellowship," *Mental Health, Religion & Culture* 1, no. 2 (1998): 139, found that out of 1,399 surveyed respondents, 55 percent reported having been "miraculously healed" at least once—including 11 percent who claimed that they had "often" had the experience.

30. Lewis, *Healing*, back cover, 44.

31. David Wilson, quoted in Lewis, *Healing*, 44–45.

32. Margaret M. Poloma, *Main Street Mystics: The Toronto Blessing and Reviving Pentecostalism* (Walnut Creek, CA: AltaMira, 2003), 112.

33. Margaret M. Poloma and John C. Green, *The Assemblies of God: Godly Love and the Revitalization of American Pentecostalism* (New York: New York University Press, 2010), 126; Poloma, *The Assemblies of God at the Crossroads: Charisma and Institutional Dilemmas* (Knoxville: University of Tennessee Press, 1989), 60.

34. Amy, interview by author, telephone, August 21, 2006.

35. Bill Johnson, interview by Margaret M. Poloma, video recording, Harrisburg, Pennsylvania, October 30, 2008.

36. See chapter 2 for further discussion of the Lakeland Outpouring; Alice Rhee, "Revivalist Claims Hundreds of Healings," Field Notes from NBC News, May 29 2008, fieldnotes.msnbc.msn.com/_news/2008/05/29/4377388-revivalist-claims-hundreds-of-healings (accessed 10/11/11).

37. Rhee, "Revivalist Claims Hundreds of Healings"; Jeffrey Kofman, Karson Yiu, and Nicholas Brennan, "Thousands Flock to Revival in Search of Miracles," *ABC News/Nightline,* July 9, 2008, abcnews.go.com/Nightline/FaithMatters /story?id=5338963&page=1 (accessed 10/11/11); Travis Reed, "Florida Revival

Drawing Criticism—and Thousands of Followers," Associated Press, July 28, 2008, www.pantagraph.com/lifestyles/faith-and-values/article_0fe92491-afdd-51ee-9ccf -2f2d39d3b52a.html (accessed 10/11/11); Stephen Hunt, "The Florida 'Outpouring' Revival: A Melting Pot for Contemporary Pentecostal Prophecy and Eschatology?" *PentecoStudies* 8, no. 1 (2009): 37–57; informants listed in "Fresh Fire Media Packet," interviews by author, telephone, July 10–20, 2008. Apparently there were two versions of the media binder. One contained "a few pages of incomplete medical records, and the doctors' names were crossed out," to quote from the *Nightline* article cited above. But the version mailed to me shortly after the release of the *Nightline* story omitted even these records.

38. Stephen R. Strader, e-mail to author, September 17, 2008 (ellipses and capitalization in original).

39. Stephen R. Strader with Mary Achor, *The Lakeland Outpouring: The Inside Story!* (Windermere, FL: Legacy Media Group, 2008), 65–68.

40. Ibid.; U.S. Department of Health and Human Services Office for Civil Rights, "HIPAA Administrative Simplification," February 16, 2006, section 164.514, 66.

41. For background on the IAHR, see chapter 2; Cal Pierce, *Imparting the Anointing for Healing: Ministry Team Training,* vol. 1 (Spokane, WA: Healing Rooms Ministries, 2004). I offered the options that IAHR staff could distribute the surveys while I was on site (preferred) or that I would mail copies to be distributed by IAHR staff. The IAHR staff agreed to the latter, but never returned any of the 500 survey copies provided despite repeated follow-up efforts. I made similar attempts with the Indiana state coordinator of IAHR-affiliated healing rooms—and the outcome was the same. Cal Pierce, interview by author, Lancaster, Pennsylvania, October 20, 2011.

42. Harvey, interview by author, Spokane, Washington, January 11, 2005.

43. Romans 10:17 (AV); Candy Gunther Brown, "Touch and American Religions," *Religion Compass* 3, no. 4 (July 2009): 770–783.

44. Field notes, Santa Maria, California, November 15, 2007.

45. Ralph, interview by author, telephone, January 15, 2008. The reference to the "law and the prophets" alludes to Luke 16:31 (NIV), in which Jesus says: "If they do not listen to Moses and the Prophets, they will not be convinced even if someone rises from the dead."

46. Martin E. Marty, "Religion and Healing: The Four Expectations," in *Religion and Healing in America,* ed. Linda L. Barnes and Susan S. Sered (New York: Oxford University Press, 2005), 500, 502; Marty, "Proof-Shroud," *The Christian Century* 97 (April 2, 1980): 391.

47. Joy, e-mails to author, November 18, 2009, June 28, 2011. Given that the distance refractive prescription, not counting the prism, is small, it is likely that in 2006 Joy could see 20/20 with each eye separately. When she used both eyes together, the heterophoria caused her to strain her eyes (triggering migraines) to fight double vision (vertical diplopia). By treating the double vision, the prism lenses allowed Joy to see well enough to drive a car. Clifford Brooks, O.D., e-mail to author, July 15, 2011; David Miller, O.D., e-mail to author, June 27, 2011.

48. Joy, "Story of Healing," Facebook posting, May 16, 2009.

49. Arthur Manning, letter to author, April 24, 2009; Manning, *Why the Sad Countenance?* (Zellwood, FL: author, n.d.), 15–17; Manning, e-mail newsletter, November 1, 2011.

50. Rolland Baker, sermon at Voice of the Apostles conference, Harrisburg, Pennsylvania, November 3, 2005.

51. Darren Wilson, *Finger of God* (Chicago: Wanderlust Productions, 2007). The title references Jesus's statement in Luke 11:20 (NIV): "But if I drive out demons by the finger of God, then the kingdom of God has come to you."; Wade Clark Roof, *A Generation of Seekers: The Spiritual Journeys of the Baby Boom Generation* (San Francisco: HarperSanFrancisco, 1993), 135.

52. R. Andrew Chesnut, *Born Again in Brazil: The Pentecostal Boom and the Pathogens of Poverty* (New Brunswick, NJ: Rutgers University Press, 1997); Fion De Vletter, *Migration and Development in Mozambique: Poverty, Inequality, and Survival* (Cape Town, South Africa: Idasa, 2006).

53. Patty, e-mail to Global Awakening, forwarded with permission to author, June 22, 2010; Patty, e-mail to author, July 20, 2010. As in the case of Patty, all subjects were informed about the research study and gave their consent before GA released their contact information.

54. Bethany, e-mail to author, July 30, 2011.

55. Bethany, e-mail, July 30, 2011.

56. Daisy, e-mail to Global Awakening, forwarded with permission to author, May 26, 2011.

57. Daisy, e-mail, May 26, 2011.

58. Fresh Fire Ministries conference DVD, Seattle, Washington, March 2004; Stan, interview by author, Londrina, Paraná, Brazil, June 10, 2008; Mimi, interview by author, Londrina, Paraná, Brazil, June 12, 2008.

59. Silva frequently described his alleged healing—and displayed his palmar creases (which are commonly associated with Down's)—during public talks, for instance in Harrisburg, Pennsylvania, November 6, 2003, and in Londrina, Paraná, Brazil, June 17, 2007 and June 11, 2008.

60. Davi Silva's retraction was removed from Casa de Davi's website sometime between June and October 2011; Até o Fim, www.myspace.com/davisilvao ficial, and Asaph Borba e a Restauração de Davi Silva, tiagolinno.wordpress.com /2011/05/16/asaph-borba-e-a-restauracao-de-davi-silva/ (both accessed 10/11/11).

61. Amos Tversky and Daniel Kahneman, "Judgments under Uncertainty: Heuristics and Biases," *Science* 185 (1974): 1124–1131.

62. Frank, interviews by author.

63. For discussions of Martin Luther King, Jr.'s plagiarism, see Clayborne Carson, "Editing Martin Luther King, Jr.: Political and Scholarly Issues," in *Palimpsest: Editorial Theory in the Humanities*, ed. George Bornstein and Ralph G. Williams (Ann Arbor: University of Michigan Press, 1993), 305–315; and "Becoming Martin Luther King, Jr.—Plagiarism and Originality: A Round Table," *Journal of American History* 78, no. 1 (June 1991): 11–123. On Kenneth Hagin's plagiarism, see Catherine Bowler, "Blessed Bodies: Healing within the African American Faith Movement," in *Global Pentecostal and Charismatic Healing*, ed. Candy Gunther Brown (New York: Oxford University Press, 2011), 100.

64. Dan, interview by author, São Paulo, São Paulo, Brazil, September 26, 2007.

65. George, trip journal, Belém, Pará, Brazil, September 12, 2004; George, trip journal, Joineville, Santa Catarina, Brazil, June 10, 2007; George, interview by author, Pemba, Cabo Delgado, Mozambique, June 4, 2009.

66. "Del Nickels—Construction," in Global Awakening, "Mission to Rio de Janeiro and Imperatriz, Brazil," September 18, 2007, www.globalawakening.com /Publisher/ArticlePrintable.aspx?id=1000025019 (accessed 10/11/11); GA testimony form, September 27, 2007.

67. Global Awakening, "Mission to Rio de Janeiro and Imperatriz, Brazil."

68. See the discussion of biblical healings in chapter 5; Randy Clark, interview by author, Imperatriz, Maranhão, Brazil, September 22, 2007; GA testimony form, September 27, 2007.

69. Global Awakening posts trip reports and testimonies from international trips at www.globalawakening.com/Groups/1000016876/Global_Awakening /Global/International/Testimonies/Testimonies.aspx (accessed 10/11/11); Mark, interview by author, Londrina, Paraná, Brazil, June 14, 2008; Mark, e-mail to author, June 18, 2010.

70. Amanda Porterfield, *Healing in the History of Christianity* (New York: Oxford University Press, 2005), 161; GA testimony form, September 27, 2007.

71. Meredith B. McGuire and Debra Kantor, *Ritual Healing in Suburban America* (New Brunswick, NJ: Rutgers University Press, 1988), 15; Poloma, *Assemblies of God*, 57; Lenoir, "Inscription Practices," 12.

4. How Do Sufferers Perceive Healing Prayer?

1. "George: Brain Tumor Victim Turned Victor," in *Changed in a Moment,* ed. Randy Clark (Mechanicsburg, PA: Global Awakening, 2010), 93–127.

2. Ibid., 112.

3. Ibid., 119.

4. Ibid., 117.

5. John R. Platt, "Strong Inference: Certain Systematic Methods of Scientific Thinking May Produce Much More Rapid Progress than Others," *Science* 146 (October 16, 1964): 352; Thomas C. Chamberlin, "The Method of Multiple Working Hypotheses," *Science* 148 (1897; May 7, 1965): 754–756; Albert Einstein, "On the Method of Theoretical Physics," *Philosophy of Science* 1.2 (April 1934): 165.

6. Charlotte Aull Davies, *Reflexive Ethnography: A Guide to Researching Selves and Others* (New York: Routledge, 1999), 213.

7. Victor W. Turner, "An Essay on the Anthropology of Experience," in *The Anthropology of Experience,* ed. Turner and Edward M. Bruner (Chicago: University of Chicago Press, 1986), 33.

8. I made minor modifications to the survey questions between conferences as I learned from responses received. The appendix supplies the most recent version of the English survey. The conference locations and dates were: Toronto, Ontario (August 17–20, 2005); Harrisburg, Pennsylvania (November 2–5, 2005); St. Louis, Missouri (February 28–March 3, 2006); Rio de Janeiro, Rio de Janeiro, Brazil (September 15–19, 2007); Imperatriz, Maranhão, Brazil (September 21–25, 2007); Londrina, Paraná, Brazil (June 10–15, 2008); and Pemba, Cabo Delgado, Mozambique (June 3–15, 2009). Surveys were included in North American conference registration packets and hand circulated by GA staff in Brazil and Mozambique; I could not track how many of the 3,500 total copies made it into the hands of participants, but my impression is that many did not. A highly conservative response rate estimate is 26 percent for the preconference questionnaires and 17 percent for the postconference questionnaires. Although such apparently low percentages may raise questions about sample bias, the response rate among those who actually received copies of the survey was likely higher. Those who needed and perceived healing were probably more likely to return surveys. This does not create a major problem for the analysis, because the primary goal was to understand perceptions of illness and healing rather than making a statistical argument about the percentage of conference attendees who typically experience healing. Because literacy is extremely limited in Mozambique, I attempted to survey only students enrolled in an IM Bible college. Even so, responses were so incomplete and confusing that I excluded this data from quantitative analyses.

9. I used Microsoft Excel as a database and SPSS statistical software for multivariate regression analysis. Because I performed all data coding, there are no measures of interrater reliability. I frequently referred back to the wording of responses (in English and Portuguese) to perform qualitative analyses and to check coding choices.

10. George Marsden, *Religion and American Culture,* 2nd ed. (New York: Harcourt College, 2001), 278; Grant Wacker, "The Pentecostal Tradition," in *Caring and Curing: Health and Medicine in the Western Religious Traditions,* ed. Ronald L. Numbers and Darrel W. Amundsen (New York: Macmillan, 1986), 527.

11. On Word of Faith, see Arlene Sánchez Walsh, "Santidad, Salvación, Sanidad, Liberación: The Word of Faith Movement among Twenty-First-Century Latina/o Pentecostals," in *Global Pentecostal and Charismatic Healing* [hereafter *GPCH*], ed. Candy Gunther Brown (New York: Oxford University Press, 2011), 151–168; Catherine Bowler, "Blessed Bodies: Healing within the African American Faith Movement," in *GPCH,* 81–105. On healing and cure, see Pamela E. Klassen, "Textual Healing: Mainstream Protestants and the Therapeutic Text, 1900–1925," *Church History* 75, no. 4 (2006): 809–810; Susan S. Sered and Linda L. Barnes, introduction to *Religion and Healing in America* (New York: Oxford University Press, 2005), 10.

12. David Hilborn, ed., *"Toronto" in Perspective: Papers on the New Charismatic Wave of the Mid-1990's* (Waynesboro, GA: Acute, 2001); Margaret M. Poloma, *Main Street Mystics: The Toronto Blessing and Reviving Pentecostalism* (New York: Rowman & Littlefield, 2003). I did not ask Brazilians (or Mozambicans) for education and income information to avoid causing embarrassment, at the request of Brazilian GA staff, who assert that most Brazilians who attend GA conferences have very low education and income levels. This claim is consistent with the findings of R. Andrew Chesnut, *Born Again in Brazil: The Pentecostal Boom and the Pathogens of Poverty* (New Brunswick, NJ: Rutgers University Press, 1997), 6. Most Brazilians surveyed either did not answer the race/ethnicity question or simply indicated that they were Brazilian *(Brasilero/a),* so it may be that Caucasians are overrepresented in the data.

13. I used multiple regression analysis to evaluate four dependent variables: healing need, healing expectation, healing claim (less restrictive), and healing experience (more restrictive). I analyzed all surveys together, and the Brazilian and North American (and other non-Brazilian) surveys separately. In addition to the seven demographic measures, I examined fifteen health-related independent variables: past healings, healing need, physical versus mental/emotional/spiritual need, seriousness of problem, symptom severity, problem duration, physical versus mental/emotional/spiritual healing reported, degree of healing, expecta-

tion of healing, past prayer, past doctor visits, past alternative medical visits, future intentions to use prayer, future intentions to use medical doctors, future intentions to use alternative medicine. In a given multiple regression analysis, only one dependent variable was modeled, and the remaining dependent variables were included (where possible) as independent variables to clarify the relationships among them. Standardized beta values (β) are measures of the strength of influence of each predictor variable, with higher values indicating stronger influence. Statistical significance is claimed where $p < 0.05$; a trend is noted where $p < 0.1$; $p < 0.01$ indicates a "highly significant" effect. I generally chose not to report results where $p > 0.1$ in order to avoid unnecessarily cluttering the text. Adjusted R square (R^2) values indicate the percentage of variance explained by each corresponding regression model taking into account all dependent variables included in the model. For All Subjects, three models were significant: Need, $R^2 = 0.26$; Less Restrictive, $R^2 = 0.80$; More Restrictive, $R^2 = 0.69$; Expectation was not significant. For Brazilian subjects, three models were significant: Need, $R^2 = 0.43$; Less Restrictive, $R^2 = 0.61$; More Restrictive, $R^2 = 0.32$; Expectation was not significant. For North Americans, all models were significant: Need, $R^2 = 0.96$; Less Restrictive, $R^2 = 0.88$; More Restrictive, $R^2 = 0.93$; Expectation, $R^2 = 0.18$. Several of the R^2 values are exceptionally high. This is because there were very strong correlations in North American subjects between reporting physical versus mental/emotional/spiritual needs or healings and needing or experiencing healing. Specifically, in the North American Need model, the zero order correlation between physical versus mental/emotional/spiritual need and needing healing was 0.97. Similarly, in the North American More Restrictive model, the zero order correlation between physical versus mental/emotional/spiritual healing and experiencing healing was 0.88. Given the high R values of some health-related independent variables, it could be that demographic factors would have accounted for significant variance if other factors were excluded from the model. To investigate this further, I ran multivariate regression models that included only the demographic independent variables, but not the health-related independent variables. The R values of the resulting models were so low that none of the models were significant, confirming my original conclusion that the demographic factors did not predict the dependent variables.

14. Older North Americans were significantly more likely to need healing ($\beta = 0.06$, $p = 0.01$), and to experience improvement ($\beta = 0.08$, $p = 0.006$).

15. For the deprivation thesis, see Robert Mapes Anderson, *Vision of the Disinherited: The Making of American Pentecostalism* (New York: Oxford University Press, 1979), 228; Chesnut, *Born Again in Brazil*, 6, challenges the adequacy of

the deprivation model to account for pentecostal healing in Brazil; Lewis, *Healing*, 63, 332.

16. The original survey did not include a question about past healings; I added the question after five GA conference attendees wrote unsolicited descriptions in their surveys. The percentage of IMT members who reported past divine healings is significantly larger than the percentage of Brazilians (84 percent versus 59 percent, $p = 0.000016$, Fisher's Exact Test, hereafter abbreviated as FET). This finding led me to wonder whether the disparity reflects a difference between Brazilians and North Americans (especially because large-scale surveys show higher percentages of Brazilians than North Americans reporting divine healing) or between IMT members—who may have been motivated by their healing experiences to travel to another country to pray for other people's healing—and those simply attending services in their own country. If IMT participants had unusually memorable past healing experiences, this might help to account for the inverse relationship between IMT past and current healings ($\beta = -0.07$, $p = 0.01$). One may conjecture that IMT members recalling past healings constructed a higher standard for what counts as an improvement in symptoms. This would be consistent with the psychological tendency of people to anchor memories of past events in present understandings, which can make past occurrences appear more significant in retrospect than at the time; Hartmut Blank, Jochen Musch, and Rüdiger F. Pohl, eds., special issue on "Hindsight Bias," *Social Cognition* 25.1 (2007). Throughout this chapter, I used a FET for comparing two groups by two categories. I used a one-tail significance test in several cases where previous research predicted the direction of difference. Where I do not specify that a one-tail test was used, I employed the more conservative two-tail test.

17. Reporting a physical problem was the factor that best predicted need for healing ($\beta = 0.56$, $p < 0.001$); Gary Langer, "Poll: Americans Searching for Pain Relief," *ABC News*, May 9, 2005, abcnews.go.com/Health/PainManagement/story?id=732395 (accessed 10/12/11).

18. $t(516) = 2.93$, $p = 0.004$. I used t-tests to assess whether the means of two groups were statistically different. All p-values reported for t-tests are two-tailed.

19. Compared with Brazilians, North Americans reported 88 percent versus 82 percent non-life-threatening, 4 percent versus 2 percent life-threatening, and 8 percent versus 16 percent serious conditions, $\chi^2 (2) = 8.121$, $p = 0.02$. I used a chi-square test (χ^2) to determine whether there was a significant difference in frequencies when comparing two or more groups by two or more categories.

20. Thomas J. Csordas, "The Rhetoric of Transformation in Ritual Healing," *Culture, Medicine and Psychiatry* 7 (1983): 337.

21. Six percent of North Americans versus 17 percent of Brazilians sought mental, emotional, or spiritual, but not physical healing, p < 0.001, FET.

22. Chesnut, *Born Again in Brazil.*

23. R. Andrew Chesnut, "Exorcising the Demons of Deprivation: Divine Healing and Conversion in Brazilian Pentecostalism," in *GPCH,* 171; Meredith B. McGuire and Debra Kantor, *Ritual Healing in Suburban America* (New Brunswick, NJ: Rutgers University Press, 1988), 5; Margaret M. Poloma, *Main Street Mystics: The Toronto Blessing and Reviving Pentecostalism* (Walnut Creek, CA: AltaMira Press, 2003), 105.

24. Two hundred forty-five people reported healing, which is 27 percent of the total returning a preconference survey and 37 percent of those who indicated a need for healing.

25. Csordas, "Rhetoric of Transformation in Ritual Healing," 337.

26. Eighty-four percent of North Americans versus 80 percent of Brazilians reported physical problems, p = 0.02, FET.

27. Physical healings were more prevalent when judged by both less and more restrictive inclusion criteria; North American Less Restrictive, $\beta = 0.42$, p < 0.001; Brazilian Less Restrictive, $\beta = 0.45$, p < 0.001; North American More Restrictive, $\beta = 0.12$, p = 0.04; Brazilian More Restrictive, $\beta = 0.34$, p = 0.03). Variations in survey wording may account for some of the difference in findings between this and previous surveys; this survey's use of the terms *pain, illness,* and *disability* may have encouraged respondents to emphasize physical problems more than they would have given a more open-ended question.

28. Deborah C. Glik, "The Redefinition of the Situation: The Social Construction of Spiritual Healing Experiences," *Sociology of Health and Illness* 12, no. 2 (1990): 151, 154.

29. Lewis, *Healing,* 63. For an explanation of words of knowledge, see chapter 1.

30. Marsden, *Religion and American Culture,* 278.

31. This analysis included t-tests and Pearson correlations.

32. Lewis, *Healing,* 125; r = 0.13, t(174) = 1.75, p = 0.08. I used Pearson correlations to test the degree of linear relationship between two variables; all p values reported are two-tailed. There was not a significant difference in pre-post Likert ratings for those with life-threatening versus non-life-threatening conditions. Respondents reporting a higher severity of symptoms before prayer tended to report a greater degree of improvement after prayer, judging from Likert ratings (r = 0.89, t(192) = 27.16, p = $5.1*10^{-68}$), but this result is confounded by the *ceiling effect,* whereby when people report the highest symptom severity, there is nowhere to go but down. Moreover, judging from people's answer to the question of how completely they were healed, the correlation is not significant. Peter C. Austin and

Lawrence J. Brunner, "Type I Error Inflation in the Presence of a Ceiling Effect," *American Statistician* 57, no. 2 (May 1, 2003): 97–104, doi:10.1198/0003130031450.

33. Margaret M. Poloma and Lynette F. Hoelter, "The 'Toronto Blessing': A Holistic Model of Healing," *Journal for the Scientific Study of Religion* 37 (1998): 257–272.

34. North American respondents were more likely to report healing by the more restrictive criterion if the healing was physical ($\beta = 0.12$, p = 0.04), they had more severe symptoms ($\beta = 0.19$, p < 0.001), and they experienced a higher degree of healing ($\beta = 0.64$, p < 0.001). Brazilians were more likely to report healing by the more restrictive criterion if the healing was physical ($\beta = 0.34$, p = 0.3) and they had had the problem for a long time ($\beta = 0.25$, p = 0.03). All respondents were more likely to report healing by the less restrictive criterion if the healing was physical ($\beta = 0.39$, p < 0.001) and they indicated a higher degree of healing ($\beta = 0.17$, p = 0.002).

35. Twenty-two percent of Brazilians versus 6 percent of North Americans claimed healing based on faith and/or spiritual experience without improvement in symptoms, p = 0.0007, FET; 15 percent of Brazilians versus 2 percent of North Americans claimed healing by faith alone, p = 0.0005, FET.

36. Randy Clark, sermon in Carmi, Illinois, April 17, 2010.

37. Mark 5:34; Matthew 17:20.

38. In the North American Expectation model, plans to visit a doctor correlated negatively ($\beta = -0.37$, p = 0.03), and there was a trend toward more restrictive healing as a predictor of expectation ($\beta = 0.74$, p = 0.052). In the North American More Restrictive model, there was a trend toward expectation of healing ($\beta = 0.63$, p = 0.052).

39. Brazilian high faith = 84 percent versus North American high faith = 56 percent, p = 4.15×10^{-13}, FET. I changed the expectation question mid-research. North American conference attendees answered "Do you expect to receive healing of the condition you described during this conference?" (yes, no, not sure). Brazilians and IMT members answered "How likely do you think it is that you will receive healing of the condition during this conference?" (0-to-10 Likert scale). For comparison purposes, I coded 0–2 Likert responses as "no," 3–7 as "not sure," and 8–10 as "yes." Coded in this way, the percentage of North American conference attendees and IMT members falling into each category was almost identical, confirming this coding decision. Moreover, comparing Brazilians with only IMT members, I still found a highly significant difference, 84 percent versus 56 percent, p = 7.73×10^{-7}, FET.

40. p = 4.0×10^{-24}, FET.

41. McGuire and Kantor, *Ritual Healing*, 188.

42. Leon Festinger, *A Theory of Cognitive Dissonance* (Stanford: Stanford University Press, 1957).

43. Causes of healing identified by Brazilians were: 33 percent = faith, 66 percent = God, 2 percent = faith and God; North Americans: 21 percent = faith, 64 percent = God, 15 percent = faith and God , χ^2 (2) = 10.207, p = 0.006.

44. Norman Gevitz, *Other Healers: Unorthodox Medicine in America* (Baltimore: Johns Hopkins University Press, 1988), 256; Andrew Weil, *Health and Healing* (Boston: Houghton Mifflin, 1988), 28.

45. Francis MacNutt, *The Power to Heal* (Notre Dame, IN: Ave Maria Press, 1977), 28.

46. In the North American More Restrictive model, past prayer ($\beta = 0.13$, p = 0.01) and future prayer ($\beta = 0.45$, p < 0.001) predicted improvement in symptoms.

47. Forty-two percent of North Americans versus 35 percent of Brazilians reported making more than five doctor visits for the same problem; χ^2 (2) = 5.269, p = 0.07.

48. In the North American More Restrictive model, fewer past doctor visits ($\beta = -0.07$, p = 0.048) and future doctor plans ($\beta = 0.22$, p < 0.001) predicted improvement in symptoms. In the North American Expectation model, future doctor plans ($\beta = -0.37$, p = 0.03) predicted diminished expectation of healing.

49. One explanation for the disparity between Brazilian and North American responses to the alternative medicine question is that there is a taboo in Brazilian pentecostal culture against using many of the alternatives listed on the Portuguese survey because they are viewed as false religions, whereas many of the alternatives listed in the English version have been defined in North American pentecostal culture as compatible with Christianity. Chesnut, *Born Again in Brazil*, 3; Candy Gunther Brown, "Chiropractic and Christianity: The Power of Pain to Adjust Cultural Alignments," *Church History* 79, no. 1 (March 2010): 1–38. The Portuguese survey includes Macumba, Umbanda, Candomblé, Quimbanda, Xangô, Para, Kardecist spiritism, spiritualism, Catholic folk healers, curandeiros, African-Brazilian priests/priestesses, herbalists, shamans, psychic surgery, Caecó, metaphysics, Santeria, yoga, homeopathy, and chiropractic. The English survey catalogues chiropractic, massage, meditation, acupuncture, herbal medicine, yoga, Reiki, naturopathy, homeopathy, Therapeutic Touch, Christian Science, Native American, Unity, Santeria, curanderos/as, and psychic. It may be that Brazilians were in fact more likely than they were willing to admit even on an anonymous survey to have used and to plan to continue using culturally common alternatives. Conversely, North Americans may have underreported use of alternatives because some, such as chiropractic, have become so

culturally mainstream that respondents viewed them as conventional "health care professionals" rather than as "alternative" providers. Further comparative work is definitely in order, but I have reserved this project for another book (in progress).

5. Can Health Outcomes of Prayer Be Measured?

1. Field notes, Impiri, Cabo Delgado, Mozambique, June 4, 2009.

2. Field notes, June 4, 2009.

3. Michel Cahen, "L'État Nouveau et la diversification religieuse au Mozambique, 1930–1974: II. La portugalisation désespérée (1959–1974)" [The New State and Religious Diversity in Mozambique, 1930–1974: The Desperate Portugalization (1959–1974)], *Cahiers d'Études Africaines* 40 (2000): 551–592; Tracy J. Luedke, "Healing Bodies: Materiality, History, and Power Among the Prophets of Central Mozambique" (Ph.D. diss., Indiana University, 2005); George O. Ndege, *Culture and Customs of Mozambique* (Westport, CT: Greenwood Press, 2006); João M. Cabrita, *Mozambique: The Tortuous Road to Democracy* (New York: Palgrave, 2000); Fion De Vletter, *Migration and Development in Mozambique: Poverty, Inequality, and Survival* (Cape Town: Idasa, 2006); M. Louise Fox, *Beating the Odds: Sustaining Inclusion in Mozambique's Growing Economy* (Washington, DC: World Bank, 2008); Patrick Chabal and David Birmingham, *A History of Postcolonial Lusophone Africa* (Bloomington: Indiana University Press, 2002); Gretchen Bauer and Scott D. Taylor, *Politics in Southern Africa: State and Society in Transition* (Boulder, CO: Lynne Rienner, 2005); Alice Dinerman, *Revolution, Counter-Revolution, and Revisionism in Postcolonial Africa: The Case of Mozambique, 1975–1994* (New York: Routledge, 2006); Jessica Schafer, *Soldiers at Peace: Veterans and Society after the Civil War in Mozambique* (New York: Palgrave Macmillan, 2007); Ogbu Kalu, *African Pentecostalism* (New York: Oxford University Press, 2008); Instituto Nacional de Estatística, *3° Recenseamento Geral da População e Habitação* [Third General Census of Population and Housing], 2007, www.ine.gov.mz/censo2007 (accessed 10/16/11). I thank Michael McClymond for help with background research on Mozambique and Brazil.

4. Francis Christie and Joseph Hanlon, *Mozambique and the Great Flood of 2000* (London: International Africa Institute, 2001); "Mozambique: How Disaster Unfolded," BBC News, February 24, 2000, news.bbc.co.uk/2/hi/africa/655227.stm (accessed 10/16/11); Rolland and Heidi Baker, *There is Always Enough: The Story of Rolland and Heidi Baker's Miraculous Ministry Among the Poor* (Tonbridge, Kent: Sovereign Word, 2003), 39–52, 79–103.

5. Dale A. Matthews, Sally M. Marlowe, and Francis MacNutt, "Effects of Intercessory Prayer on Patients with Rheumatoid Arthritis," *Southern Medical Journal* 93 (December 2000): 1177–1186; Thomas Csordas, *Body/Meaning/Healing* (New York: Palgrave Macmillan, 2002), 13; Amanda Porterfield, *Healing in the History of Christianity* (New York: Oxford University Press, 2005), 17. I developed the idea for this study in part by listening to a videotaped interview of Harold Koenig, M.D., M.H.Sc., in which he suggested testing the effects of prayer practices on audition; Symposium on Spiritual Healing: Spiritual and Medical Perspectives, New Haven, Connecticut, September 16, 2008; Peter Hobart Knapp, "Emotional Aspects of Hearing Loss," *Psychosomatic Medicine* 10 (1948): 202–222; Amir Raz et al., "Critique of Claims of Improved Visual Acuity after Hypnotic Suggestion," *Optometry and Vision Science* 81 (2004): 872–879; Eugene P. Sheehan, Howard V. Smith, and Derek W. Forrest, "A Signal Detection Study of the Effects of Suggested Improvement on the Monocular Visual Acuity of Myopes," *International Journal of Clinical and Experimental Hypnosis* 30 (1982): 138–146; Charles Graham and Herschel W. Leibowitz, "The Effect of Suggestion on Visual Acuity, *International Journal of Clinical and Experimental Hypnosis* 20 (1972): 169–186; Charles R. Kelley, "Psychological Factors in Myopia," *Journal of the American Optometric Association* 33 (1962): 833–837.

6. Donald R. Kantel, "The 'Toronto Blessing' Revival and its Continuing Impact on Mission in Mozambique" (D.Min. diss., Regent University, 2007); Rolland Baker and Heidi Baker, *Always Enough*, 171–174; H. Baker and R. Baker, *Expecting Miracles: True Stories of God's Supernatural Power and How You Can Experience It* (Grand Rapids, MI: Chosen, 2007), 161; H. Baker, interview by author, Impiri, Cabo Delgado, Mozambique, June 4, 2009; "Mission to Recife, Brazil," December 2006, www.globalawakening.com/Articles/1000024069/Global_Awakening/Global/International/Reports/Recife_Report.aspx (accessed 10/16/10).

7. World Health Organization, "Visual Impairment and Blindness," Fact Sheet No. 282 (October 2011), and "Deafness and Hearing Impairment," Fact Sheet No. 300 (April 2010), www.who.int/mediacentre/factsheets/en/ (accessed 10/28/11); William A. Nolen, *Healing: A Doctor in Search of a Miracle* (New York: Random House, 1974), 99, 282; Luke 7:22, Matt. 11:5. Arlene Sánchez Walsh, *Latino Pentecostal Identity: Evangelical Faith, Self, and Society* (New York: Columbia University Press, 2003), 44, comments on the tendency of pentecostals to script contemporary healings in biblical terms.

8. The study dates were: Impiri, Namuno, Chiúre, and Pemba, Cabo Delgado, Mozambique (June 3–15, 2009); Seattle, Washington (June 25–27, 2009); Barretos and São Paulo (São Paulo) and Uberlandia, Minas Gerais, Brazil (September 23–October 4, 2009); and Chicago, Illinois (October 25–26, 2009). The audiometer

is an Earscan ES3, Micro Audiometrics Corp, Murphy, N.C., calibrated three months prior to the study, with calibration valid for twelve months; we used logarithmic visual acuity charts produced by Precision Vision, La Salle, IL.

9. Candy Gunther Brown, Ph.D., Stephen C. Mory, M.D., Rebecca Williams, M.B. BChir., DTM&H, and Michael J. McClymond, Ph.D., "Study of the Therapeutic Effects of Proximal Intercessory Prayer (STEPP) on Auditory and Visual Impairments in Rural Mozambique," *Southern Medical Journal* 103, no. 9 (September 2010): 864–869. We made available study information sheets written in Portuguese (the national language), with Makua (the local tribal language) translation offered, explaining the research project and diagnostic tests. We reported visual measurements using the metric system in the *SMJ* article, but U.S. customary units in this book.

10. James W. Hall and H. Gustav Mueller, *Audiologists' Desk Reference*, vol. 1, *Diagnostic Audiology Principles, Procedures, and Practices* (San Diego: Singular, 1996), 82.

11. The sound meter is a Tenma model 72–935.

12. $t(10) = 3.93$, $p < 0.003$; all statistical results are two tailed unless otherwise noted. See chapter 4 for a discussion of t-tests and other statistical methods.

13. $t(10) = -0.48$, $p = 0.64$.

14. The population statistics on hearing improvement following PIP included samples of both ears from some individuals, which may constitute nonindependent samples. To correct for this, the reported paired t-test was performed on data from all ears individually, but the probability was evaluated by conservatively assuming only 1 degree of freedom for each individual.

15. Wilcoxon signed rank test $z = 2.49$, $p < 0.02$.

16. In Brazil, however, the 20' vision chart was used for all subjects. All subjects who were tested both before and after PIP were included in the analysis.

17. Todd L. Edwards, *Brazil: A Global Studies Handbook* (Santa Barbara: ABC-CLIO, 2008); Francisco Vidal Luna and Herbert S. Klein, *Brazil Since 1980* (New York: Cambridge University Press, 2006); R. Andrew Chesnut, *Born Again in Brazil: The Pentecostal Boom and the Pathogens of Poverty* (New Brunswick, NJ: Rutgers University Press, 1997); Gabriel Ondetti, *Land, Protest, and Politics: The Landless Movement and the Struggle for Agrarian Reform in Brazil* (University Park, PA: Pennsylvania State University Press, 2008); Kia Lilly Caldwell, *Negras in Brazil: Re-envisioning Black Women, Citizenship, and the Politics of Identity* (New Brunswick, NJ: Rutgers University Press, 2007); Robin E. Sheriff, *Dreaming Equality: Color, Race, and Racism in Urban Brazil* (New Brunswick, NJ: Rutgers University Press, 2001); Livio Sansone, *Blackness Without Ethnicity: Constructing Race in Brazil* (New York: Palgrave Macmillan, 2003); James H. Sweet, *Recreating*

Africa: Culture, Kinship, and Religion in the African-Portuguese World, 1441–1770 (Chapel Hill: University of North Carolina Press, 2003); R. Andrew Chesnut, *Competitive Spirits: Latin America's New Religious Economy* (New York: Oxford University Press, 2003); Roger Bastide, *The African Religions of Brazil: Toward a Sociology of the Interpenetration of Civilizations* (Baltimore: Johns Hopkins University Press, 2007); David Lehman, *Struggle for the Spirit: Religious Transformation and Popular Culture in Brazil and Latin America* (Cambridge, MA: Polity, 1996); Jose Oscar Beozzo and Luis Carlos Susin, *Brazil: People and Churches* (London: SCM, 2002); Instituto Brasileiro de Geografia e Estatística, *População Residente, por Sexo e Situação do Domicílio, Segundo a Religião* [Resident Population by Sex and Place of Residence, According to Religion], 2000, www.ibge.gov.br/home/estatistica/populacao/censo2000/populacao/religiao_Censo2000.pdf (accessed 10/16/11).

18. t(35) = 3.25, p = 0.0013, one tail.

19. t(17) = 3.84, p < 0.001, one tail.

20. r = 0.17; t(14) = 0.63, p = 0.27.

21. Mean = 2.94, range 1 to 14.8.

22. t(22) = 2.66, p = 0.007, one tail.

23. WHO, "Visual Impairment and Blindness," and "Deafness and Hearing Impairment."

24. Sheehan, Smith, and Forrest, "Signal Detection Study"; Graham and Leibowitz, "Effect of Suggestion"; Kelley, "Psychological Factors in Myopia"; Kenneth Sterling and James G. Miller, "The Effect of Hypnosis upon Visual and Auditory Acuity," *American Journal of Psychology* 53 (1940): 269–276; Raz, "Critique of Claims."

25. Ambient noise measured 76.3–103.1 dBSPL; Martine responded to tones in her left ear: 500 Hz, 60 dBHL; 1 kHz, 50 dBHL; 2 kHz, 45 dBHL; 3 kHz, 40 dBHL; 4 kHz, 35 dBHL; 6 kHz, 55 dBHL; 8 kHz, 65 dBHL; right ear: 500 Hz, 55 dBHL; 1 kHz, 45 dBHL; 2 kHz, 35 dBHL; 3 kHz, 30 dBHL; 4 kHz, 30 dBHL; 6 kHz, 60 dBHL; 8 kHz, 55 dBHL; during posttests at 6 and 8 kHz, a strong wind was making high-frequency noise. A potential confound is that AN was also reduced, from 79.1–98.7 dBSPL to 57.9–68.6 dBSPL.

26. Catherine Bowler, "Blessed Bodies: Healing within the African American Faith Movement," in *Global Pentecostal and Charismatic Healing* [hereafter GPCH], ed. Candy Gunther Brown (New York: Oxford University Press, 2011), 86; Arlene Sánchez Walsh, "Santidad, Salvación, Sanidad, Liberación: The Word of Faith Movement among Twenty-First-Century Latina/o Pentecostals," in GPCH, 152.

27. Gabriel, interview by Michael McClymond, Uberlandia, Minas Gerais, Brazil, September 28, 2009; Gabriel, interview by author, Lancaster, Pennsylva-

nia, October 20, 2011. For Gabriel, in the left ear at 500 Hz, the thresholds were reduced from 35 dBHL to 10 dBHL; 3 kHz, 15 dBHL to 5 dBHL; 6 kHz, 20 dBHL to 10 dBHL. In the right ear at 500 Hz, the threshold was reduced from 30 dBHL to 15 dBHL; at 3 kHz, the threshold was 60 dBHL before and after PIP; at 6 kHz, the threshold went from 35 dBHL to 20 dBHL.

28. Maria's responses to tones in the left ear were reduced from 500 Hz 100 dBHL to 85 dBHL; 3 kHz 95 dBHL to 65 dBHL; 6 kHz 85 dBHL to 75 dBHL (80 dBHL in first retest); right 500 Hz >100 dBHL to 80 dBHL (85 dBHL in first retest); 3 kHz >100 dBHL to >100 dBHL; 6 kHz >100 dBHL to >100 dBHL. AN was reduced from 60–67 dBSPL to 29–65 dBSPL.

29. Richard J. Herrnstein, "Relative and Absolute Strength of Responses as a Function of Frequency of Reinforcement," *Journal of the Experimental Analysis of Behaviour* 4 (1961): 267–72; Cephas N. Omenyo, "New Wine in an Old Wine Bottle? Charismatic Healing in the Mainline Churches in Ghana,", in *GPCH*, 231.

30. Luedke, "Healing Bodies," viii; Kathleen E. Sheldon, *Pounders of Grain: A History of Women, Work, and Politics in Mozambique* (Portsmouth, NH: Heinemann, 2002); Jennifer Leigh Disney, *Women's Activism and Feminist Agency in Mozambique and Nicaragua* (Philadelphia: Temple University Press, 2008).

31. The *Southern Medical Journal* posted a series of podcast interviews with me and also with the Harvard Medical School professor Dr. John Peteet, a physician unrelated to the study who wrote an editorial commentary that responds briefly to questions raised about the study. "Study of the Therapeutic Effects of Proximal Intercessory Prayer on Auditory and Visual Impairments in Rural Mozambique, Parts 1–3," and "Proximal Intercessory Prayer," journals.lww.com /smajournalonline/Pages/podcastepisodes.aspx?podcastid=1 (accessed 10/16/11). For critical responses, see for instance, P. Z. Meyers, "Templeton Prayer Study Meets Expectations," *Pharyngula,* August 4, 2010, scienceblogs.com/pharyn gula/2010/08/templeton_prayer_study_meets_e.php (accessed 10/16/11); Steven Novella, "Proximal Intercessory Prayer," NEUROLOGICAblog: Your Daily Fix of Neuroscience, Skepticism, and Critical Thinking, August 5, 2010, theness. com/neurologicablog/index.php/proximal-intercessory-prayer/ (accessed 10/16/11); "Prayer: Proximity Could be Key to Success of Healing Prayer," *Skeptic's Dictionary,* www.skepdic.com/prayer.html (accessed 10/16/11).

32. Dale A. Matthews et al., "Physical Health," in *Scientific Research on Spirituality and Health: A Report Based on the Scientific Progress in Spirituality Conferences,* ed. David B. Larson, James P. Swyers, and Michael E. McCullough (Rockville, MD: National Institute for Healthcare Research, 1998), 38, 40; Carol Thoresen et al., "Religious/Spiritual Interventions," in *Scientific Research on Spirituality and*

Health, ed. Larson, Swyers, and McCullough, 117; limitations to the commonly employed method of null-hypothesis testing are noted by Paul E. Meehl, "Appraising and Amending Theories: The Strategy of Lakatosian Defense and Two Principles that Warrant It," *Psychological Inquiry* 1, no. 2 (1990): 108–141.

33. Anthony G. Greenwald, "Within-subjects Designs: To Use or Not to Use?" *Psychological Bulletin* 83 (1976): 314–320; Tomas Knapen et al., "The Reference Frame of the Tilt Aftereffect," *Journal of Vision* 10 (2010): 1–13; Celeste McCollough, "Color Adaptation of Edge-detectors in the Human Visual System," *Science* 149 (1965): 1115–1116; Dennis P. Phillips and Susan E. Hall, "Psychophysical Evidence for Adaptation of Central Auditory Processors for Interaural Differences in Time and Level," *Hearing Research* 202 (2005): 188–199.

34. Ruth R. Faden, Tom L. Beauchamp, and Nancy M. P. King, *A History and Theory of Informed Consent* (New York: Oxford University Press, 1986), 302–303; Dónal O'Mathúna, "The Subtle Allure of Therapeutic Touch," *Journal of Christian Nursing* 15 (Winter 1998): 4–13.

35. Jacob Cohen, *Statistical Power Analysis for the Behavioral Sciences,* 2nd ed. (Hillsdale, N.J.: Erlbaum, 1988), 6–14.

36. See chapter 2 for a discussion of Hawthorne, placebo, empathy, hold-back, and demand effects. Rob McCarney et al., "The Hawthorne Effect: A Randomized Controlled Trial," *BMC Medical Research Methodology* 7 (2007): 30; Harold S. Zamansky, Bertram Scharf, and Roger Brightbill, "The Effect of Expectancy for Hypnosis on Prehypnotic Performance," *Journal of Personality* 32 (1964): 236–248; Mariangela Di Lillo et al., "The Jefferson Scale of Physician Empathy: Preliminary Psychometrics and Group Comparisons in Italian Physicians," *Academic Medicine* 84 (2009): 1198–1202; Raz, "Critique of Claims"; see essays in *GPCH.*

37. John H. Taylor, "Practice Effects in a Simple Visual Detection Taks [sic]," *Nature* 201 (1964): 691–692.

38. John R. Platt, "Strong Inference: Certain Systematic Methods of Scientific Thinking May Produce Much More Rapid Progress than Others," *Science* 146 (October 16, 1964): 347–353.

39. Historically, valid empirical results have been reported before mechanisms were understood. For example, Joseph Lister (1827–1912) reported effects of antiseptic treatment, without modern controls or statistical methods before the germ theory of disease was fully accepted; Lister, "On the Effects of the Antiseptic System of Treatment upon the Salubrity of a Surgical Hospital," *Lancet* (1870): 40–42.

40. Walter Moczynski, "Spiritual Healing as Alternative, Complementary and Integrative Therapy: A Potential Slippery Slope," in *Medical Ethics in Health Care Chaplaincy: Essays,* ed. Moczynski, Hille Haker, and Katrin Bentele (Berlin:

Lit Verlag, 2009), 175–206; John R. Peteet, "Proximal Intercessory Prayer," *Southern Medical Journal* 103, no. 9 (September 2010): 853.

6. Do Healing Experiences Produce Lasting Effects?

1. Randy Clark, *Lighting Fires* (Lake Mary, FL: Creation House, 1998), 10–11.

2. Clark, *Lighting Fires*, 7, 12; Clark, interview by Margaret M. Poloma and Matthew T. Lee, tape recording, Mechanicsburg, Pennsylvania, August 28, 2008.

3. Elaine J. Lawless, *Handmaidens of the Lord: Pentecostal Women Preachers and Traditional Religion* (Philadelphia: University of Pennsylvania Press, 1988), 60, 65; Stanley Hauerwas and L. Gregory Jones, eds., introduction to *Why Narrative? Readings in Narrative Theology* (Grand Rapids, MI: Eerdmans, 1989), 14; Nicholas Lash, "Ideology, Metaphor, and Analogy," in *Why Narrative?*, 120; Louis O. Mink, "Narrative Form as a Cognitive Instrument," in *The Writing of History: Literary Form and Historical Understanding*, ed. Robert H. Canary and Henry Kozicki (Madison: University of Wisconsin Press, 1978), 131.

4. Clark, *Lighting Fires*, 15, 43; Clark, interview by author, Imperatriz, Maranhão, Brazil, September 22, 2007.

5. Clark, *Lighting Fires*, 15, 74, 78, 80, 83; Clark, interview by Poloma and Lee; Clark, *God Can Use Little Ole Me: Remarkable Stories of Ordinary Christians* (Shippensburg, PA: Revival Press, 1998), 10.

6. Clark, interview by author, Pemba, Cabo Delgado, Mozambique, June 7, 2009; Clark, interview by Poloma and Lee; Clark, interviews by author, Toronto, Ontario, August 17, 2005; Harrisburg, Pennsylvania, November 2, 2005; St. Louis, Missouri, March 4, 2006; Carmi, Illinois, April 17, 2010; Lancaster, Pennsylvania, October 21, 2011.

7. Heidi Baker, interview by Randy Clark, video recording, Pemba, Cabo Delgado, Mozambique, June 4, 2009.

8. Rolland Baker and H. Baker, *There is Always Enough* (Tonbridge, Kent: Sovereign Word, 2003), 48, 67; H. Baker with Shara Pradhan, *Compelled by Love* (Lake Mary, FL: Charisma House, 2008), 2; R. Baker and H. Baker, *Always Enough*, 68; H. Baker, interview by Clark, video recording, Harrisburg, Pennsylvania, October 30, 2008; H. Baker, quoted in Margaret M. Poloma, *Main Street Mystics: The Toronto Blessing and Reviving Pentecostalism* (Walnut Creek, CA: Alta Mira, 2003), 218; H. Baker, interview by author, Costa Mesa, California, December 20, 2010.

9. H. Baker, interview by author, 2010; H. Baker, interview by Margaret M. Poloma, video recording (made by author), Harrisburg, Pennsylvania, October 30, 2008; R. Baker and H. Baker, *Always Enough*, 26.

10. R. Baker and H. Baker, *Always Enough*, 12; Donald R. Kantel, "The 'Toronto Blessing' Revival and its Continuing Impact on Mission in Mozambique" (D.Min. diss., Regent University, 2007), 128; Heidi G. Baker, "Pentecostal Experience: Toward a Reconstructive Theology of Glossolalia" (Ph.D. diss., King's College London, 1996); R. Baker, interview by author, Costa Mesa, California, December 20, 2010. Rolland Baker began work on a dissertation but did not complete it.

11. H. Baker, interview by author, 2010; H. Baker and R. Baker, *Expecting Miracles: True Stories of God's Supernatural Power and How You Can Experience It* (Grand Rapids, MI: Chosen, 2007), 86; R. Baker, interview by author; H. Baker, sermon at Voice of the Apostles, Lancaster, Pennsylvania, October 19, 2011.

12. H. Baker, interview by Clark, 2009; H. Baker, interview by Donald Kantel, Pemba, Cabo Delgado, Mozambique, March 27, 2006, transcription in Kantel, " 'Toronto Blessing,' " 164, 195.

13. H. Baker, interview by Poloma; H. Baker, interview by Kantel, 195; H. Baker, interview by Clark, 2009; "Soaking in God's Glory," TACF conference DVD, October 20, 2005.

14. H. Baker, interview by Clark, 2009; H. Baker, interview by Kantel, 196.

15. H. Baker and R. Baker, *Expecting Miracles*, 95–96; H. Baker, interview by Kantel, 165.

16. R. Baker, interview by author.

17. H. Baker, interview by Poloma; H. Baker, interview by Clark, 2009.

18. H. Baker and R. Baker, *Expecting Miracles*, 192.

19. H. Baker, interview by Poloma; H. Baker, interview by Darren Wilson, *Finger of God*, DVD (Chicago: Wanderlust Productions, 2007); H. Baker, interview by author, 2010.

20. H. Baker and R. Baker, *Expecting Miracles*, 26; R. Baker, interview by Darren Wilson, *Finger of God;* R. Baker, "Core Values at Iris: Simple, Controversial and not Optional!," e-mail newsletter, September 17, 2010; H. Baker, interview by author, 2010.

21. H. Baker, interview by author, Impiri, Cabo Delgado, Mozambique, June 4, 2009.

22. H. Baker, interview by Clark, 2009.

23. H. Baker, interview by Clark, 2009.

24. H. Baker with Pradhan, *Compelled by Love*, 75; Francis, interview by Darren Wilson, Johannesburg, South Africa, in *Finger of God*.

25. Francis, interview by Wilson, *Finger of God*.

26. George, interview by author, telephone, February 1, 2004; "George: Brain Tumor Victim Turned Victor," in *Changed in a Moment*, ed. Randy Clark (Mechanicsburg, PA: Global Awakening, 2010), 99.

27. Subsequent to these encounters, public scandals erupted around both Silva and Bentley, as discussed in previous chapters.

28. "George," 117, 126–127; George, interview by author, Charlotte, North Carolina, July 11, 2004.

29. "Prophecy" is included in 1 Corinthians 12:8 (AV) alongside the "word of knowledge" in a list of nine gifts of the Holy Spirit; George, interview by author, July 11, 2004.

30. Mahesh Chavda, *Only Love Can Make a Miracle* (Charlotte, NC: Mahesh Chavda Ministries, 1990), 17, 21, 39, 46–50.

31. Ibid., 63–70; Hebrews 13:8.

32. Chavda, *Only Love,* 72–79.

33. Ibid., 76, 118–119.

34. Ibid., 13–14, 133–135.

35. Mulamba Manikai, quoted in Chavda, *Only Love,* 138–139; Mahesh Chavda, *Resurrection of Katshinyi,* DVD (Charlotte, NC: Mahesh Chavda Ministries, 1986); Acts 9: 36–41.

36. Chavda, *Only Love,* 139–140, 146.

37. George, interview by author, St. Louis, Missouri, March 2, 2006.

38. Lisa and Sean, interviews by author, telephone, February 1, 2004.

39. Lisa and Sean, interviews by author, Charlotte, North Carolina, July 11, 2004.

40. Lisa and Sean, interviews by author, St. Louis, Missouri, March 3, 2006.

41. Field notes, Charlotte, North Carolina, July 10, 2004; Lisa and Stan, interviews by author, July 11, 2004.

42. Mimi, Lisa, Sean, and Diana, interviews by author, telephone, January 3, 2011.

43. The reference is to 2 Corinthians 12:7–10 (NIV), in which the apostle Paul is described as having a "thorn in my flesh, a messenger of Satan" that God refused to remove despite repeated prayers. Interpolating that the thorn must have been a physical sickness (an interpretation rejected by many pentecostals), cessationist evangelicals use this verse to rebut the pentecostal argument that healing is God's will.

44. Donna, e-mail to author, June 17, 2010; Bill Johnson, interview by Margaret Poloma, video recording, Harrisburg, Pennsylvania, October 30, 2008; Donna, interview by author, Cincinnati, Ohio, January 13, 2007.

45. George, interview by author, Cincinnati, Ohio, January 13, 2007.

46. Donna, e-mail to author, June 17, 2010.

47. Donna, interview by author, 2007. See chapter 1 for a discussion of the sozo model.

48. Chavda Ministries International, *Pour Out Your Spirit Conference*, DVD, July 11, 2009.

49. Donna, e-mails to author, June 17, 2010, June 22, 2011; see Matthew 12:44 and Luke 11:26.

50. Susan, interview by author, Cincinnati, Ohio, January 13, 2007; Susan, e-mail to author, January 29, 2007.

51. Susan, e-mail to author, January 29, 2007.

52. Susan, e-mail to author, January 29, 2007; Mark 9:29.

53. Susan, e-mail to author, December 3, 2009.

54. Susan, interview by author, Kansas City, Missouri, January 4, 2011.

55. Susan, mass e-mail of written testimony, August 24, 2010; Susan's mother, e-mail to author, June 18, 2010.

56. Susan, written testimony, August 24, 2010.

57. George, interview by author, March 3, 2006; James Maloney (with a foreword by Bill Johnson), *The Dancing Hand of God* (Argyle, TX: Answering the Cry, 2008), 27–29; George, trip journal, Comayagua, Honduras, September 2, 2009.

58. Forwarded e-mail, in George, trip journal, Tegucigalpa, Honduras, June 7, 2010.

59. Ernesto, interview by George, transcription in trip journal, Managua, Nicaragua, October 17, 2010.

60. Fernando, interview by George, video recording, Estelí, Nicaragua, October 16, 2010.

61. Fernando, interview by George, 2010.

62. Antonio, interview by George, video recording, León, Nicaragua, October 9, 2010; Isaiah 53:5 (NIV).

63. Geovany, interview by George, video recording, León, Nicaragua, October 9, 2010; George, trip journal, León, Nicaragua, August 6, 2011.

Conclusion: What Science Can Show about Prayer

1. Peter Lipton, "Testing Hypotheses: Prediction and Prejudice," *Science* 397.5707 (January 14, 2005): 220; Carl Sagan, *The Demon-Haunted World: Science as a Candle in the Dark* (New York: Random House, 1996), 213.

2. Matthew T. Lee and Margaret M. Poloma, *A Sociological Study of the Great Commandment in Pentecostalism: The Practice of Godly Love as Benevolent Service* (Lewiston, NY: Edwin Mellen, 2009), 7; Margaret M. Poloma and Ralph W. Hood, Jr., *Blood and Fire: Godly Love in a Pentecostal Emerging Church* (New York: New York University Press, 2008), 4.

3. Lee and Poloma, *Sociological Study,* 44.

4. Pitirim A. Sorokin, *The Ways and Power of Love: Types, Factors, and Techniques of Moral Transformation,* rev. ed. (Philadelphia: Templeton Foundation Press, 2002), 15–16.

5. Robert Wuthnow, "Altruism and Sociological Theory," *Social Service Review* 67 (1993): 351–356; William Scott Green, "Epilogue," in *Altruism in World Religions,* ed. Jacob Neusner and Bruce Chilton (Washington, DC: Georgetown University Press, 2005), 193–194.

Acknowledgments

The proverb that it takes a village to raise a child applies equally to the writing of this book. The breadth of my subject led me to seek out advice and aid from researchers in several social and natural science disciplines. For help with survey research, I thank Ronald L. Numbers, Hilldale Professor of the History of Science and Medicine, University of Wisconsin-Madison, who consulted on survey design; Joshua W. Brown, Assistant Professor of Psychological and Brain Sciences, Indiana University, who collaborated on data collection and quantitative analysis; and research assistants Kate Netzler, Laura Lewellyn, Suzanne Lee, Leah York, and Jason Close, who worked on data collection, translation, and entry. Craig S. Keener, Professor of New Testament at Asbury Theological Seminary, was also kind enough to share primary sources. In conducting clinical research, I received help with study design, data collection, and analysis from Stephen C. Mory, M.D., psychiatrist; Rebecca Williams, M.B. BChir., DTM&H, general practitioner in South Africa; Michael M. McClymond, Ph.D., Associate Professor of Theological Studies, Saint Louis University; Joshua W. Brown, Ph.D.; Mark Reinke, M.D., otolaryngologist; Kenneth Scott, M.D., otolaryngologist; Harry Cohen, M.D., ophthalmologist; David Zaritsky, M.D., radiologist; Earl Craig, M.D., physiatrist; Clifford W. Brooks, O.D., Professor of Optometry, Indiana University; Lance Haluka, O.D., optometrist; David Miller, O.D., optometrist; Paul Cooke, Ph.D., Associate Professor of Communicative Sciences & Disorders, Michigan State University; and members of Indiana University's Statistical Consulting Center and Department of Speech & Hearing Sciences. In developing a theoretical framework, I learned from Professors Margaret M. Poloma, Matthew T. Lee, and Stephen G. Post's work on pentecostalism, "Godly Love," and altruism.

I wish to extend special appreciation to Michael McClymond, who read hundreds of my predraft pages, shared much of his work with me, and made many insightful suggestions that helped me to conceptualize and organize the book. I thank Michael Fisher and the editorial team at Harvard University Press for their skillful shepherding of this project. I am also grateful for valuable suggestions from anonymous reviewers.

This research was made possible by generous financial support from the Flame of Love Project, which was funded by the John Templeton Foundation and administered by the University of Akron and by the Institute for Research on Unlimited Love; and from Indiana University through a Lilly Endowment–funded New Frontiers in the Arts and Humanities grant, an Outstanding Junior Faculty award, and a New Frontiers traveling fellowship. The findings and conclusions do not necessarily represent the views of the funding agencies. Chapter 1 further develops some ideas from an earlier essay, "Global Awakenings: Divine Healing Networks and Global Community in North America, Brazil, Mozambique, and Beyond," in *Global Pentecostal and Charismatic Healing,* ed. Candy Gunther Brown (New York: Oxford University Press, 2011), 351–369, by permission of Oxford University Press, Inc. Chapter 5 continues the discussion of findings presented in a journal article by Candy Gunther Brown, Ph.D., Stephen C. Mory, M.D., Rebecca Williams, M.B. BChir., DTM&H, and Michael J. McClymond, Ph.D., "Study of the Therapeutic Effects of Proximal Intercessory Prayer (STEPP) on Auditory and Visual Impairments in Rural Mozambique," *Southern Medical Journal* 103.9 (September 2010): 864–869.

Index